Small Animal Surgery

An Atlas of Operative Techniques

WAYNE E. WINGFIELD, D.V.M., M.S.

Diplomate, American College of Veterinary Surgeons,
Associate Professor,
Department of Clinical Sciences,
College of Veterinary Medicine and Biomedical Sciences,
Colorado State University,
Fort Collins, Colorado

and

CLARENCE A. RAWLINGS, D.V.M., Ph.D.

Diplomate, American College of Veterinary Surgeons,
Associate Professor,
Department of Small Animal Medicine and Surgery,
and Department of Physiology and Pharmacology,
College of Veterinary Medicine,
University of Georgia,
Athens, Georgia

*Illustrated by Floyd Hosmer
and Dan Beisel*

1979   W. B. SAUNDERS COMPANY/PHILADELPHIA/LONDON/TORONTO

W. B. Saunders Company: West Washington Square
Philadelphia, PA 19105

1 St. Anne's Road
Eastbourne, East Sussex BN21 3UN, England

1 Goldthorne Avenue
Toronto, Ontario M8Z 5T9, Canada

Library of Congress Cataloging in Publication Data

Wingfield, Wayne.

Atlas of small animal surgery.

1. Veterinary surgery—Atlases.   I. Rawlings, Clarence, joint author.   II. Title. [DNLM: 1. Surgery, Operative—Veterinary—Atlases. SF911 W771a]

SF911.W73   636.089′7′00222   78-57920

ISBN 0-7216-9463-2

Atlas of Small Animal Surgery   ISBN 0-7216-9463-2

© 1979 by the University of Georgia. Copyright under the International Copyright Union. All rights reserved. This book is protected by copyright. No part of it may be reproduced, stored in a retrieval system, or transmitted in any form or by any means, electronic, mechanical, photocopying, recording, or otherwise, without written permission from the University of Georgia. Made in the United States of America. Press of W. B. Saunders Company. Library of Congress catalog card number 78-57920.

Last digit is the print number: 9   8   7   6   5   4   3   2   1

To advancements in

VETERINARY SURGERY

past, present, and future.

Contributors

CHARLES WILLIAM BETTS, D.V.M.
Diplomate, American College of Veterinary Surgeons
Associate Professor, Department of Small Animal Medicine
University of Georgia
Athens, GA

DAN BEISEL
Medical Illustrator, Educational Resources
College of Veterinary Medicine
University of Georgia
Athens, GA

TERRY L. BRIAN, A.A., B.A.
Medical Photographer, Educational Resources
College of Veterinary Medicine
University of Georgia
Athens, GA

JONATHAN N. CHAMBERS, D.V.M.
Assistant Professor
Department of Small Animal Medicine
University of Georgia
Athens, GA

THOMAS EARLEY, D.V.M.
Department of Small Animal Medicine
College of Veterinary Medicine
University of Georgia
Athens, GA

ANDREW J. FREY, D.V.M.
12543 Appleton Way
Mar Vista, CA

FLOYD E. HOSMER, B.F.A., B.S., M.S.
Medical Illustrator
Medical Graphics Department
Mayo Clinic
Rochester, MN

LINDA S. HOFMANN
Department of Small Animal Medicine
College of Veterinary Medicine
University of Georgia
Athens, GA

CONNIE C. MARSHALL, A.B.J.
Graphic Artist, Educational Resources
College of Veterinary Medicine
University of Georgia
Athens, GA

MELVYN J. POND, B.V.M.S., M.R.C.V.S.
Diplomate, American College of Veterinary Surgeons
Section of Comparative Medicine
Yale University School of Medicine
New Haven, CT

CLARENCE A. RAWLINGS, D.V.M., Ph.D.
Diplomate, American College of Veterinary Surgeons
Associate Professor, Department of Small Animal Medicine
and Surgery and Department of Physiology and
Pharmacology
College of Veterinary Medicine
University of Georgia
Athens, GA

ROGER A. REHMEL, D.V.M.
Assistant Professor
Department of Small Animal Medicine
University of Georgia
Athens, GA

EBERHARD ROSIN, D.V.M., Ph.D.
Diplomate, American College of Veterinary Surgeons
Associate Professor
Department of Small Animal Medicine
University of Georgia
Athens, GA

GRETCHEN M. SCHMIDT, D.V.M.
Diplomate, American College of Veterinary Ophthalmologists
Assistant Professor, Department of Small Animal Surgery
  and Medicine
Michigan State University
East Lansing, MI

DWIGHT STOWE
Photographer, Educational Resources
College of Veterinary Medicine
University of Georgia
Athens, GA

WAYNE E. WINGFIELD, D.V.M., M.S.
Diplomate, American College of Veterinary Surgeons
Associate Professor, Department of Clinical Sciences
College of Veterinary Medicine and Biomedical Sciences
Colorado State University
Fort Collins, CO

Preface

As the title implies, this book presents personal preferences in the performance of operative procedures. As a result of his experiences, training, natural abilities, and personality, the surgeon will inevitably modify his technique accordingly. Success in the use of these techniques will result from the perfect technical execution of the operative maneuvers.

The content of this book has been derived from our experiences in the veterinary teaching hospital and private practice. Not every operative procedure has been included. The procedures that are illustrated represent techniques that have been effectively utilized in the operative laboratory as well as for the management of surgical diseases. Whether or not the surgeon utilizing this book has performed the procedures heretofore, it is felt the techniques will prove both viable and useful.

In providing a format whereby the preoperative, operative, and postoperative techniques can be reviewed, this book should enable the surgeon to be better prepared to face complications, should they result. The procedures have been described and organized in such a way that they may be referred to during the operative procedure. In most instances the figures have associated explanations on the adjacent page.

Special thanks are extended to our students, past and present, for their review, use, and criticism of the format of the book. To the employees of the W. B. Saunders Company we express our thanks for their interest and guidance. The editorial support of Mr. Robert W. Reinhardt, Laura Tarves, Betty Richter, and Karen McFadden has been masterful.

WAYNE E. WINGFIELD
CLARENCE A. RAWLINGS

Contents

Chapter 1
SURGICAL PRINCIPLES 1
   Wayne E. Wingfield

Chapter 2
ANESTHESIA 5
   Clarence A. Rawlings
Patient Evaluation 5
Patient Preparation 5
Equipment Preparation 8
Anesthetic Considerations for Specific Diseases 8
Monitoring Anesthesia 11
Postoperative Management 12

Chapter 3
PREOPERATIVE AND OPERATIVE PATIENT MANAGEMENT 14
   Linda S. Hofmann
Patient Preparation 14
Preparation of the Surgical Environment 14
Preparations of the Operative Site 16
Preparations of the Surgical Team 20

Chapter 4
INSTRUMENTS 23
   Jonathan N. Chambers

Chapter 5
SUTURE PATTERNS 27
   Jonathan N. Chambers

Chapter 6
OPHTHALMIC SURGICAL PROCEDURES 33
   Gretchen M. Schmidt
Irrigation of the Nasolacrimal Apparatus 33
Subconjunctival Injection 35
Immobilization of the Globe 36

Superficial Keratectomy.. 38
Corneal Laceration Repair 39
Third Eyelid Flap 41
Tarsoconjunctival Resection—Lid-Splitting Procedures for Distichiasis 43

Chapter 7
SOFT TISSUE SURGERY 45

Thoracotomy.. 45
Clarence A. Rawlings

Abdominal Approach and Closure 51
Jonathan N. Chambers

Esophagotomy and Esophageal Anastomosis... 55
Eberhard Rosin

Salivary Gland Excision.. 61
Wayne E. Wingfield

Pharyngostomy... 65
Clarence A. Rawlings

Tracheotomy... 69
Clarence A. Rawlings

Chest Drains... 71
Clarence A. Rawlings

Patent Ductus Arteriosus.. 74
Clarence A. Rawlings

Pulmonary Lobectomy.. 77
Clarence A. Rawlings

Diaphragmatic Rupture.. 80
Wayne E. Wingfield

Gastrotomy 84
Wayne E. Wingfield

Permanent Gastropexy... 91
Charles William Betts

Pyloromyotomy 94
Charles William Betts

Enterotomy 97
Clarence A. Rawlings

Intestinal Anastomosis... 101
Eberhard Rosin

Anal Sac Extraction... 105
Clarence A. Rawlings

Splenectomy 106
Andrew J. Frey

Nephrotomy and Nephrectomy 109
Clarence A. Rawlings

Cystotomy.. 112
Wayne E. Wingfield

Urethrotomy... 117
Clarence A. Rawlings

Scrotal Urethrostomy... 119
Clarence A. Rawlings

Feline Perineal Urethrostomy 120
Clarence A. Rawlings

CONTENTS

Ruptured Urethra 125
   Clarence A. Rawlings

Urethral Prolapse 130
   Clarence A. Rawlings

Ovariohysterectomy 133
   Eberhard Rosin

Cesarean Section 139
   Jonathan N. Chambers

Mastectomy 143
   Andrew J. Frey

Canine Castration 145
   Charles William Betts

Feline Castration 149
   Clarence A. Rawlings

Lateral Ear Resection 151
   Wayne E. Wingfield

Chapter 8
NEUROLOGICAL SURGERY 156

Stabilization of Atlantoaxial Subluxation 156
   Jonathan N. Chambers

Bulla Osteotomy 160
   Wayne E. Wingfield

Cervical Disk Fenestration 165
   Wayne E. Wingfield

Cervical Ventral Decompression 169
   Charles William Betts

Thoracolumbar Hemilaminectomy and Intervertebral Disk Fenestration 172
   Charles William Betts

Chapter 9
ORTHOPEDIC SURGERY 177

Approach to the Shoulder 177
   Roger A. Rehmel

Intramedullary Pinning of the Humerus 182
   Thomas Earley

Fractured Humerus—Cerclage Wiring 184
   Thomas Earley

Transolecranon Approach—Tension Band Wiring 186
   Thomas Earley

Fractured Humerus—Lateral Condyle: Lag Screw Application 188
   Thomas Earley

Intramedullary Pinning of the Radius 190
   Thomas Earley

Femoral Head Ostectomy 192
   Roger A. Rehmel

Intramedullary Pinning of the Femur 198
   Thomas Earley and Melvyn J. Pond

Luxating Patella: Trochlear Arthroplasty and Tibial Crest Transplantation 202
   Roger A. Rehmel

Intramedullary Pinning of the Tibia 204
    Thomas Earley

Fractured Tibia—Full Kirschner Application 206
    Thomas Earley

Feline Onychectomy 208
    Clarence A. Rawlings

Caudectomy 210
    Roger A. Rehmel

Appendix 1
ANESTHETIC DRUG DOSAGES 213
    Clarence A. Rawlings and John I. Taylor

Appendix 2
SUTURE MATERIALS 218

Index 225

SURGICAL PRINCIPLES CHAPTER 1

WAYNE E. WINGFIELD

Asepsis is acknowledged to be preferable in the performance of surgery in veterinary medicine. A full discussion of patient and surgical preparation will be noted in Chapters 2 and 3. Even in the presence of asepsis, the healing of wounds will occasionally be delayed. In assessing the reasons for such a delay, rough handling of tissue, misuse of instruments, prolonged operative times, and contamination of the wounds with powders or bandages are often indicated as the probable causes.

The various organs manipulated by the surgeon are sensitive to abuse. The abuse is usually caused by unskillful handling, excessive trauma, or injudicious use of instruments.

Through the disruption of tissue integrity by trauma or the use of the surgeon's knife, a series of morphologic changes occurs. These morphologic changes are associated with the healing of a wound. With the initiation of a traumatic episode, the blood vessels undergo transient vasoconstriction. This is rapidly replaced by vasodilatation, and there is a release of proteins and plasma. Endothelial permeability to white blood cells increases, and the wound (traumatic or surgical) rapidly fills with a cellular exudate composed of white blood cells, proteins, fibrin, and red blood cells. White blood cells rapidly begin to engulf cell fragments and debris. The duration and intensity of this inflammatory response depends upon the amount of local tissue damage. During an operative procedure, the degree of local tissue damage should be minimized in order to lessen the early inflammatory reaction.

Manipulation of tissues with the fingers and hands of the surgeon creates more diffuse cellular trauma than careful manipulation with instruments. In utilizing instruments, great care should be exercised continuously in order to maintain normal vascularity to tissues. Excessive undermining of skin, stripping of periosteum from bone, or dissection of organs such as the esophagus will lessen the vascularity to the structure and thus prolong the initial phases of healing in a wound. Additionally, misuse of instruments will disrupt the healing of tissues. Allis tissue forceps applied to skin with excessive trauma will cause additional injury, producing more cellular debris to be cleaned up by phagocytosis. The use of traumatic, crushing forceps on tissues will lead to cellular death. In applying these instruments, a minimum of tissue should be grasped. In so doing, the inflammatory phase is reduced, and the wound heals in more normal time intervals. Pinpoint ligation of bleeding vessels will minimize tissue trauma and should be utilized for this purpose.

The addition of foreign matter also affects the rate at which a tissue heals. With asepsis, the surgeon can avoid the introduction of bacteria, hair, and other debris. Close, careful shaving of the hair within the operative field is an absolute necessity in veterinary surgery.

Talcum powder or starch from the surgeon's gloves should be carefully rinsed away before initiating the incision in order to avoid the tendency for the body to phagocytize this debris. Likewise, antibacterial powders or caustic antiseptics must also be removed from the site prior to normal healing.

Suture materials are recognized by the body as foreign matter. With sutures of absorbable material (e.g., plain catgut), the inflammatory response may be increased. Some other responses by the body may lessen the inflammation (i.e., fibrous encapsulation of stainless steel). Suture materials are necessary but must be applied correctly. The minimum number of stitches required to achieve the desired surgical result should be used. In the application of suture material, the knots employed should minimize tissue trauma. If tied too tightly, the suture material will disrupt vascularity and may even destroy cells. With the normal inflammatory response associated with healing, some swelling of surrounding tissue will result. This swelling will produce increased cellular trauma if the initial suture is tied too tightly.

Prolonged operative times increase the risk of the procedure. The risk is not only from arrhythmias during anesthesia but from wound complications. Surgical lamps, air conditioning, heaters, and exposure to air all tend to dry tissues. Once these tissues are dried from exposure, it is safe to assume that the cells involved are dead. Constant attention to moistening of exposed tissues will reduce this problem. With preoperative planning and effective usage of surgical assistants, the duration of the operation will be reduced. This duration can also be lessened through use of sharp needles and dissecting instruments. Thus, not only will the operation take less time, but tissue trauma will be reduced.

Suture Material

An ideal suture material for the veterinary surgeon must have adequate strength, be sterile, cause minimal tissue reactivity, have complete and measured absorbability, provide secure knot-tying characteristics, and be monofilamentous and economical. Needless to say, the ideal suture material does not exist!

In choosing a suture material, the surgeon must consider the type of wound and the chemical and physical characteristics of the suture. With an awareness of the biologic reactions of the various suture materials, a suture as strong as the normal tissues or one that looses strength in proportion to the gain in wound strength must be selected.

The suture size need be no greater than the strength of the tissue on which it is used. All too often, the veterinarian utilizes suture of far greater size than required. It must be recognized that this merely increases the inflammatory phase of the wound healing and adds little to the strength of the repaired wound. In utilizing smaller sized sutures, there will be less tissue trauma and smaller knots. Furthermore, the surgical skill of the surgeon will be called upon in order to handle the material and tissues more gently, and the small suture will be less likely to strangulate tissues (Table 1–1).

Table 1–1 GENERAL GUIDELINES FOR SELECTION OF SUTURE SIZES IN SMALL ANIMAL SURGERY

Tissue	Suture Size
Skin	3-0 to 4-0
Subcutaneous tissues	3-0 to 4-0
Thin skin, skin grafts, ligation of small vessels	4-0 to 6-0
Gastrointestinal or urogenital	3-0 to 5-0
Cardiovascular	3-0 to 6-0
Ligation of large pedicles or blood vessels > 2.0 mm	2-0 to 3-0
Nerves	5-0 to 10-0

Suture materials are categorized as two groups: absorbable sutures and nonabsorbable sutures.

Absorbable sutures are digested and assimilated by the body during the healing process. Through the action of macrophages, the suture material will be replaced by healthy tissue. Absorbable sutures (i.e., catgut or polyglycolic acid) will be more rapidly absorbed in the presence of an abundant blood supply, sepsis, or naturally occurring enzymes. Both catgut and polyglycolic acid have a place in the surgeon's armamentarium. They are especially useful where recurrence of stone formation with nonabsorbable suture might be encountered (urinary bladder), where contamination cannot be eliminated (small intestine), where it is desirable to have the body remove the suture (liver), or where subcutaneous sutures are employed. Absorbable sutures are contraindicated in the infected wound, in grossly contaminated areas, and in the skin.

Nonabsorbable sutures are not digested or absorbed by the tissue. When buried, these sutures usually become encapsulated by fibrous tissues. Because they are nonabsorbable, these sutures have high tensile strength and cause low tissue reactivity. Sutures made of metal (e.g., stainless steel), natural materials (e.g., silk), or synthetic materials (e.g., polyester fibers) are nonabsorbable.

When the surgeon desires a suture material of high tensile strength and/or low tissue reactivity, the nonabsorbable material is selected. These sutures are especially useful in the presence of infection. In these cases, a monofilamentous, nonabsorbable suture material (stainless steel or polypropylene) would preferably be chosen. These materials are somewhat more difficult to handle and knot tying is more difficult, but they have distinct advantages over multifilamentous materials (e.g., braided silk). With the multifilamentous material, there is a tendency to harbor bacteria and greater tissue reactivity. Generally, the nonabsorbable material is more economical than the absorbable.

In the application of suture materials, it is well to recall certain principles propounded by Halsted in 1893:

1. Only interrupted sutures should be used to close wounds (minimal tissue trauma).

2. Silk of greater diameter than 4-0 should not be used (small suture size).

3. Sutures should not bridge a dead space as a chord subtends an arc (accurate apposition of tissue layers without undue tension).

4. Transfixion sutures should be employed in ligation because finer material can be used.

5. A greater number of fine sutures provides better closure than a few coarse ones.

6. Meticulous hemostasis should be maintained and minimal trauma should be exerted on the tissue.

ANESTHESIA

CHAPTER 2

CLARENCE A. RAWLINGS

Just as successful performance of asepsis is required prior to successful surgery, so the choice and techniques of anesthesia are vital to proper surgical procedures. Improperly delivered anesthesia can either kill the patient or markedly complicate the surgical procedure and recovery from surgery. Many surgical procedures are not performed because of the veterinarian's reluctance to anesthetize the patient. A thorough evaluation of the patient combined with preoperative preparation of the patient, knowledgeable selection of the anesthetic regimen, careful monitoring, and thorough postoperative care can permit the practitioner to successfully anesthetize many diseased and debilitated surgical patients.

Patient Evaluation

The surgical candidate should be evaluated by performing a history, physical examination, and laboratory tests. Questions during a preanesthetic history session should concentrate on the cardiopulmonary, hepatic, and renal systems. Topics should include exercise tolerance, degree of physical activity, fainting, dyspnea, coughing, cyanosis, volume of urination and water intake, appetite, defecation, seizures, and peculiar behavior. Prior patient experience with anesthesia and exposure to drugs provide important information. Treatment with drugs such as organophosphates, antibiotics, and corticosteroids can have a marked impact on the patient's ability to tolerate anesthesia.

The physical examination should be thorough, with emphasis placed upon the cardiovascular and pulmonary systems. The thorax should be auscultated, the femoral pulses palpated, mucous membranes examined, and skin tonicity examined for elasticity. Abnormalities that are detected during either the history or the physical examination should be studied until the clinician has a good appreciation of their effect on the patient's tolerance for anesthesia. Complete diagnostic studies are ideal for all patients, but many surgical procedures are sufficiently urgent that such studies are not practical.

Veterinarians should develop a minimum data base for all animals in preparation for anesthesia and surgery. Animals in a higher risk category (over 4 or 5 years of age) or with disease should be more thoroughly evaluated than young adults presented for elective procedures (e.g., castration). Minimal evaluation of young animals presented for elective procedures should include a packed cell volume, total solids, microfilaria examination, fecal flotation, and urinalysis. With older animals and animals with a history of disease, the veterinarian should add a hemogram and chemistry profile. Other function studies, such as coagulograms and hepatic function tests, may be desirable. The evaluation of traumatized animals frequently includes thoracic radiographs and electrocardiograms.

Patient Preparation

Preparation of the nonemergency patient should be initiated only after thorough evaluation. Preparation should correct or minimize abnormal physiology of the patient. Dogs and cats should be fasted from food for at least 6 hours and from water for at least 2 hours prior to surgery. Care must be taken not to limit the fluid intake in the old animal with potential renal failure and not to produce hypoglycemia in the debilitated patient. The urinary bladder should be empty, especially prior to a laparotomy. Preinduction medications should be considered for all patients. Atropine is commonly used by many clinicians and is indicated when vagally mediated bradycardia is anticipated, e.g., in response to xylazine, narcotics, ocular surgery, and drugs that increase salivation, such as phencyclidine derivatives. The use of sedative agents can allow for reduction of the dosage of the inducing anesthetic agent and ease of induction. Excitement, with its catecholamine release, should be avoided.

Many patients have received drug therapy that could alter their response to the stress of anesthesia and surgery. Those animals that have received regular treatments with corticosteroids are prone to developing adrenal gland dysfunction. Some of the animals will demonstrate adrenal hyperactivity, but others may not reveal abnormalities until stressed by anesthesia and surgery. All animals that are currently being administered corticosteroids should have preoperative administration of corticosteroids, unless the procedure can be planned far enough in advance to attempt withdrawing the patient from corticosteroid therapy. Patients requiring medication for congestive heart failure, i.e., digitalis type drugs and diuretics, should also have these drugs continued. Many animals receiving digitalis type drugs do not require them. These animals should have the digitalis type drugs discontinued for several days prior to surgery, as these drugs potentiate ventricular arrhythmias. Another drug type that should be continued is the anticonvulsant drug in animals with a history of epileptiform seizures. The use of these drugs may also allow for reduction of the dosage of the anesthetic agents.

Many drugs, such as antibiotics, vitamins, and antihistamines, generally have a limited impact on anesthesia. Some antibiotics (streptomycin, neomycin, and polymyxin) potentiate the effect of the nondepolarizing muscle relaxants. Cholinergic drugs should be withdrawn several hours prior to anesthesia, as they can produce excessive respiratory tract secretions and bronchospasms and can alter cardiac reflexes. The phenothiazine tranquilizers should generally be discontinued because of their alpha-blockade effect, which can produce hypotension, and their tendency to lower seizure threshold. In contrast to this rationale for withdrawal, many clinicians routinely preanesthetize their patients with a phenothiazine tranquilizer. Organophospate insecticides should be withdrawn several days prior to anesthesia, utilizing the depolarizing muscle relaxants, as organophosphates reduce the level of cholinesterase.

The most common abnormalities of preanesthetized patients are associated with fluid, electrolyte, and acid-base derangements. These should be totally, or at least partially, corrected by treatment prior to the additional stresses of anesthesia and surgery. Common routes for fluid loss are vomiting, diarrhea, and polyuria. Respiratory losses during pyrexia and prolonged anorexia may complicate fluid homeostasis. Electrolyte losses during vomiting include hydrogen, chloride, sodium, and potassium ions. If the fluid loss is from distal to the pylorus, bicarbonate is also lost, resulting in metabolic acidosis. Most vomiting animals have metabolic acidosis due to this loss of duodenal contents and/or to the decreased tissue perfusion that is produced by dehydration. Diarrhea and polyuria both produce deficits of sodium, potassium, and bicarbonate. Evaluation of fluid loss can be based on weight loss, skin tonicity, tackiness of mucous membranes, and general appearance. The packed cell volume, total solids, and urine specific gravity (if the kidneys can concentrate urine) should be elevated. The electrolyte levels (sodium, potassium, and chloride) and acid-base status (arterial or venous blood gases and pH or venous total carbon dioxide) are good aids in characterizing electrolyte losses. Serum levels of an electrolyte, such as potassium, may be normal despite a significant whole-body deficit of that electrolyte. These serum levels are used to indicate the direction of electrolyte abnormalities and to monitor replacement therapy.

The primary therapy for the fluid and electrolyte losses discussed in the previous paragraph is to administer an isotonic, polyionic fluid. Fluid deficits should be estimated as a percentage of body weight and this volume of fluid calculated. Eighty per cent of the fluid deficit should be administered within the first 24 hours, and the remainder should be administered during the second 24-hour period. Continuing fluid losses must be estimated and their volume replaced. Daily maintenance should be provided at a rate of 20 to 25 ml/lb or 30 ml/lb if pyrexia is present. An intravenous route by a catheter is preferred for this high volume of fluid administration. Adequacy of fluid administration is evaluated by frequent physical examinations and determination of packed cell volume, total solids, central venous pressure, and urine output. A mild diuresis should be the objective in most patients receiving fluid replacement. A more rapid administration of fluid frequently only increases the volume of diuresis and may not accelerate fluid shifts into extravascular spaces. In contrast to rehydration, a brisk diuresis is desired in the treatment of uremia. Preoperative administration of either blood or packed cells should be considered when the packed cell volume is less than 25 per cent. Blood should be available for transfusion for animals with low hematocrits and those with anticipated blood loss and hemodilution.

A few animals will have severe enough deficits of either potassium or bicarbonate to require specific supplementation. Metabolic acidosis in debilitated, diseased animals, as indicated by a lowered plasma bicarbonate, is frequently associated with dehydration, and this metabolic acidosis can be corrected by fluid replacement. Metabolic acidosis may also be corrected with bicarbonate administered according to calculated bicarbonate deficit. This deficit is determined by either arterial blood gas acid-base studies or venous bicarbonate levels or is estimated by means of empirical formulae. The total bicarbonate dosage can be calculated as follows:

$(HCO_3^- = 0.6 \times BW (Kg) \times HCO_3^-$ deficit, where HCO_3^- deficit = normal HCO_3^- − patient's HCO_3^-).

One half of the calculated bicarbonate is given as a slow intravenous bolus, and the balance is slowly administered according to later plasma HCO_3^- levels. Empirical dosages can be determined by equating the animal's condition to either mild, moderate, or severe acidosis. The initial and total dosages, respectively, are mild (1 mEq/lb, 3 mEq/lb), moderate (2 mEq/lb, 6 mEq/lb), and severe (3 mEq/lb, 9 mEq/lb). Bicarbonate administration must be slow and to effect in order to avoid paradoxical cerebrospinal acidosis and depression. The rapid administration of HCO_3^- can produce a rapid movement of carbon dioxide across the cerebrospinal fluid membrane. The movement of HCO_3^- is a slower process, and, consequently, the elevated CO_2 level in the cerebrospinal fluid is not buffered sufficiently to prevent local acidosis. When the potassium level is low (less than 3 mEq/l), supplementation may be provided intravenously at 0.25 mEq/lb/hour or by adding 35 mEq/l of subcutaneous fluid. Potassium is most safely administered orally, but this method is frequently not sufficient for preanesthetic preparation. Volume diuresis can markedly lower the potassium level to a hypokalemic range and can also be used to correct the hyperkalemia (7 to 8 mEq/l) produced in some cases of postrenal obstruction. Severe hyperkalemia (greater than 10 mEq/l) may require treatment with insulin and glucose therapy. Rapid alterations of the potassium level should be monitored with an electrocardiogram, as both potassium deficits and excesses have profound cardiac effects.

Prior to surgery, antibiotic therapy should be considered for many patients. This is particularly important in patients that have diseases which could produce septic shock. Prophylactic antishock dosages of corticosteroids are indicated if hypotensive shock is likely. All patients except those too fractious for restraint should have an intravenous route established prior to induction. This provides a route for fluids and emergency drugs during the critical periods of induction and recovery.

Complete restoration of normal physiology is not possible or realistic in many patients prior to anesthesia. Surgery may be an emergency or may be required to correct continuing alterations in body functions. These patients are a more critical anesthetic risk and preanesthetic preparation should be as complete as possible.

Equipment Preparation

The equipment and the expendable supplies for anesthesia should be made available prior to positioning the animal on the table for induction. The anesthesia machine must be checked in a repetitive, thorough fashion. Check points include (1) adequate oxygen supply, functional valves, and properly operating flowmeter; (2) adequate volatile anesthetic, (3) carbon dioxide absorber; (4) one-way valves; (5) pop-off valves; (6) anesthetic scavenger system; (7) hoses and Y-pieces; and (8) connecting tubes. Endotracheal tubes should be examined for correct size, patency, cuff inflation, and cuff leak. Several sizes should be available. Supplies of alcohol swabs, intravenous catheters, gauze, tape, ophthalmic ointment, intravenous administration set, intravenous fluids, lubricating jellies, and calculated dosages of anesthetic agents should be prepared for use. Emergency drugs and equipment should be checked regularly.

Anesthetic Considerations for Specific Diseases

Animals with disease conditions frequently have surgical problems. The disease conditions may be so serious that general anesthesia should not be used. Sedation and/or local anesthetic techniques should be considered as alternatives to general anesthesia. The following considerations are based upon diagnoses that the clinician has determined by establishing the minimum data base or by pursuing the diagnostic algorithm for clinical signs of disease. Anesthetic recommendation peculiar to the surgical procedure will be discussed with that procedure. Disease severity and patient-drug interactions markedly alter the importance of anesthetic regimens to a successful anesthesia experience. The suggestion of anesthetic regimens does not insure that these regimens are without disadvantages or that other regimens are incorrect.

CARDIAC DISEASE

Many patients with cardiac disease (congenital cardiac disease, cardiomyopathy, valvular insufficiency, and heartworm disease) have a decreased cardiac reserve. Congestive heart failure may be present or may develop during the anesthetic episode. Other patients with heart murmurs or circulating microfilariae have little decrement of cardiac reserve and can be treated by routine methods. A history of decreased exercise tolerance and reduced physical activity, when combined with examination findings of cardiac disease, dictate a more thorough diagnostic study. Thoracic radiographs and electrocardiograms are useful aids in quantifying cardiac disease. Animals receiving digitalis drugs should have electrocardiograms. A "P—R" interval equal to 130 msec has historically been considered typical of adequate digitalization.

Cardiac output and contractility are markedly reduced by many anesthetic agents, especially the thiobarbiturates, halothane (Fluothane), and methoxyflurane (Metofane). Cardiac patients are prone to develop arrhythmias (atrial fibrillation, ventricular tachycardia, premature ventricular contractions), and drugs that potentiate ventricular arrhythmias, e.g., thiamylal sodium (Surital) or halothane (Fluothane), should not be used or should be used with extreme caution. Some experimental work would suggest that acepromazine maleate (Acepromazine) has an antiarrhythmic effect. Local anesthetics (lidocaine), oxygen, and other cardiac resuscitation drugs should be available for all cardiac cases. When left heart failure is present, pulmonary edema results and needs to be treated with diuretics (furosemide), reduction of blood volume, high fractions of oxygen, and possibly anti-edema dosages of corticosteroids. When these patients have a high heart rate (175 beats per minute or greater), atropine should not be administered, as more severe tachycardia may result.

When the patient will tolerate them, atropine and possibly acepromazine maleate (Acepromazine) are administered prior to a narcotic or neuroleptanalgesic induction. The animal should be administered oxygen by face mask. Induction can be with an intravenous administration of a combination of fentanyl and droperidol (Innovar-Vet) or oxymorphone (Numorphan) given over a 2- to 4-minute period. After intubation, anesthesia can be maintained by additional administration of the narcotic (oxymorphone) and nitrous oxide. The inhalant anesthetics may be added, but extreme caution should be exercised. Muscle relaxation by succinylcholine (Sucostrin) or pancuronium bromide (Pavulon) can reduce the amount of anesthetic agent required. Monitoring would ideally include indirect blood pressure, an electrocardiogram, and urine output. The narcotic agents can be chemically reversed at the end of anesthesia and the nitrous oxide is rapidly exhaled. Supplemental oxygen and an intravenous route should be available during the early postoperative period.

Pulmonary Disease

Pulmonary diseases generally produce difficulty in ventilation (upper airway obstruction or extrapleural restrictive disease such as hydrothorax), difficulty in blood gas exchange (pneumonia, pulmonary edema), or a combination of both conditions. In patients with difficulty in exchanging blood gases, hypoxemia with respiratory alkalosis may be present. This respiratory alkalosis may be compensated by a metabolic acidosis, and a period of respiratory acidosis during anesthesia often produces severe acidemia. The period from induction to intubation and positive pressure ventilation must be extremely short and without excessive excitement of the patient. When decreased pulmonary function produces hypoxemia or acidemia, either can produce ventricular arrhythmias. When possible, the pulmonary disease should be treated prior to anesthesia. Many pulmonary patients can have their function markedly improved by anesthetic techniques that include positive pressure ventilation with 50 per cent or higher levels of oxygen. This is particularly true in patients with acute ventilatory problems such as a diaphragmatic hernia.

Preanesthesia by a sedative and atropine can be administered. Care must be taken to prevent excitement of the patient. The patient should be administered 100 per cent oxygen for 5 minutes by face mask or induction chamber. Induction to the point of intubation must be rapid and done with a minimum of cardiac depressive agents. Partial induction with either nitrous oxide and halothane (Fluothane), thiobarbiturates, or intravenous narcotics can be used to rapidly sedate the patient prior to paralysis with succinylcholine (Sucostrin). Intubation must be rapid, with positive pressure ventilation being instituted. When the succinylcholine (Sucostrin) is excluded, more induction agent is required. All patients require ventilatory assistance with a high concentration (at least 50 per cent) of oxygen. Following anesthesia, oxygen should be continued by oxygen cage, endotracheal tube, face mask, or tracheostomy tube.

Hepatic Disease

Patients with decreased liver function can have difficulty metabolizing anesthetic agents and providing substances, such as albumin, glucose, and fibrinogen, that are required for successful anesthesia and surgery. Barbiturates and phenothiazine tranquilizers seem to be poorly tolerated by hepatic cases and produce prolonged depression. Since the halogenated hydrocarbons, especially halothane, have been incriminated as producing centrolobular necrosis, the use of halothane in these patients is questionable. Other drugs, especially methoxyflurane, markedly decrease hepatic blood flow during anesthesia.

Clinical pathology tests of increased bromsulphalein dye, elevated bilirubin, and/or high ammonia level suggest decreased liver function. The ability of an individual patient to tolerate anesthesia seems to be poorly correlated with function tests, possibly because of the multiple and unrelated functions performed by the liver. Hepatocellular necrosis is indicated by an elevated serum glutamic-pyruvic transaminase (SGPT), and serum alkaline phosphatase is a reflection of biliary stasis. These enzymes are elevated in many traumatized dogs, and patients receiving corticosteroids frequently have an elevated alkaline phosphatase. Since the half-life of these enzymes is approximately four days, an acute insult can increase their levels for several days. Enzyme levels of greater than 2 or 3 times a high normal range are a serious concern when anesthesia is being considered.

The patient can be preanesthetized with narcotics, such as meperidine and atropine. Anesthesia can be induced by either inhalant (nitrous oxide and halothane) or intravenous narcotics (Numorphan). Intubation may be aided by muscle relaxation with succinylcholine (Sucostrin). Anesthesia may be supplemented with gas anesthesia.

Renal Disease

The renal medulla and its blood flow are affected by the arteriolar constriction and hypotension that frequently develop during anesthesia. Blood pressure to the renal tubules is decreased during its flow through two arteriolar resistors that are in series (preglomerular arterioles and postglomerular arterioles) and the glomerular capillaries. A decrease in systemic arterial blood pressure can reduce medullary flow sufficiently to produce ischemia and hypoxia. Medullary flow must be maintained to prevent postoperative tubular failure to concentrate glomerular filtrate (urine). If medullary flow is reduced, diuresis by either hypervolemia or diuretics in the presence of hypervolemia can increase tubular flow sufficiently to prevent cast obstruction of nephrons.

Most noninhalant anesthetics or their metabolic end-products are eliminated by the kidneys. A functional renal system should be present to eliminate these drugs, maintain acid-base balance, and regulate fluid balance.

Preanesthetic evaluation of all patients should include a urinalysis, and either a blood urea nitrogen or creatinine should be obtained on older patients. Any patient whose specific gravity is less than 1.025 or who has proteinuria should be considered to have decreased renal function. If the specific gravity of a random urinalysis is less than 1.025, the specific gravity measurement should be repeated. If a second random sample is less than 1.025, the kidneys should be challenged by either a controlled dehydration or an antidiuretic hormone. If the patient cannot concentrate urine, intensive renal management should be undertaken. Many of these patients are geriatric dogs that also have chronic cardiac disease. This system should be critically evaluated, as a volume overload can produce cardiac failure.

Prior to preanesthesia, the patient should be rehydrated and then prehydrated with approximately 20 ml/lb of isotonic, polyionic fluids. The animal may then be sedated, possibly with acepromazine maleate. Excitement with catecholamine discharge during induction should be avoided. Anesthesia can be induced by inhalant drugs (halothane and nitrous oxide), intravenous narcotics, neuroleptanalgesics, or possibly one of the thiobarbiturates. Maintenance can be done with inhalant anesthesia. Monitoring should include urine output and indirect arterial blood pressure. Diuresis of 4 to 8 ml/lb/hour should be attained, and urine flows less than 1 ml/lb/hour are inadequate. Lower urine outputs should be treated initially by increasing the fluid administration rate or possibly by either furosemide or osmotic diuresis. Fluid administration is best monitored by central venous pressure in order to prevent fluid overload and congestive heart failure with pulmonary edema.

Monitoring Anesthesia

The mortality rate among animals subject to improperly administered anesthetics is probably greater than that due to improper selection of an anesthetic regimen. Alert and thorough monitoring of the anesthetized patient should detect physiologic alterations prior to death. All anesthetized patients should be monitored by reflexes, heart rate, respiratory rate, and body temperature. Level of consciousness, response to painful stimuli, swallowing, and palpebral, pedal, and corneal reflexes are especially useful parameters during induction of anesthesia. Corneal reflex, jaw muscle tone, pupil size, eye position, and response to surgical stimuli should be monitored during maintenance, but cardiopulmonary changes are more discriminating indicators of plane of anesthesia. The cardiac and ventilatory frequency and the character of the pulse and breathing should be monitored during all anesthetic episodes. An esophageal stethoscope should be used routinely. It may be connected to a monoaural fitting for the surgeon or to an amplifier. Hypothermia is one indication of inadequate tissue perfusion. Early decrements of peripheral perfusion can be detected by skin temperature, such as that between the toes. Core (rectal) and skin temperatures can be measured by either a mercury thermometer or an electronic thermistor.

The anesthetized patient whose condition is more critical than that of the routine patient should also be monitored by indirect arterial blood pressure measurements. Pressure measurements seem to be a more accurate reflection of anesthetic stage than is heart rate. Hypertension may be produced as an animal begins to awaken sufficiently to feel painful stimuli. Hypotension is frequently the result of hypovolemia or of cardiac depression by an excessive amount of anesthetic agent. Two other useful and economical means of evaluating fluid volume are urinary output and central venous pressure. These are particularly useful in managing renal and/or cardiac patients. Urinary output should be greater than 1 ml/lb/hr; this level is an indirect indication of adequate renal blood flow. Central venous pressure is transduced from a catheter positioned near the right atrium and is measured with a saline manometer zeroed to the level of the right atrium. A rapid increase in the height of the water column or a water level greater than 15 cm above the right atrium suggests that the blood volume is greater than the heart can effectively circulate. Fluid and anesthetic administration should cease, and drug-induced diuresis should be considered. A low central venous pressure (less than 5 cm H_2O) or a falling pressure is an indication that more fluid can be safely administered.

Several other monitoring devices are useful in better defining an animal's anesthetic and physiologic status. Some of the more useful devices and tests are a volumeter, arterial blood gases, an electrocardiogram, thermodilution cardiac output, and a peripheral nerve stimulator. A volumeter within the circuitry of the anesthetic machine will measure minute ventilation and tidal volume and is a much better indicator of ventilatory depression than is respiratory frequency. The combined effectiveness of the cardiopulmonary systems can be objectively determined by arterial blood gases. Carbon dioxide retention (respiratory acidosis) indicates insufficient ventilation, and a low bicarbonate level (metabolic acidosis) indicates insufficient tissue perfusion. The cause of metabolic acidosis should be determined, and treatment usually includes decreasing the anesthetic level and replenishing the blood volume. Total compliance of the lungs and chest wall can be roughly determined by the tidal volume of air moved during inflation to 10 cm H_2O airway pressure. This compliance should be rechecked during anesthesia. Decreases of compliance are commonly due to atelectasis, pulmonary edema, and extrapleural restrictive disease (gastric distention or head in a dependent position with elevation of the rear half of the body). The electrocardiogram is another means of determining cardiac rate. It can also detect difficulty in repolarization (altered S–T segment or large "T" waves) that may be the result of either myocardial ischemia or hypoxia. The heart can be normally activated and have a normal electrocardiogram but not be effectively pumping blood. Thermodilution cardiac output, which has recently been used to monitor anesthesia for larger animals, is a better measure of cardiac function. Animals with ventilatory depression after muscle relaxants can be evaluated by a nerve stimulator. The ability of stimulated skeletal muscles to contract suggests that ventilatory depression is not due to the muscle relaxant, and an etiology such as hyperventilation-induced hypocarbia, severe hypercarbia, anesthetic depression, or neurologic disease should be considered.

Good management of the anesthetized patient should include adequate maintenance of oxygen, fluids, and heat. Oxygen supply should be provided based upon nomogram-determined oxygen requirement. These amounts should be supplied if oxygen flow rates are as follows: (1) Vaporizer — in-circuit: 10 to 40 pounds = 500 ml/min; 40 to 100 pounds = 750 to 1000 ml/min; over 100 pounds = 1.5 l/min; (2) Vaporizer — out-of-circuit: 10 to 100 pounds = 1 l/min; over 100 pounds = 1.5 l/min; and (3) Nonrebreathing system (Ayres T-piece) for animals less than 10 pounds = 1 to 2 l/min. The anesthetic bag for the nonrebreathing system should be slightly distended, or the oxygen flow rate should be adjusted.

Fluid administration should provide at least 12 hours of the maintenance requirement, as the preoperative fasting and postoperative abstinence from water is at least this long. Daily maintenance requirement is 20 to 25 ml/lb, or greater if either polyuria or fever is present. Most dogs can tolerate fluid volume of up to 40 ml/lb being administered in a one-hour period. Fluid administration should replace continuing losses produced by the surgery and should produce a mild diuresis. These factors should be satisfied by an administration rate of 5 ml/lb/hour to a maximum of 40 ml/lb. Further supplementation is indicated if excessive bleeding is present or if the monitoring determines a volume deficit. Maintenance of a normal body temperature is difficult in small patients, and the degree of hypothermia can be reduced by a warm water circulating blanket, covering the body with warm towels, and warming fluids for intravenous administration and surgical lavages.

Postoperative Management

Postoperative management and monitoring should be continued as during surgery, until the animal has recovered sufficiently that monitoring is no longer as critical. Vital signs, especially pulse and respiration, should be determined every 5 minutes until the animal is extubated, then every 10 minutes until the animal is sternal, and then every 15 minutes until the animal is able to stand. Body and skin temperature should be measured every 30 minutes until the animal is standing. Other measurements should be performed as indicated by the patient's condition, and these should be similar to those performed during surgery. Animals should be extubated once a swallowing reflex has returned and when there is no longer a need for either ventilatory support or oxygen administration. Intravenous fluid administration may be indicated after surgery.

Special management such as aspiration of chest tubes and collection of urine may be required. To reduce hypostatic congestion, animals should be turned every 30 minutes, unless this manipulation is contraindicated by the surgical procedure.

The recovery facility should provide comfort for the animal and be available for frequent monitoring. Small and young animals should recover in a pediatric incubator that warms, humidifies, and increases the oxygen content in the patient's environment. All animals should be kept warm by a warm water circulating blanket and body wraps. They should be made comfortable and kept dry and clean of their excreta and hemorrhage.

Postoperative medications are generally a continuation of the fluid and antibiotic therapy. Analgesics of either pentazocine or meperidine hydrochloride should be given to the animal in obvious pain. Animals with a violent recovery may require sedation, and animals prone to seizures (postmyelogram) may require anticonvulsant therapy.

Anesthesia may be associated with a wide variety of complications: excessive pain, seizure, hypothermia, hyperthermia, paralysis, ventilatory depression, dyspnea, airway obstruction, prolonged recovery, hemorrhage, pulmonary edema, renal shutdown, arrhythmias, vomiting, cyanosis, hypotension, and death. An effort should be made to detect these changes early in their course, and an aggressive course of diagnosis and treatment should be initiated.

PREOPERATIVE AND OPERATIVE PATIENT MANAGEMENT

CHAPTER 3

LINDA S. HOFMANN

Patient Preparation

After a thorough physical examination and analysis of laboratory data, the routine surgical patient should be prepared for surgery by withholding food for at least 6 hours prior to surgery. Water should be allowed until preoperative medication is given. Animals are frequently admitted to the hospital infested with fleas, ticks, or lice. A bath should be given whenever practical, but the elimination of external parasites is essential to prevent contamination of the operative site. The animal may be sprayed with an insecticide to remove the parasites. An hour before surgery, the animal should be exercised to encourage voiding. If the animal fails to urinate, the bladder can be expressed or catheterized when the animal is anesthetized.

Preparation of the Surgical Environment

The room and environment in which surgery is performed play a significant part in creating and maintaining an aseptic surgery. Preparations of the surgeon, patient, and supplies are wasted without specific preparations of the environment. A cleaning and disinfecting protocol must be established and maintained at regular intervals. Equipment, walls, floors, vents, and even the air itself must be as free from bacteria as possible.

CLEANING AND DISINFECTION OF THE OPERATING ROOM AND ITS EQUIPMENT

Prior to Surgery

Each morning prior to surgery, the operating room should be damp dusted with a disinfectant solution. Walls, table surfaces, kick buckets, chairs, and surgery lights should receive a thorough disinfection. The surgery lights should not be overlooked, for in their position directly over the surgical field they can be a prime source of contamination. Wheels of equipment and various foot pedals (i.e., power equipment, suction, electrosurgical unit) should be cleaned and disinfected. Places such as door ledges, cabinet tops, towel dispensers, view boxes, and the underside of equipment should not be overlooked.

Equipment such as the heating pad, the ECG, and the suction unit should be checked and ready for use. Instrument packs and supplies should be assembled. A wheeled cart can be used for transporting packs and supplies if they are stored outside of the operating room.

Between Cases

Soiled instruments and discarded materials should be promptly removed from the operating room. Tables, kick buckets, stands, and heating pads should be cleaned and disinfected after each case. Suction tubing and bottles should be replaced with clean units. The floors should be mopped or wet vacuumed with a disinfectant.

Post Surgery

All furniture and equipment in the operating room should be moved at the end of the day for cleaning and disinfecting. Wet vacuuming of the floor is superior to mopping; however, mopping may be used. The mop and bucket should be reserved for the operating room and marked "surgery only." The mop should be cleaned and disinfected daily by being laundered or soaked in a clean disinfectant for 30 minutes. Wet vacuuming involves flooding the floor with a disinfectant and vacuuming the floor dry. Dry mopping, sweeping and dry dusting should not be done in the operating room as they tend to increase air currents and the spread of organisms. After surgery, the scrub sinks should be thoroughly cleaned and disinfected to remove oily deposits that are left by the scrubbing process. The soap dispensers and foot pedals should also be included in the cleaning and disinfecting procedure. If the scrub brushes are reusable, they should be cleaned and resterilized.

Weekly

Air filters to the operating rooms should be changed once a week or more often if necessary. Wheels on equipment and suction unit motors should be lubricated. Electrical cords and foot pedals should be checked for fraying and to insure good operating condition.

Monthly

Sterile supplies should be dated at the time of sterilization, and this dating should be inventoried each month. All cloth or paper articles are double wrapped and considered sterile for one month. Articles in heat-sealed plastic are considered sterile for one year.

OPERATING ROOM ATTIRE

The operating room is an area of utmost cleanliness, and constant effort is required in maintaining asepsis. As persons entering the operating room are potential sources of contamination, policies regulating attire must be maintained. Surgical caps and masks must be worn whether surgery is being performed or not. Cleanliness and good personal hygiene should be habits of all who enter the operating room.

Visitors

Visitors should be given clean observation gowns and disposable shoe covers to be worn over their street clothes and shoes. Outer articles of clothing, without additional gowns, should not be permitted in the operating room.

Operating Room Personnel

The clothing of operating room personnel should be simple in design and comfortable. Scrub tops and pants or scrub dresses are acceptable; however, tops should be tucked in and dresses should fit closely. Loose clothing can accidently touch sterile surfaces. Cotton clothing is preferred over silk, nylon, or other synthetics because of the explosive hazard created by static electricity. Light blue, jade green, or misty green colors produce less glare than white. If a separate pair of shoes for surgery is impractical, shoe covers should be worn. All shoes must be cleaned of blood and debris daily.

Hat

All hair must be covered. The type of hat worn is determined by the amount of hair that needs to be covered. Those with short hair may wear the standard cap. Others with fuller and longer hair should wear the bouffant hat. Beards and sideburns can be effectively covered by a surgeon's hood.

Mask

A properly applied mask should fit snugly around the nose and chin. Loosely fitting or improperly worn masks are of little value in preventing exhaled organisms from entering the operating room. The mask should be comfortable and easy to breathe through. Coughing, sneezing, and talking increase moisture in the mask, and moisture decreases the filtration of organisms and allows their escape into the operating room. A moist mask is ineffective and must be replaced by a dry one.

Preparations of the Operative Site

The operative site should be prepared for surgery in order to remove as many bacteria as possible without harming the skin or interfering with wound healing. Skin cannot be sterilized; however, bacteria can be reduced to a relatively safe level for surgery by removal of hair, mechanical scrubbing, and the effective use of surgical scrub and germicidal solutions. The best solution and technique remain controversial. Hair removal and initial skin preparation should take place outside the operating room.

HAIR REMOVAL

Hair should be clipped well beyond the margins of the incision. If the animal is cooperative, the hair can be removed prior to anesthesia. A number 40 clipper blade will remove most hair satisfactorily. If additional hair needs to be removed, moisten the area with a soap solution and shave with a straight razor. Hair can be removed close to the skin when clipped in a direction opposite to that in which it grows. The clipper blade should be checked prior to use for broken teeth, as these cut and abrade the skin. The blade should be held flat and not used in a raking motion, as this can injure the skin (Fig. 3–1). Occasionally, the blade will become hot, and it should be checked frequently to prevent clipper burns. This is especially important in use on white poodles with delicate pink skin. Several products are available to cool and lubricate the blades. When the hair has been

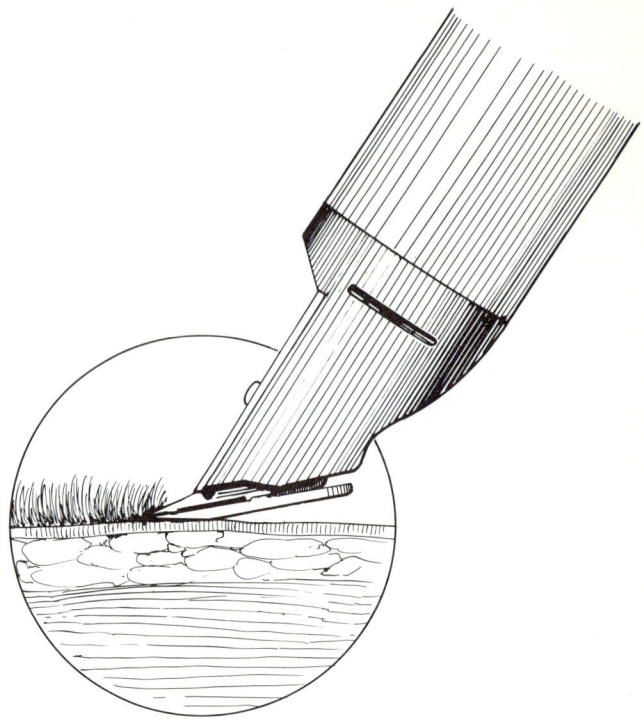

Figure 3–1

removed, the animal should be thoroughly vacuumed.

PREPARATION SOLUTIONS

A selection of compatible scrub and germicidal solutions is important to achieve maximum effectiveness. The limitations of the solutions need to be recognized. For example, hexachlorophene loses its effectiveness when regular soap or alcohol is applied afterwards. Quaternary ammonium compounds (Zephiran) lose their effectiveness when used as a germicidal agent in the presence of soap. A commonly used surgical scrub and germicidal solution combination is providone-iodine and 70 per cent ethyl alcohol.

SURGICAL PREPARATION

The initial cleansing of the operative site should take place outside the operating room. Povidone-iodine scrub should be applied with friction, followed by a thorough rinsing with warm water. A more thorough preparation should be performed after the animal is

PREOPERATIVE AND OPERATIVE PATIENT MANAGEMENT

positioned on the operating table. The preparation solutions should be applied with sterile gloves or sterile sponge forceps. The surgical preparation should begin at the incision line and in a circular motion proceed outward toward the periphery (Fig. 3–2). The technique of prepping an orthopedic and perineal case differs slightly from an abdominal prep.

Discard the sponge when reaching the periphery or when either hair or rectum has been touched. Alternate surgical scrub and germicidal solutions at least three times and until the sponge with germicidal solution remains clean after prepping. The last application of germicide should be allowed to dry on the operative site for maximum effectiveness.

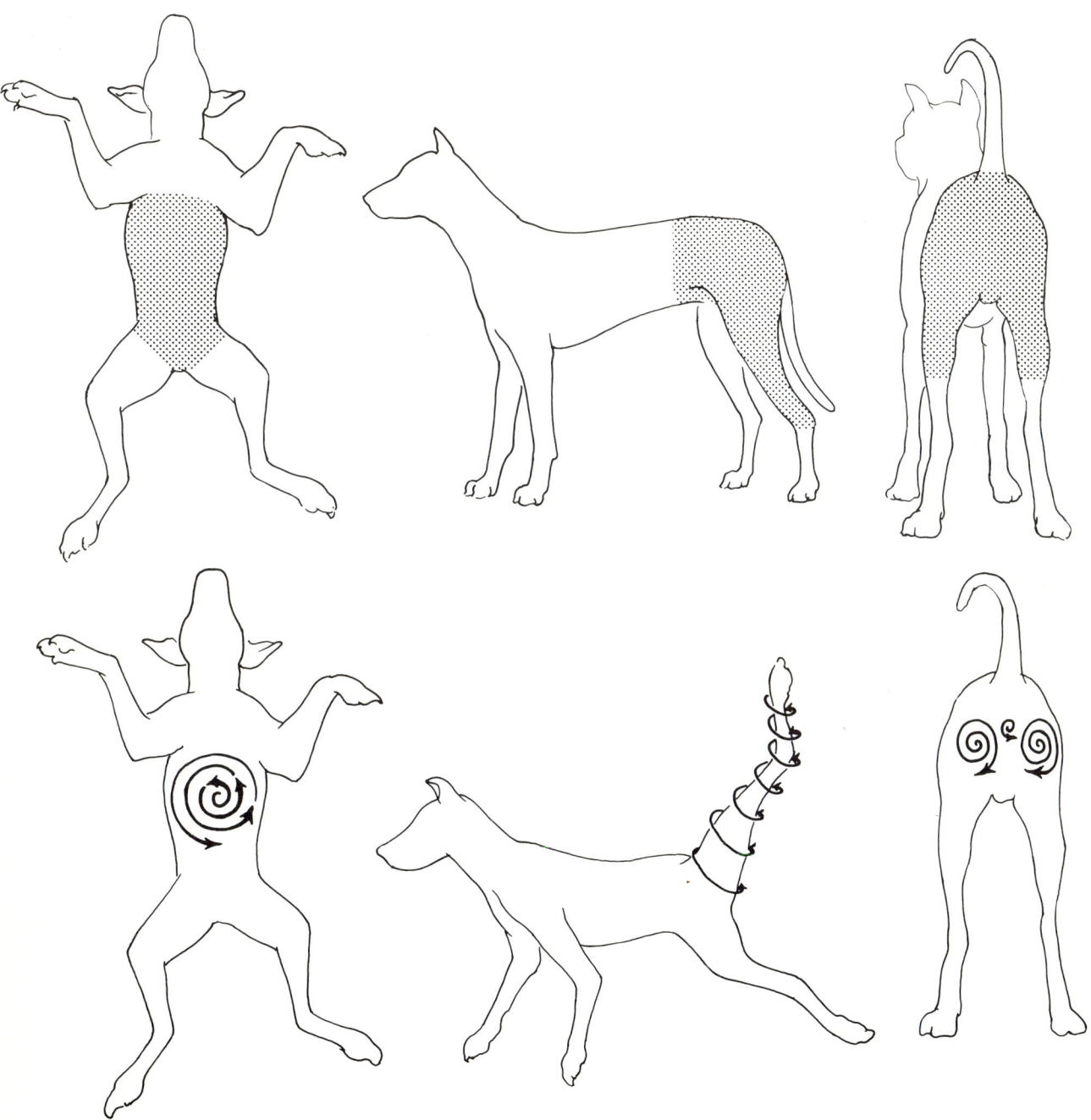

Figure 3–2

DRAPING THE PATIENT

The patient is draped by the surgeon after scrubbing, gowning, and gloving. Draping materials include cloth, waterproof paper, and plastic. The latter two types have the advantages of providing a complete barrier against bacteria and of being lint-free and disposable. Cloth drapes can absorb moisture and could therefore contaminate the sterile field. The patient should be draped prior to other preparation responsibilities (i.e., arranging instruments, accepting sterile supplies, and so on) in order to prepare a sterile field in which to work. This prevents contamination of the gown by brushing up against the unsterile table edge.

Fenestrated Drape

Fenestrated drapes are used quite often in elective surgeries such as ovariohysterectomy, castration, and onychectomy. The drape should be large enough to cover the table and the opening should be slightly larger than the length of the incision (Fig. 3–3). A single drape is unfolded and, by looking through the opening, is placed directly over the incision site. Regardless of the method used, drapes should never be dragged to the incision site.

Four Corner Draping

In four corner draping, four drapes are applied with a double thickness of about 10 inches toward the line of incision, with two drapes parallel to the patient and two perpendicular to the patient. The first and second drape should be placed parallel to the patient, with the first drape applied closest to the person draping in. A towel clamp may be used to temporarily secure the drape to the patient (Fig. 3–4A). The third drape should

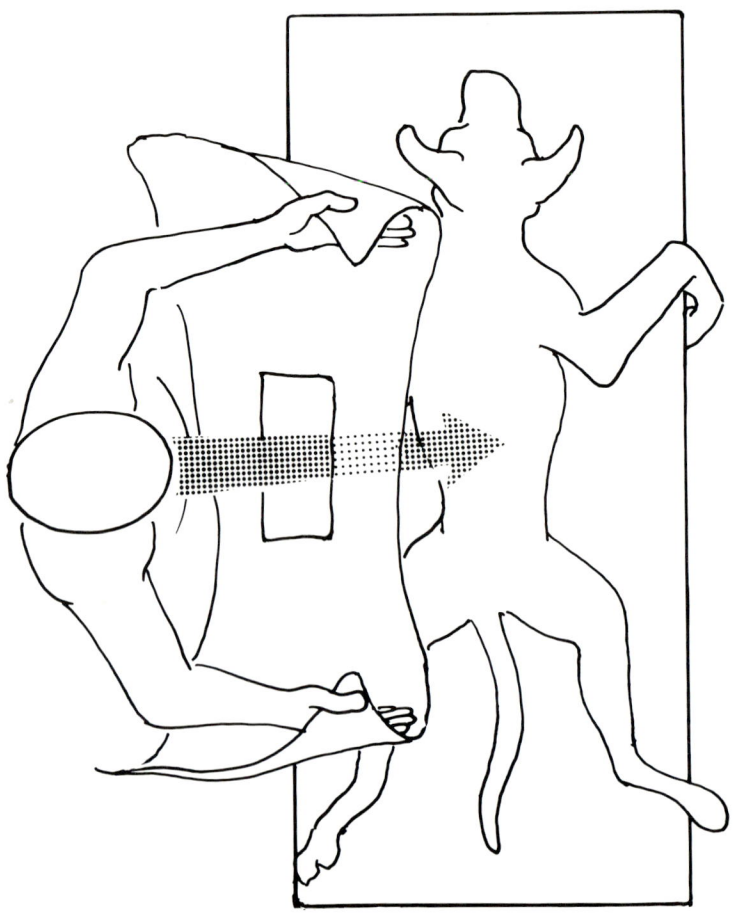

Figure 3–3

PREOPERATIVE AND OPERATIVE PATIENT MANAGEMENT

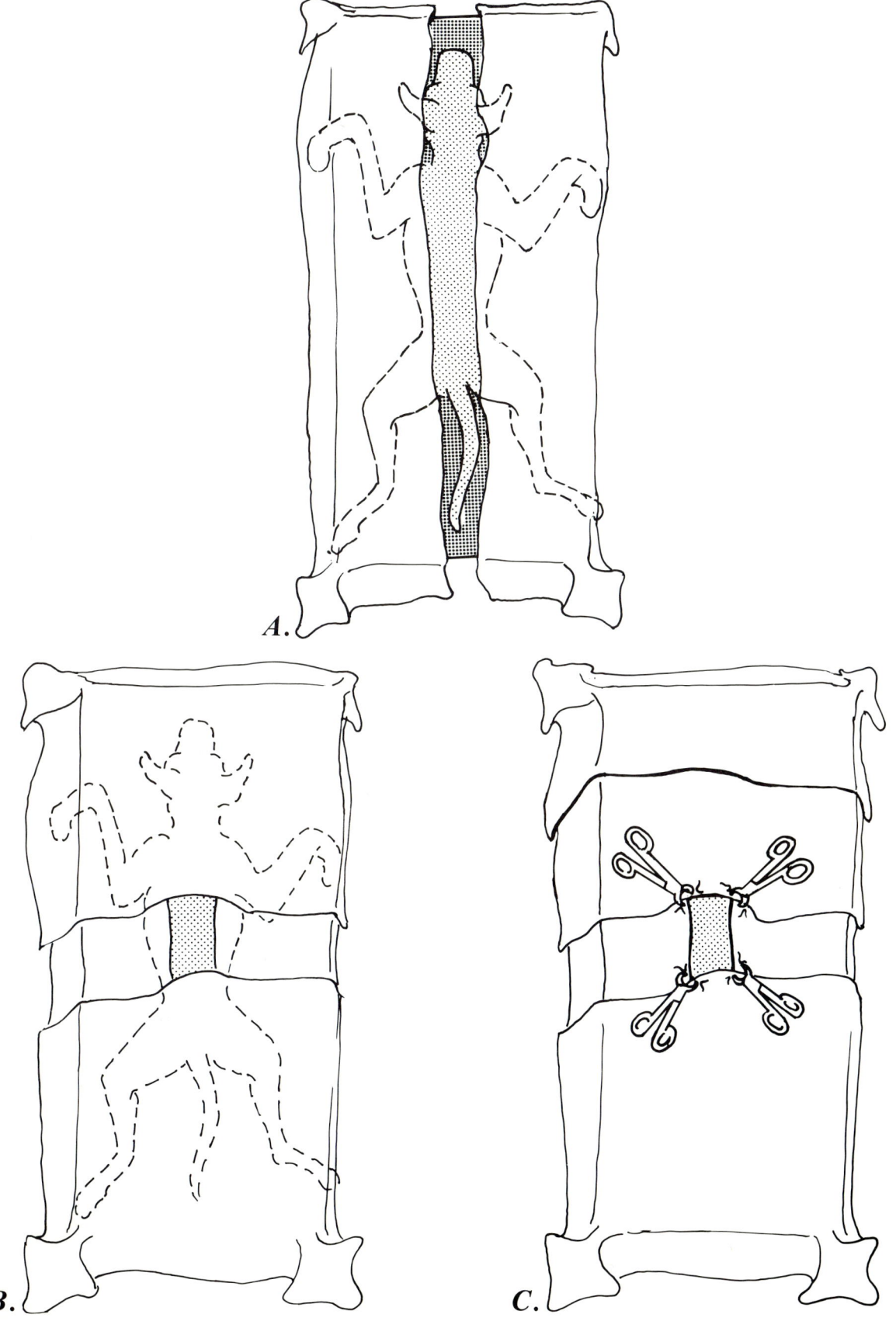

Figure 3-4

be placed perpendicular and cranial to the patient and secured with towel clamps. The fourth drape should be placed perpendicular and caudal to the patient, with the end of the drape connecting to the Mayo stand. Towel clamps should be used to secure the fourth drape to the patient and the Mayo stand (Figs. 3–4B and 3–4C).

Preparations of the Surgical Team

The objective of any scrub is to remove as many bacteria as possible by mechanical scrubbing and the use of chemical antiseptics without harming the skin. Many techniques are used so that every surface from the nails to the elbow is thoroughly scrubbed.

EQUIPMENT

A deep sink with either knee or foot controls for regulation of water flow is preferred. This eliminates the need for controlling the water supply by using the hands while performing a surgical scrub. Soap dispensers should also be operated by either foot or knee. Disposable nail cleaners should be available for cleaning under the fingernails. The scrub brush should be sterile and dispensed from a sterile, covered container or wrapped individually. Nylon-bristled brushes are preferred for their firmness and durability.

SCRUB SOLUTIONS

The two most commonly used scrub solutions are povidone-iodine and hexachlorophene. Povidone-iodine, an iodophor scrub, has been found to be three times more effective in maintaining low postscrubbing bacterial levels than is hexachlorophene.

TECHNIQUE

The technique for a complete surgical scrub remains controversial. The time and number of brush strokes may vary depending on previous scrubs and on the type of solutions used. Scrubbing times of 5 to 15 minutes and 10 to 20 brush strokes per surface have been advocated. The combination of scrubbing time and thorough brush strokes is the key to an effective surgical scrub. A guideline for the thoroughness is 10 minutes or 10 brush strokes per surface. Each scrub, however, should include two scrubs and rinses.

Fingernails should be short and free of nail polish. Rings and jewelry should be removed. The scrub begins with a general soaping and rinsing with warm water. The nails should be cleaned with a disposable nail pick. the hands should be held higher than the elbows to prevent contamination from water running off the elbows and dripping onto the hands. The scrub suit top should be tucked in and the body bent slightly at the waist to allow dripping to run off into the sink and not onto the scrub suit.

Skin surfaces should be scrubbed in a definite pattern of strokes in order to reach all surfaces. Start the scrub at the fingertips, proceeding to the surfaces of the fingers, the palms, the top of the hands, and then to the arm surfaces. After one scrub is complete, the hands and arms should be thoroughly rinsed. Discard the brush and acquire a new one for the second scrub. The process is then repeated.

GERMICIDAL RINSE

Even after thorough scrubbing, many resistant bacteria remain on the skin and continue to multiply after gloving. A germicidal rinse helps to further reduce the bacterial flora on the skin, thus reducing the chances of contamination during surgery.

Communal basins have been used but their effectiveness is reduced after repeated dippings and consequent dilution. Germicide applied from a dispenser and with mechanical rubbing is a superior method. Some solutions used for this purpose are quaternary ammonium compounds (Zephiran), 1 per cent iodine in 70 per cent ethyl alcohol, or 95 per cent ethyl alcohol followed by 70 per cent alcohol. It must be noted, however, that alcohol nullifies the action of hexachlorophene.

TOWELING

Drying the hands and forearms is necessary to prevent moisture from penetrating the gown and becoming a possible source of contamination. With dried surfaces, gloves can be donned more easily. The towel should be grasped at the top and allowed to unfold. The body should be bent at the waist to prevent the loose end of the sterile towel from brushing against the scrub suit. Toweling should start at the fingers, then proceed to the hand, and, with a twist motion, dry the wrist and forearm up to the elbow. The dried hand should grasp the free end of the towel and proceed to dry the opposite hand and arm. It is important that a clean portion of the towel be used for each section (i.e., right hand and arm, left hand and arm).

GOWNING

The sterile gown should be opened prior to scrubbing by the surgeon or other operating team members. The gown should be fan folded with the inside facing outward. The entire gown should be grasped by holding the inside edge of the neckband and allowed to unfold. Care should be taken to prevent contamination of the gown by brushing against the counter edge or other unsterile objects. The hands should now be slipped into the armholes in an upward motion. Avoid standing too close to the counter edge or near a wall, as the sleeve edges and gown front could easily be contaminated. Once the gown has been slipped on, it should be tied at the neck by an assistant.

GLOVING (CLOSED METHOD)

Closed method gloving reduces the potential for contamination, because the bare hands never touch the gloves or gown sleeve

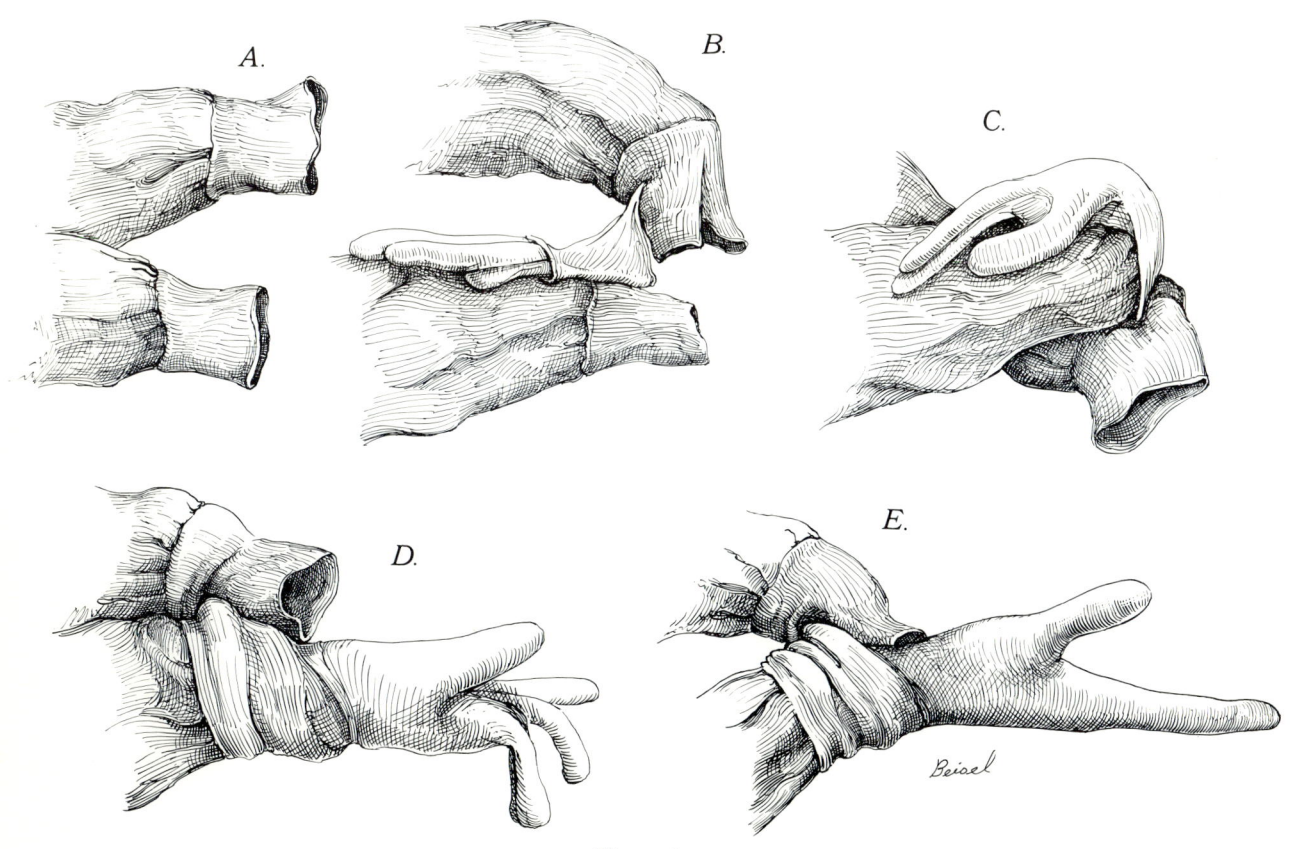

Figure 3–5

edge. Before gloving, lubricants can be applied to the hands to allow gloves to slide on more easily. Powders have been replaced by gloving cream in an effort to minimize dust particles in the operating room. Gloves are commercially prepowdered to make additional lubricants unnecessary.

Bare hands do not touch the gloves or the gown; therefore, when gowning do not allow fingers to go beyond the sleeve edge. Pick up the right glove through the gown with left hand. Place right glove on the arm with the *fingers* pointing *toward* the *shoulder* and the *thumb down*. Through the gown, use fingers to spread the cuff of the glove around the entire right gown sleeve edge. Pull cuff back over sleeve edge. Slide hand into glove by grasping the gown and pulling back. Repeat for the left glove (Fig. 3–5).

Suggested Reading

Archibald J (ed): Canine Surgery. Santa Barbara, California, American Veterinary Publications, Inc., 1965.

Catcott EJ: Animal Health Technology. Santa Barbara, California, American Veterinary Publications, Inc., 1965.

Ginsberg F, Brunner LS, and Cantilin VL: A Manual of Operating Room Technology. Philadelphia, JB Lippincott Co., 1966.

Knecht CD, Welser JR, Allen AR, and Williams DJ: Fundamental Techniques in Veterinary Surgery. Philadelphia, WB Saunders Company, 1975.

Perkins EW: Aseptic Technique for Operating Room Personnel, 2nd ed. Philadelphia, WB Saunders Company, 1964.

INSTRUMENTS CHAPTER 4

Jonathan N. Chambers

The student should be well versed in identification and proper use of the common surgical instuments.

Figure 4–1A. The Bard-Parker scalpel handle with interchangeable blades is the primary instrument for sharp dissection. The scalpel is held in the palm of the hand, with the index finger extended on the back of the blade. Incisions are made in long smooth strokes.

Figure 4–1B. Brown-Adson tissue forceps, like all tissue forceps, are held like a pencil, between the thumb and index finger. The smallest amount of tissue possible is grasped to avoid excessive trauma.

Figure 4–1C. Backhaus towel clamps afix drapes to the skin. Only a small amount of skin need be grasped to secure the drape.

Figure 4–1D. The Mathieu retractor is a hand-held, soft-tissue retractor.

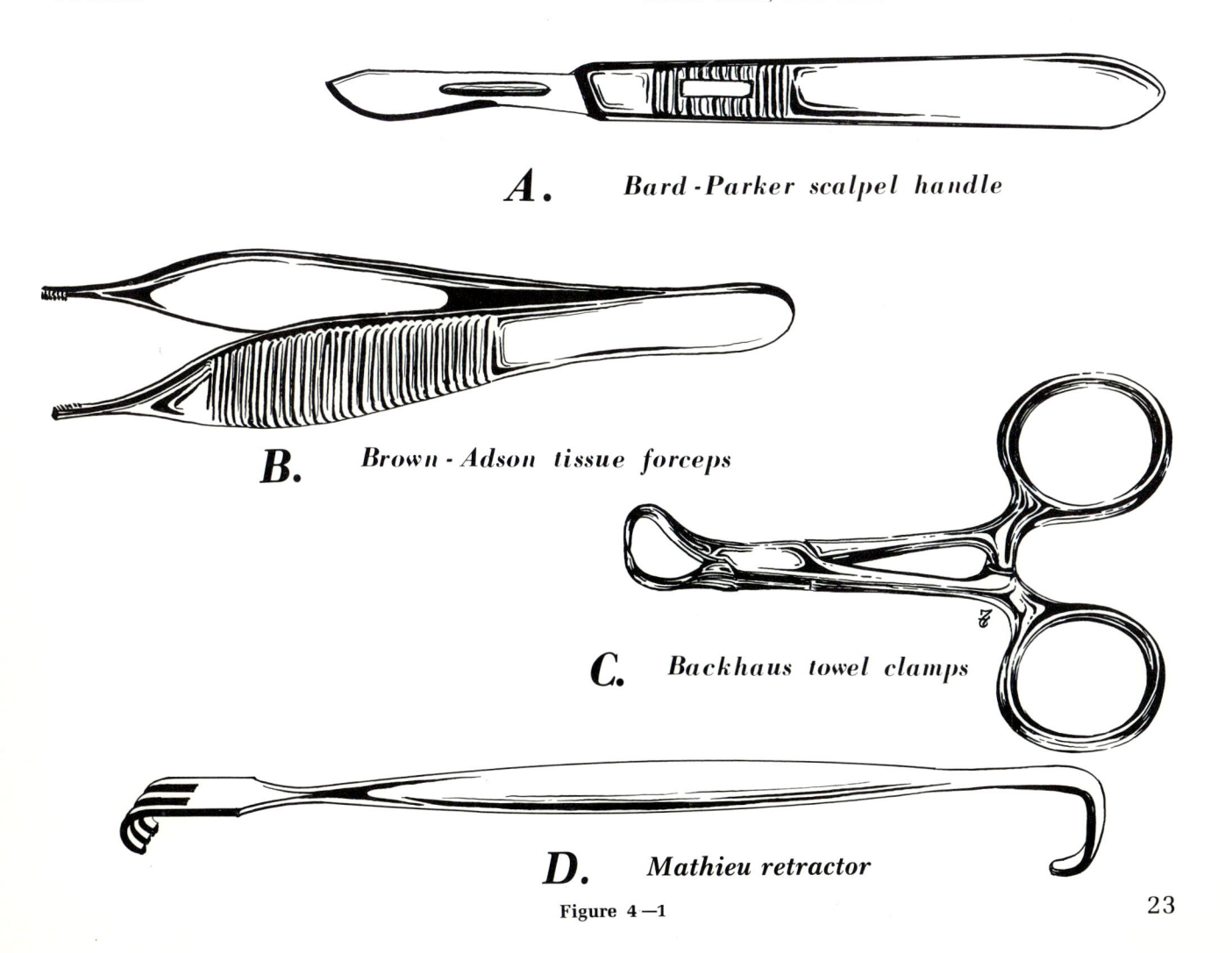

A. *Bard-Parker scalpel handle*

B. *Brown-Adson tissue forceps*

C. *Backhaus towel clamps*

D. *Mathieu retractor*

Figure 4–1

Figure 4–2A. Sharp-Sharp scissors are used for cutting all suture materials except wire.

Figure 4–2B. Wire suture scissors should be used for cutting small gauge stainless steel suture.

Figure 4–2C. Metzenbaum scissors are used for light soft-tissue dissection and should not be used on heavy fascia, skin, or suture material.

Figure 4–2D. Mayo scissors are used for general soft-tissue dissection and may be used on dense soft tissue when a knife incision is undesirable.

Figure 4–3A. The Halsted mosquito hemostat is used to control small bleeding vessels. Only the vessel is grasped to avoid trauma to surrounding tissue.

Figure 4–3B. The Kelly hemostat is used to grasp large bleeding vessels.

Figure 4–3C. Carmalt forceps are used to grasp tissue pedicles. These are "crushing" forceps and should be used judiciously.

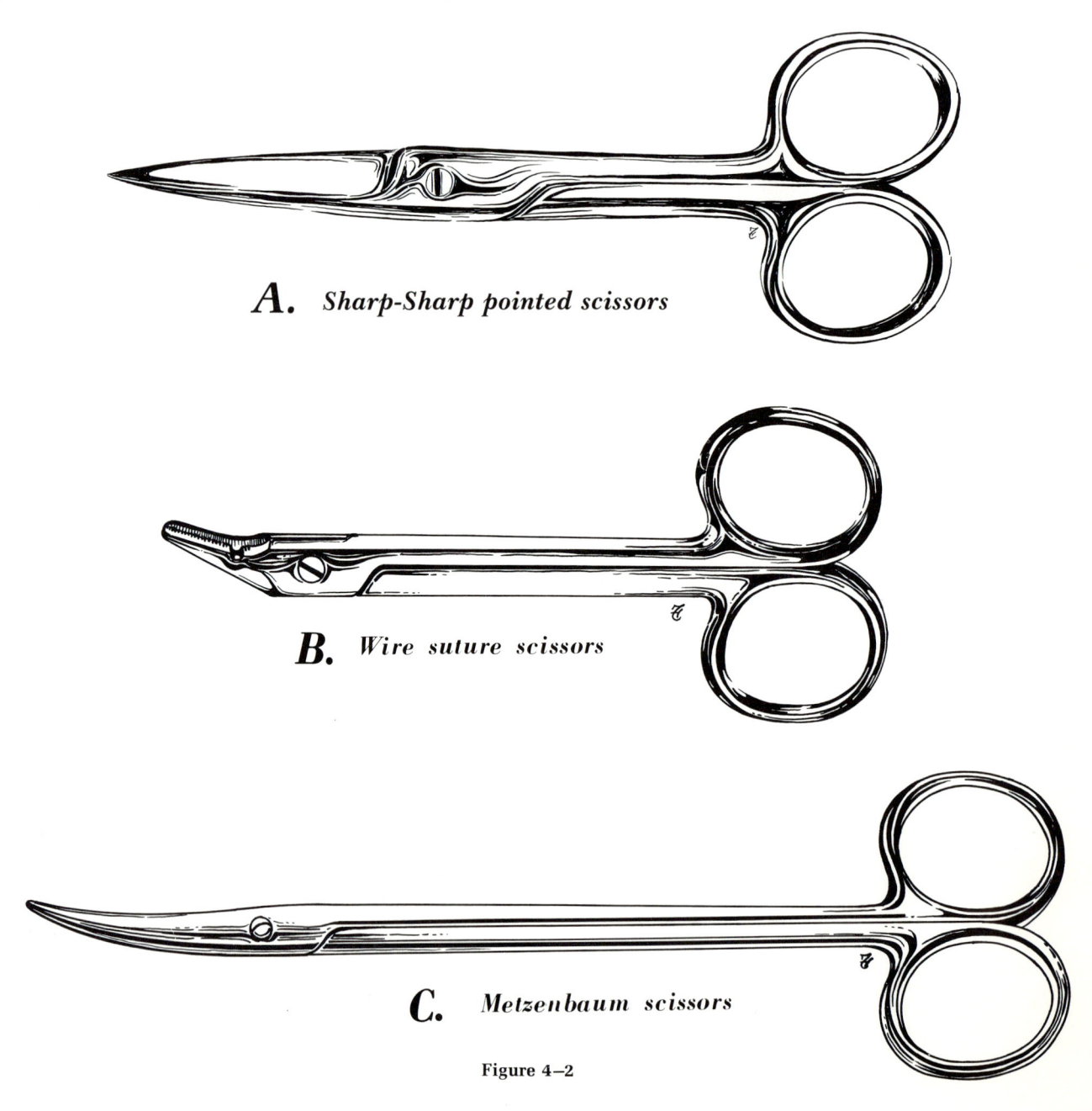

A. *Sharp-Sharp pointed scissors*

B. *Wire suture scissors*

C. *Metzenbaum scissors*

Figure 4–2

INSTRUMENTS 25

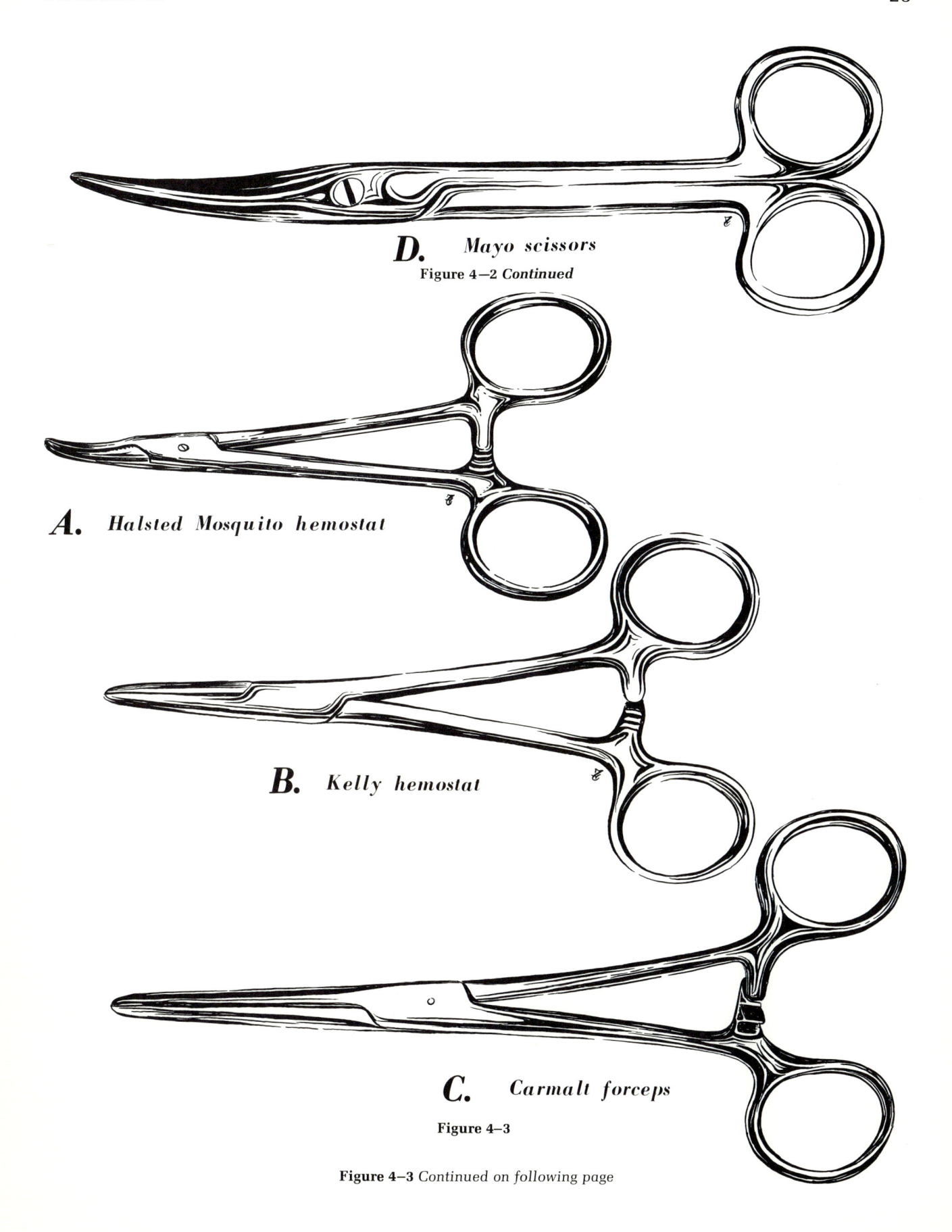

D. *Mayo scissors*
Figure 4–2 Continued

A. *Halsted Mosquito hemostat*

B. *Kelly hemostat*

C. *Carmalt forceps*
Figure 4–3

Figure 4–3 Continued on following page

Figure 4–3D. Allis tissue forceps afford a firm grip but are "traumatic." In general, they should be used only on tissue that is to be resected.

Figure 4–3E. The Mayo-Heger needle holder facilitates passage of the suture needle through the tissue. Needles should be grasped at their midpoint (away from the eye and point). Needles are withdrawn from the tissue with the needle holder to avoid damage to the delicate thumb forceps or the surgeon's glove.

D. *Allis tissue forceps*

E. *Mayo-Hegar needle holder*

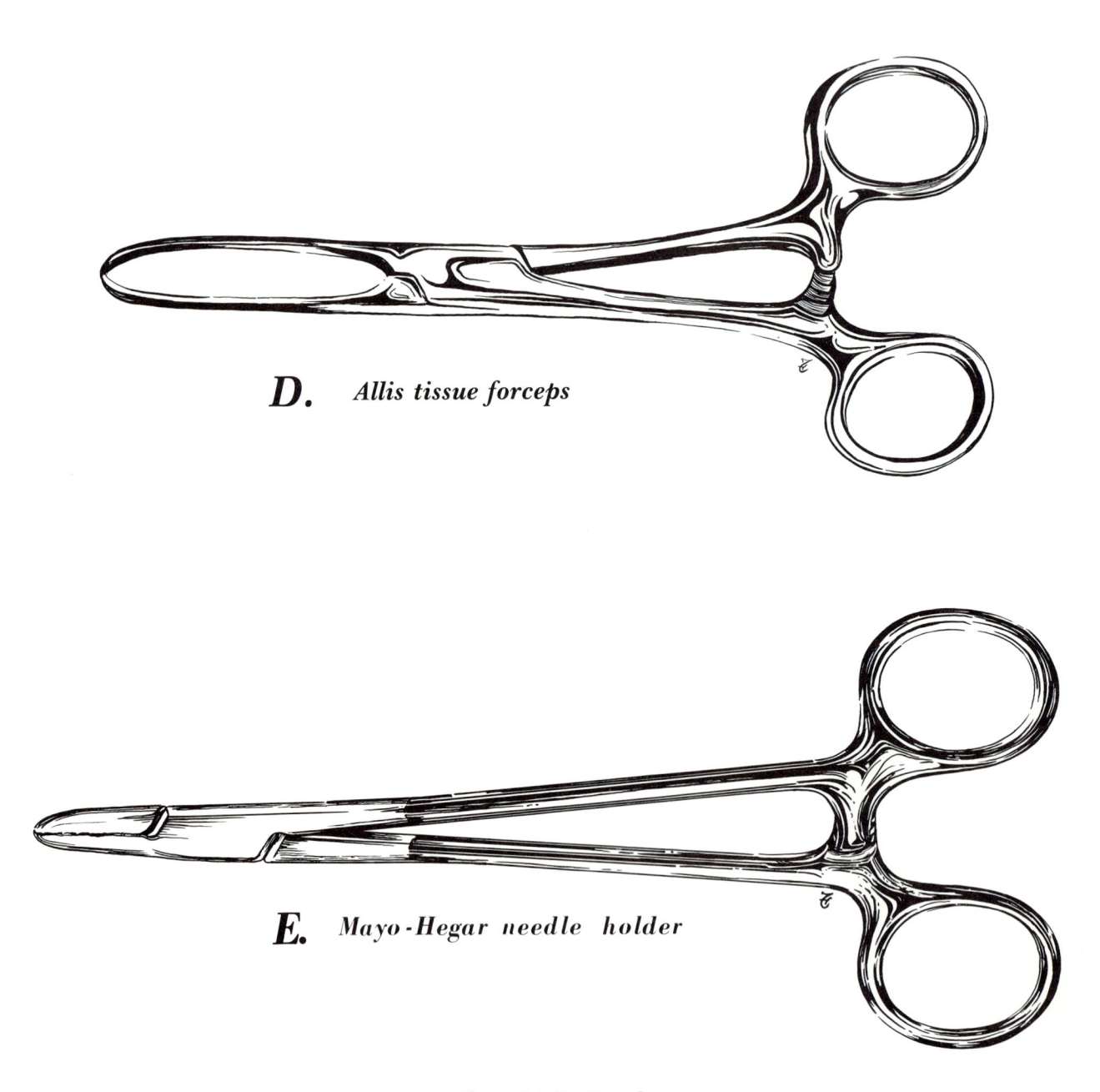

Figure 4–3 Continued

SUTURE PATTERNS   CHAPTER 5

JONATHAN N. CHAMBERS

Figure 5–1. The simple continuous pattern is an appositional stitch. The disadvantage of any continuous pattern is the need for integrity throughout the suture line. (If the suture breaks, the entire suture line fails.) Its principal advantage is speed of application. Note the proper angle at which the needle passes through the tissue (approximately 45 degrees).

Figure 5–2. This illustrates the preferred method of placing a simple continuous suture pattern, affording even, perpendicular tension at the epidermal surface.

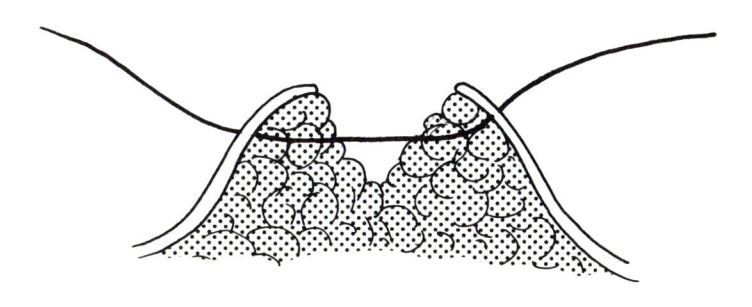

Simple Continuous

Figure 5–1

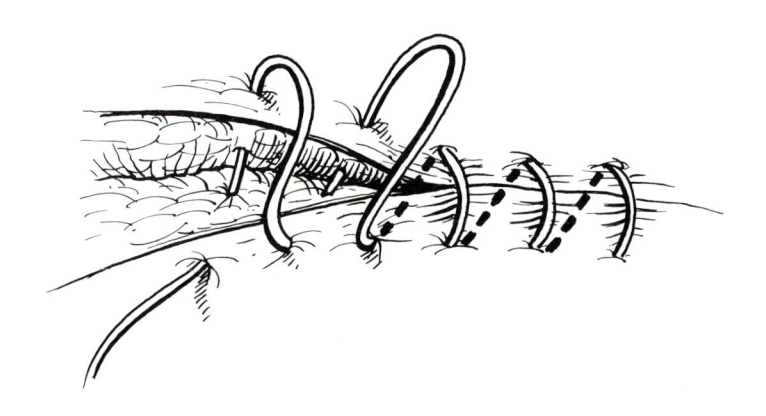

Simple Continuous · preferred

Figure 5–2

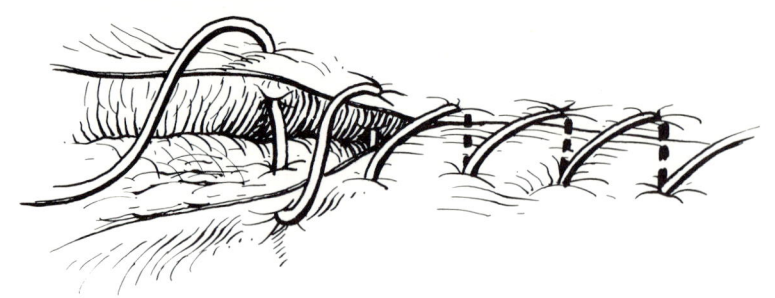

Simple Continuous (Alternative)
Figure 5-3

Figure 5-3. This illustrates the continuation of the simple continuous suture pattern of Figure 5-1.

Figures 5-4 and 5-5. The finishing knot for a simple continuous pattern may vary depending on the type of needle used.

Figure 5-6. The simple interrupted suture is the pattern most often used during surgery. The suture ends are pulled precisely parallel for maximum knot security.

Figure 5-7. The Lembert pattern inverts the tissue edge as the sutures are tied. This pattern may be in either a continuous or interrupted fashion.

Figure 5-8. The interrupted Lembert pattern acts to invert the tissue edges.

Atraumatic Needle

Closure knot   simple continuous continuous mattress

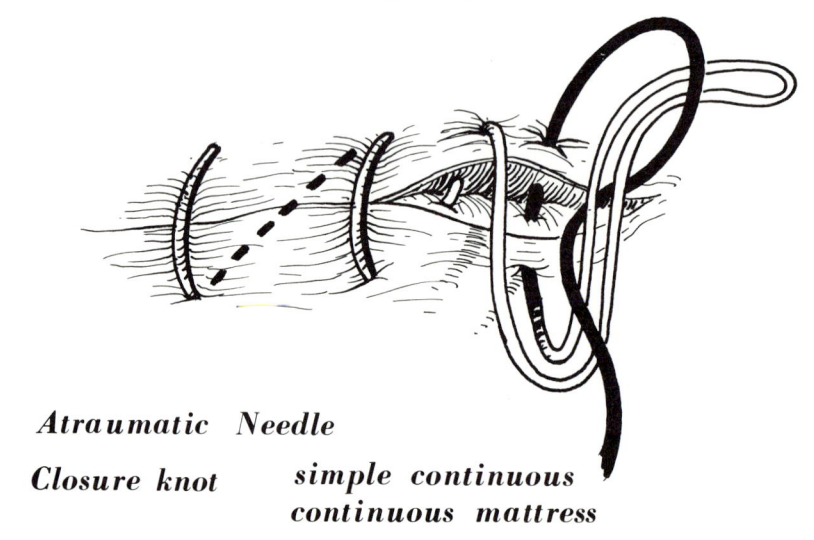

Figure 5 — 4

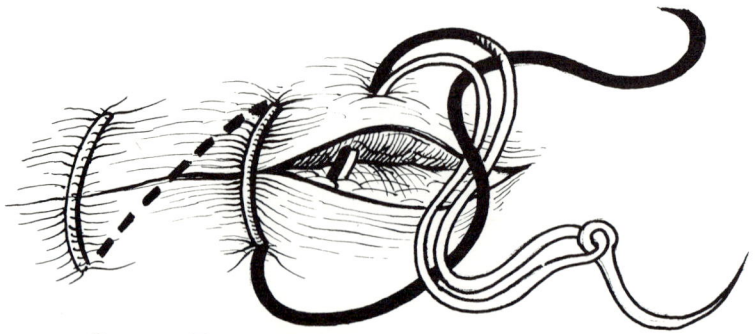

Open Eye Needle

Closure knot · simple continuous continuous mattress

Figure 5 — 5

SUTURE PATTERNS

Simple Interrupted

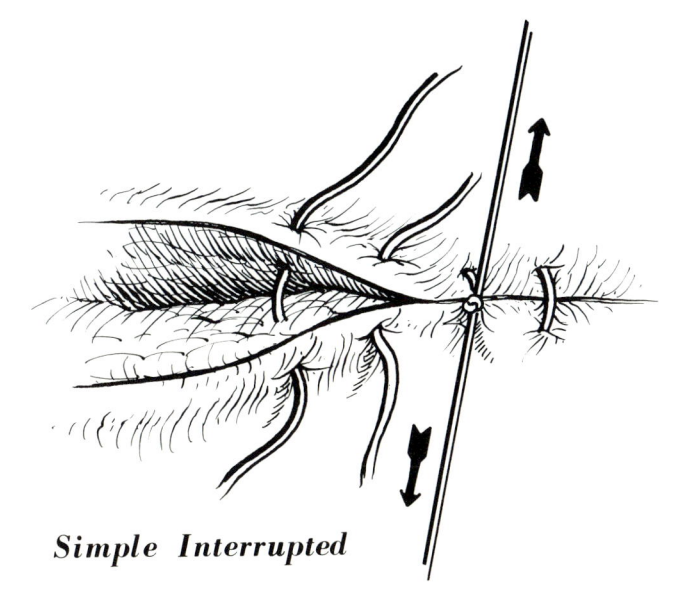

Figure 5–6

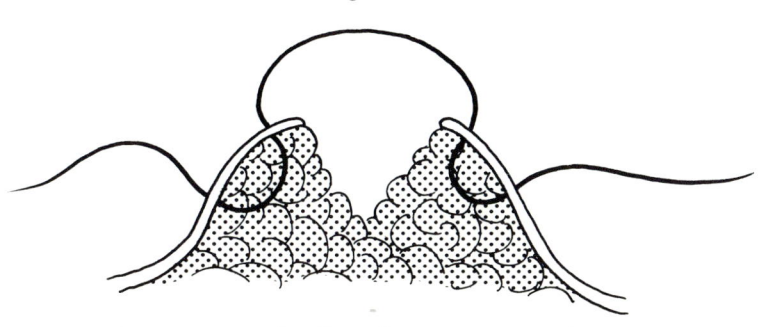

Interrupted · Lembert · inverting

Figure 5–7

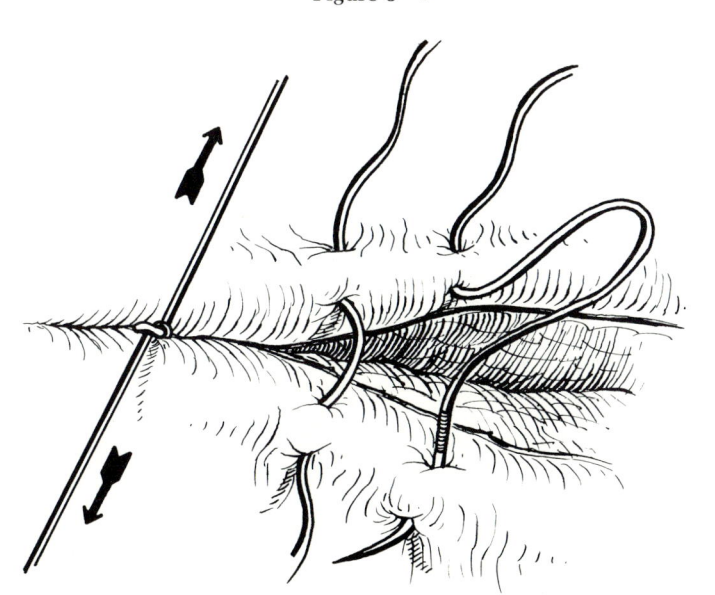

Interrupted Lembert · inverting

Figure 5–8

Figure 5–9. The mattress pattern will appose or evert the tissue edge depending on the tightness of the stitches. The continuous mattress pattern is illustrated.

Figure 5–10. The proper method of simple ligation of a vessel is illustrated.

Figure 5–11. The square knot is the standard method to secure a ligature. Unless dictated by special circumstances, all knots should be tied in this fashion.

Figure 5–12. The half-hitch knot results from an unevenly or loosely tied square knot. The half hitch can be "cinched" tight and protected from slipping by a square knot. It is especially useful when using fine monofilament suture to appose tissue edges that require tension for apposition.

Figure 5–13. The granny knot is less secure than a square knot and should not be used. This knot results when the same throw is used twice in succession.

Figure 5–14. The surgeon's knot is a double throw reinforced by at least one square knot. The double throw increases the hold of the knot. This knot should be reserved for use when suturing tissue edges under tension.

Figure 5–15. The Miller's knot is used to ligate tissue pedicles such as the ovarian pedicle and body of the uterus. This knot is extremely secure and will not be forced open by expansion of the tissue pedicle. This throw is reinforced by a square knot.

Figure 5–16. Many suture types and sizes are available, and the one chosen should be appropriately matched to the incision.

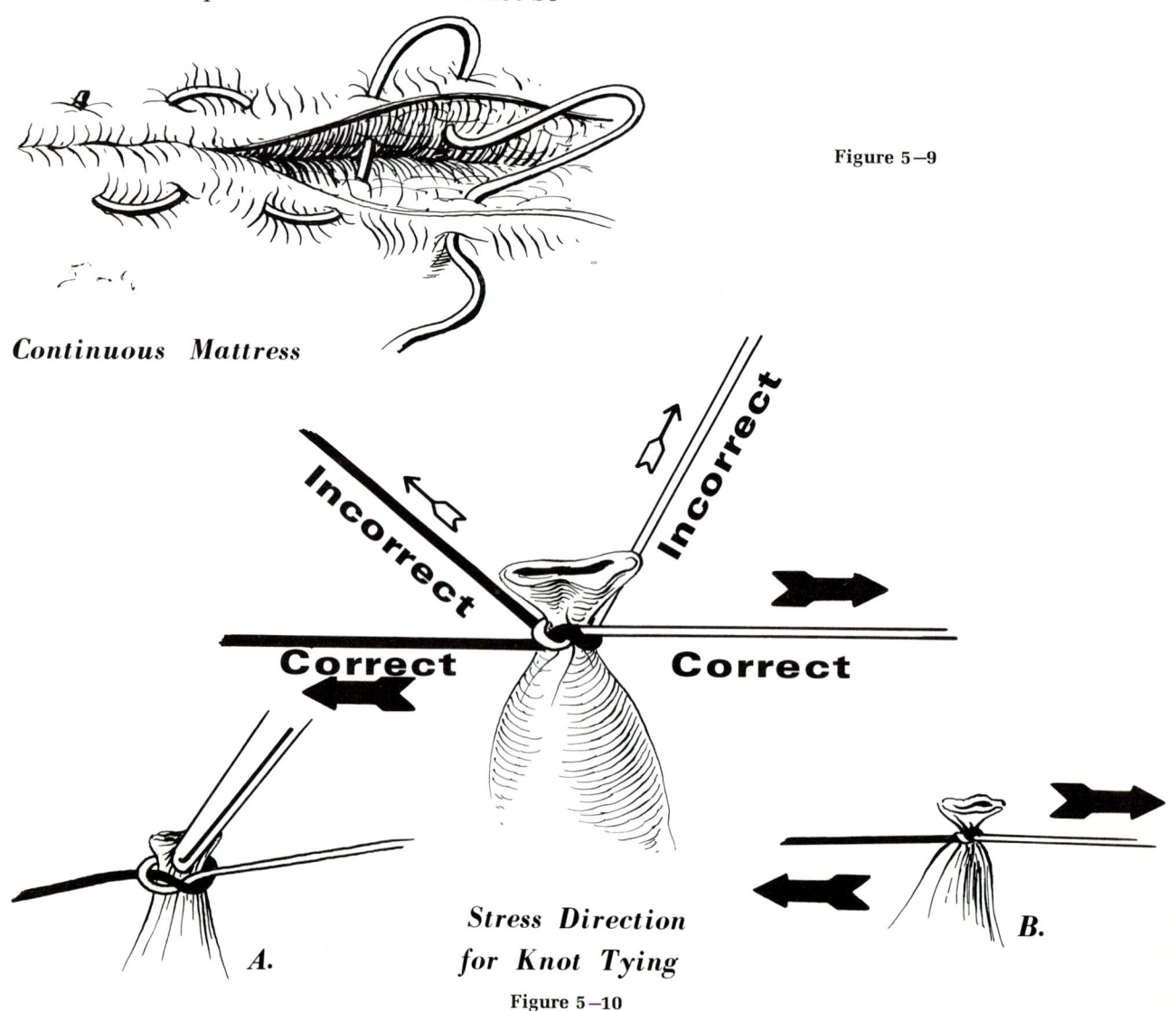

Continuous Mattress

Figure 5–9

Stress Direction for Knot Tying

A.   B.

Figure 5–10

SUTURE PATTERNS 31

Figure 5–11. Square knot.

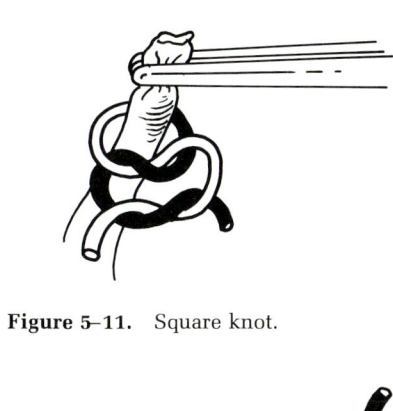

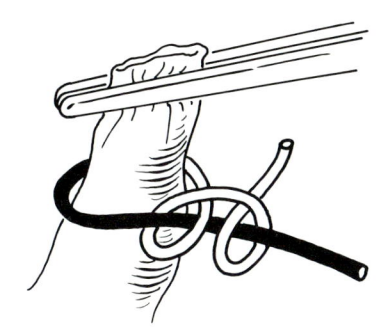

Figure 5–12. Half hitch.

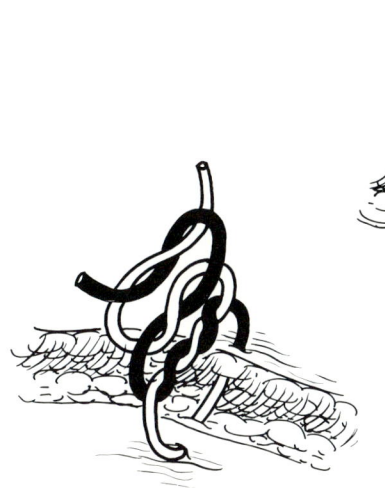

Figure 5–13. Granny knot.

Figure 5–14. Surgeon's knot.

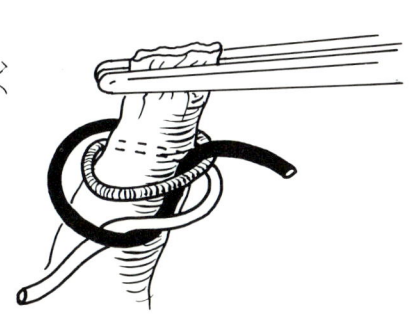

Figure 5–15. Miller's knot.

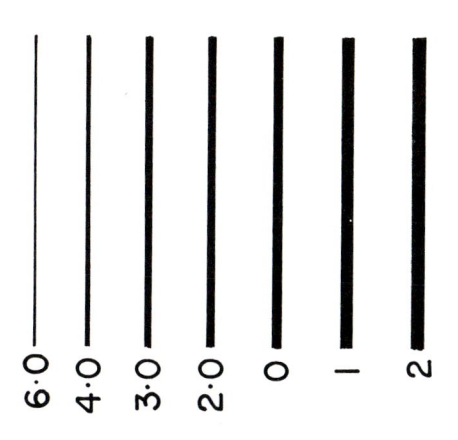

Suture Sizes

Figure 5–16

OPHTHALMIC SURGICAL PROCEDURES

CHAPTER 6

GRETCHEN M. SCHMIDT

The following procedures are designed for the surgical practice laboratory. The objectives of these procedures are to acquaint the student with basic ophthalmic surgical instrumentation and tissue handling. The order of procedures is designed for laboratory use. For a more thorough description of ophthalmic surgery, the student is referred to Bistner, Aquirre, and Batik: Atlas of Veterinary Ophthalmic Surgery (Philadelphia, W. B. Saunders Co., 1977).

6–1 IRRIGATION OF NASOLACRIMAL APPARATUS

Indications

Flushing the lacrimal excretory apparatus is both the diagnostic and therapeutic procedure for the problems of epiphora, dacryocystitis, and chronic conjunctivitis.

Anesthesia

Topical anesthesia of the conjunctiva with 0.5 per cent proparacaine hydrochloride is satisfactory in cooperative animals.

Patient Positioning

This procedure may be accomplished in the awake, cooperative patient.

Operative Preparation

A 20- or 22-gauge curved lacrimal cannula or blunted polyethylene tubing with appropriate size B-D tubing adapter is used for cannulation. Saline, eye wash, or therapeutic solutions (e.g., antibiotics, steroids) are used for irrigation.

Exposure

The medial canthus is held open manually so that the lid margins are slightly everted.

Ophthalmic Surgical Techniques

A.

B.

C.

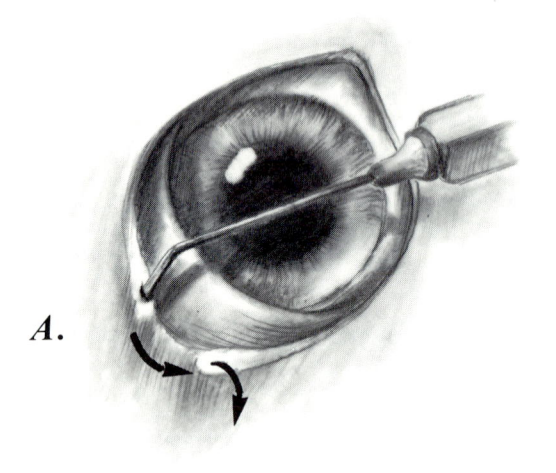

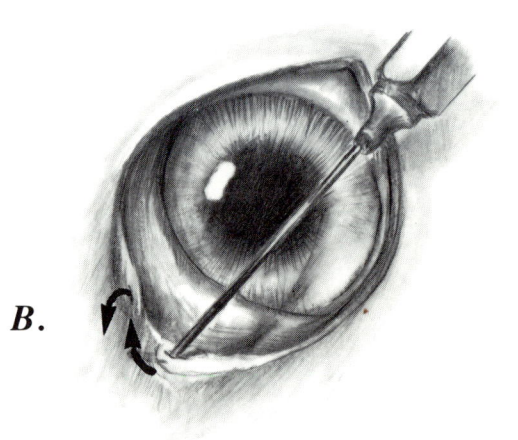

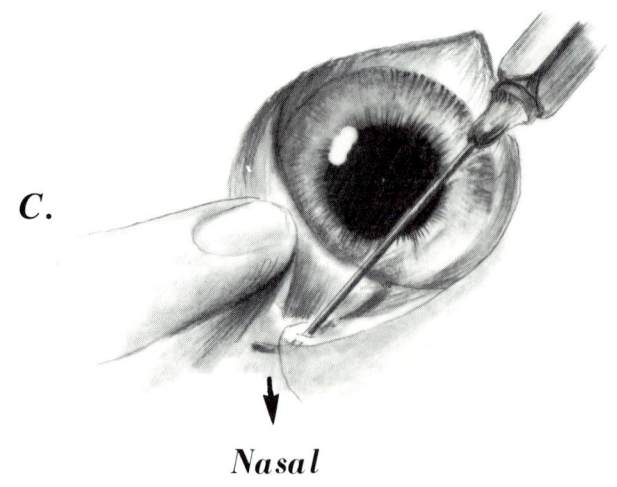

Nasal

Figure 6–1

Details of Procedure

Figure 6–1A. The cannula is inserted into the upper punctum in a line parallel to the lid margin and directed toward the caruncle. Irrigation is complete when the fluid is seen exiting from the lower punctum.

Figure 6–1B. The lower punctum is cannulated in a similar manner.

Figure 6–1C. The upper punctum is obstructed with the forefinger so that the irrigating solution passes into the nasolacrimal duct. Indications that the system is patent are observation of the fluid at the nostril and/or gagging or sneezing of the animal.

NOTES:

6–2 SUBCONJUNCTIVAL INJECTION

Indications

The subconjunctival injection is an effective means of achieving high levels of drugs in the anterior segment of the eye. Antibiotics and corticosteroids are the drugs administered most frequently by this route. The volume of drug injected subconjunctivally usually does not exceed 1 ml. Commonly used drugs and dosages are:

Chloramphenicol sodium succinate	50–100 mg
Gentamicin	20 mg
Kanamycin	10–40 mg
Triamcinolone acetonide suspension	10–40 mg
Methylprednisolone acetate suspension	10–80 mg

Anesthesia

Topical anesthesia of the conjunctiva with 0.5 per cent proparacaine hydrochloride is sufficient in a cooperative patient.

Patient Positioning

The head is firmly restrained, and the upper eyelid is retracted so as to expose the dorsolateral bulbar conjunctiva.

Operative Preparation

The medication is drawn into a tuberculin syringe with a 25- or 26-gauge needle.

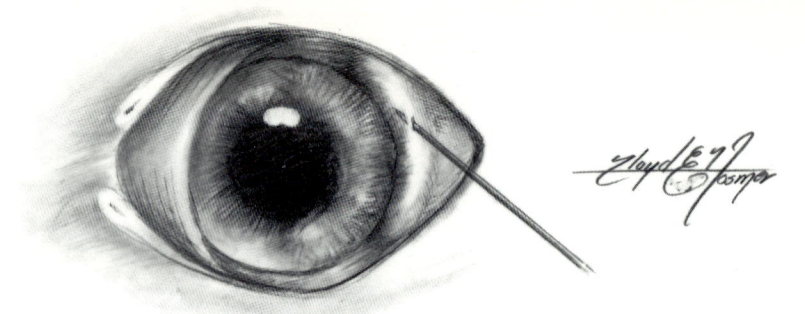

Figure 6–2

Details of Procedure

The lid is retracted with the left hand (or with the right hand if left-handed), and the tip of the needle is inserted under the bulbar conjunctiva with a short, quick motion. The needle is directed parallel to the limbus and slightly dorsad so that if the animal should move his head, an intraocular injection is prevented.

<u>Figure 6–2</u>. The drug is instilled under the bulbar conjunctiva so as to form a bleb. With absorption of the drug, this bleb dissipates, except one of methylprednisolone acetate suspension, which will remain as a visible yellow-white plaque indefinitely.

NOTES:

6–3 IMMOBILIZATION AND EXPOSURE OF GLOBE

Indications

Under general anesthesia, the animal's eye rotates down and into the orbit, allowing prolapse of the third eyelid and making exposure difficult. Exposure should be maximum and immobilization complete for corneal or intraocular surgery.

Patient Positioning

The animal is positioned in lateral recumbency. The head is positioned by sand bags so that the eye is accessible.

Operative Preparation

The periocular hair is carefully clipped to avoid skin abrasions. The cilia are cut with scissors. The conjunctival cul-de-sac and cornea are flushed with an ophthalmic irrigating solution to remove any hair or debris. The lids and periocular skin are surgically prepared in a standard manner. Care should be taken that none of the scrub solutions contact the conjunctiva or cornea. If this should occur, profuse irrigation is indicated immediately to prevent irritation and ulceration.

Self-retaining lid retractors, fine-toothed ophthalmic forceps, 4-0 silk with swaged-on ophthalmic cutting needle, and delicate needle holders are needed to immobilize and expose the globe.

OPHTHALMIC SURGICAL PROCEDURES

A.

B.

Figure 6–3

Details of Procedure

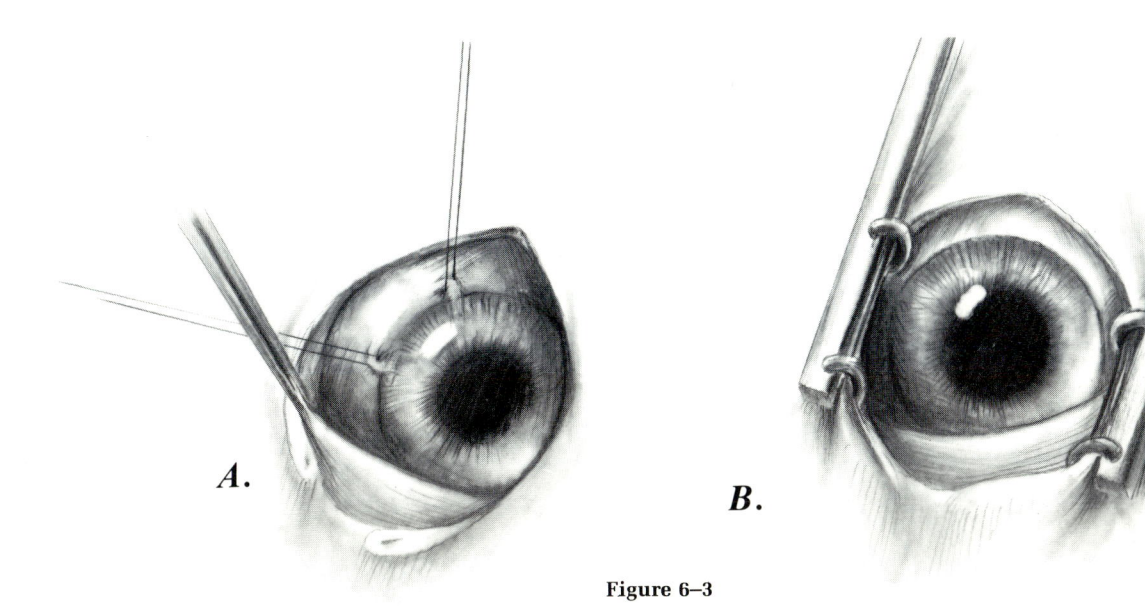

Figure 6–3A. A self-retaining lid retractor is placed under the upper and lower lids and tightened so that the lid openings are maximized. If this is not enough exposure, the retractor is removed, and a lateral canthotomy is performed. The lateral canthus is incised with scissors placed into the conjunctival cul-de-sac. The incision is made through the conjunctiva and eyelid up to the lateral orbital ligament in a line parallel to the lid margins. The retractor is then replaced.

Figure 6–3B. Two stay sutures are placed at 10 and 12 o'clock, 1 to 2 mm from the limbus. The sutures should engage episcleral tissue so that with traction, the globe can be lifted out of the orbit. When the globe is pulled forward, the third eyelid retracts into the near normal position, exposing the cornea. The ends of the sutures are fixed so that the eye is positioned properly for the procedure to be done.

When the surgery is completed, the stay sutures and the retractor are removed. If a lateral canthotomy was made, this is closed with a two-layer closure of 6-0 absorbable suture in the conjunctiva and 4-0 nonabsorbable suture in the skin. Care in apposing the lid margin is necessary to avoid malpositioning of the eyelids.

NOTES:

6–4 SUPERFICIAL KERATECTOMY

Indications

Lesions irritating the eye (dermoid cysts, corneal necrosis), causing blindness (corneal dystrophy, pigmentary keratitis), or invading the cornea (neoplasia) that are located in the superficial third of the corneal stroma may be removed by superficial keratectomy.

Anesthesia

General anesthesia is indicated.

Patient Positioning

The patient is placed in lateral recumbency, with the head positioned by sandbags.

Operative Preparation

Because the cornea and conjunctiva cannot be prepared by standard surgical scrub techniques, this procedure is regarded as "clean" surgery. Preparation of the periocular region is the same as that described in Procedure 6–3. Preoperative, topical ophthalmic, broad-spectrum antibiotics are often used to reduce the conjunctival flora. The eye is exposed and immobilized as described in Procedure 6–3.

Instruments needed for a superficial keratectomy are a self-retaining lid retractor, fine ophthalmic corneal forceps, a small surgical blade, Castroviejo corneal trephine (10 to 14 mm in diameter), and a means of irrigation of the surgical field. The corneal trephine is not absolutely necessary for this procedure, but it is helpful for the surgeon inexperienced in corneal surgery.

Suture material is needed for immobilization of the globe and closure of the lateral canthotomy, if made for added exposure. In case of perforation of the cornea during the keratectomy, 6-0 to 9-0 suture material with a swaged-on ophthalmic needle should be on hand. See section on corneal laceration repair.

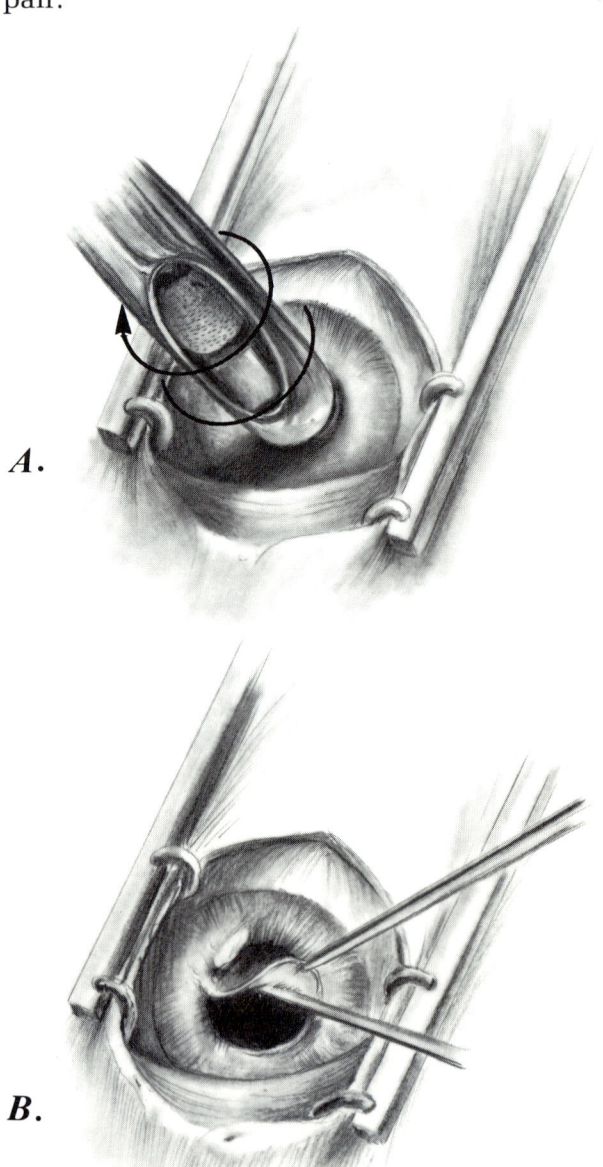

A.

B.

Figure 6–4

Details of Procedure

Figure 6-4A. The corneal trephine, with the depth guard set at 4, is placed over the corneal lesion. With firm pressure, the trephine is rotated so as to maintain the position of the trephine blades on the cornea. The trephine is rotated until the superficial cornea is evenly incised to the desired depth. The depth guard helps to control the amount of cornea incised and is helpful for surgeons inexperienced in this part of the procedure.

Figure 6-4B. The cut edge of the cornea to be removed is gently grasped with corneal forceps, and with a surgical blade, the isolated cornea is dissected free, maintaining the same lamellar plane as the trephine incision. More cornea may be removed using the trephine incision as a guide for depth of a free-hand incision.

During the surgery, the cornea is kept moist with an appropriate irrigating solution (saline, BSS). Hemorrhage is a problem only when removing a vascularized lesion and should not be extensive if the depth of the incision is correct. Hemorrhage is controlled with the use of cotton-tipped applicators.

Postoperative management is the same as for a corneal ulcer. Epithelialization time of the keratectomy site depends on the diameter. A 10 mm lesion is usually epithelialized within 72 hours.

NOTES:

6-5 CORNEAL LACERATION REPAIR

Indications

Suturing of the cornea is indicated in acute, full-thickness corneal lacerations and in chronic corneal wounds that continue to leak aqueous humor. Alternatives to suturing the cornea are conjunctival flaps, which are not discussed in this text.

Anesthesia

General anesthesia is necessary to suture the cornea.

Patient Positioning

The patient is positioned as described in Procedure 6-3.

Operative Preparations

The preparation of the operative site is the same as that described for "Superficial Keratectomy."

Instruments needed to repair a corneal laceration are a self-retaining lid retractor, fine ophthalmic corneal forceps, ophthalmic needle holders, a means of irrigating the exposed cornea, and tenotomy scissors if a prolapsed iris must be excised.

The following suture material may be used to close a corneal laceration: ophthalmic silk, gut, collagen, monofilament nylon, or polyglycolic acid. Spatula or reverse cutting needles with ⅜ or ½ circle curvature are used for corneal surgery.

Incision and Exposure

In acute corneal lacerations, the full extent of the injury often is not appreciated until the eye can be fully examined under general anesthesia. If the eye is to regain function, emergency surgery is necessary. The eye is immobilized and exposed as described in Procedure 6–3. A lateral canthotomy is usually necessary. Any prolapsed intraocular structures are gently removed from the wound edges. A fibrin clot has usually formed at the site of the laceration. This may also be removed but not at the expense of creating more trauma to the intraocular structures.

Ophthalmic Surgical Techniques

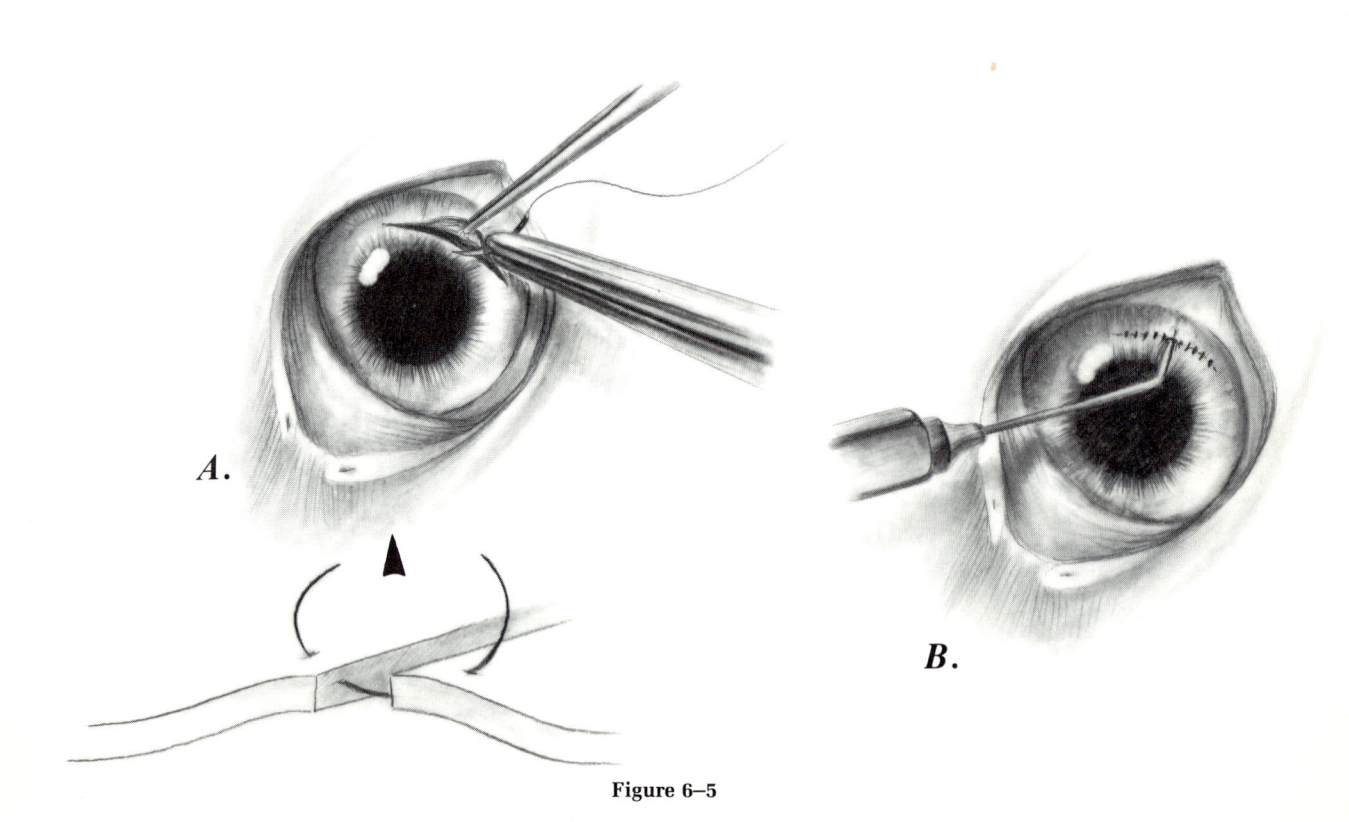

A.

B.

Figure 6–5

Details of Procedure

Figure 6–5A. The edges of the cornea are apposed with minimal handling of the corneal tissue. A simple interrupted suture pattern is used. The suture should not pass through the entire corneal thickness.

Figure 6–5B. With an air cannula or blunted 25-gauge needle, air is injected through the wound to reconstitute the anterior chamber and assess closure of the wound. Postoperatively, the eye is treated with antibiotics and mydriatics. After several days, steroids are often used to control the associated intraocular inflammation. Systemic therapy may also be used.

NOTES:

6–6 THIRD EYELID FLAP

Indications

The third eyelid flap is employed as a corneal bandage. Suturing the third eyelid so that it covers the entire cornea is indicated for exposure keratitis, keratitis caused by mechanical trauma from the eyelids, and ulcerative keratitis. Once the third eyelid is in place, the cornea cannot be examined, but topical medication is as effective when applied to the surface of the third eyelid as when applied to the cornea itself.

Anesthesia

In extremely debilitated animals, a third eyelid flap can be performed with topical anesthesia (0.5 per cent proparacaine hydrochloride). However, in most cases, a short-acting general anesthetic is used.

Patient Positioning

Lateral recumbency, with the affected eye up, is the most common position when suturing a third eyelid flap.

Operative Preparation

Any necrotic cornea or nonadherent corneal epithelium is removed from the surface before the third eyelid is sutured in place. The conjunctival cul-de-sacs are thoroughly irrigated to remove any debris. No clipping or surgical scrub is necessary. A self-retaining lid retractor, fine tissue forceps, and a needle holder are required for the procedure. Four-0 nonabsorbable suture material is adequate for most small animals.

Details of Procedure

With the lid retractor in position, the third eyelid is grasped with thumb forceps and pulled over the cornea to approximate its position when sutured in place. At least two mattress sutures are evenly spaced in the medial and lateral aspects of the third eyelid. Figure 6–6 shows the placement of the medial suture. All sutures are placed first and then tied snugly so that no suture material contacts the corneal surface. The suture is first placed through the entire thickness of the third eyelid, engaging the cartilage along the margin, starting at the palpebral surface of the third eyelid. The suture is then anchored to firm episcleral tissue about 2.5 mm from the limbus. To complete the mattress pattern, the suture is passed through the third eyelid again, engaging cartilage from the bulbar surface.

The flap is left in place for 7 to 10 days. Suture removal is done with topical anesthesia. It may take several days for the third eyelid to return to its normal position.

NOTES:

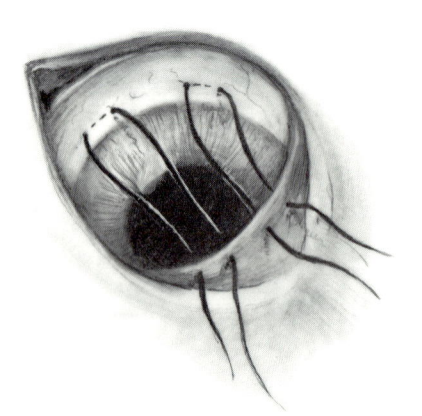

Figure 6–6

6–7 TARSOCONJUNCTIVAL RESECTION – LID-SPLITTING PROCEDURES FOR DISTICHIASIS

Indications

Ectopic eyelashes originating from the meibomian glands of the eyelid and contacting the cornea may cause no ocular irritation, conjunctivitis, blepharospasm, chronic superficial keratitis, or ulcerative keratitis. If many lashes are present and an ocular problem exists that can be related to the presence of the lashes, removal is warranted. Epilation is one means, and excision of the hair follicle by tarsoconjunctival resection is another.

Anesthesia

General anesthesia is indicated.

Patient Positioning

The patient is positioned in lateral recumbency, with the head elevated with sand bags.

Operative Preparation

The conjunctival cul-de-sac is irrigated to remove any debris. Clipping and surgical scrubbing are not necessary.

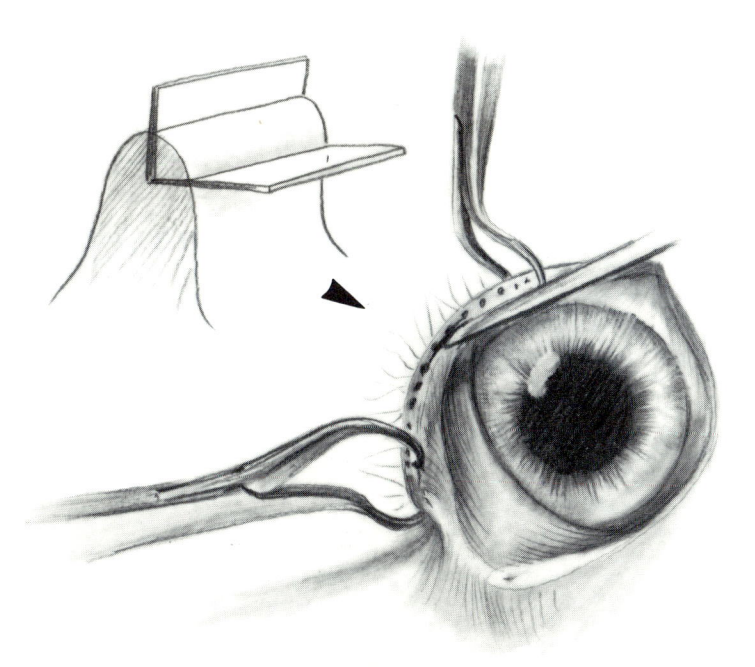

Figure 6–7

Two small towel clamps, a No. 64 Beaver blade and handle or a No. 15 Bard-Parker blade and handle, small, fine thumb forceps, tenotomy scissors, and an optivisor loupe or other means of magnification are needed for the procedure.

Exposure

The towel clamps are engaged at the medial and lateral aspects of the eyelid and held by an assistant so that the eyelid margin is everted and immobilized.

Details of Procedure

Figure 6-7. The tarsal incision is made in the eyelid margin parallel to the palpebral conjunctiva to the depth of the hair follicle (4 to 5 mm). Hemorrhage is controlled by pressure on the lid margin. If more than one half of the eyelid margin must be resected to remove the cilia, a second parallel incision is made on the other side of the hairs, and only a thin strip is resected. If less than one half of the eyelid margin needs to be resected to remove the cilia, a perpendicular incision with tenotomy scissors is made on the conjunctival side. At least one half of the eyelid margin should remain to prevent entropion. The incision is not sutured. Topical, antibiotic-steriod ophthalmic medication is used for 3 to 5 days following the surgery. Recurrence of the ectopic cilia is common, especially if the hair follicle was not removed. Repeated tarsoconjunctival resections usually lead to entropion.

NOTES:

SOFT TISSUE SURGERY CHAPTER 7

7-1 THORACOTOMY

CLARENCE A. RAWLINGS

Indications

A left or right thoracotomy at the fourth or fifth intercostal space is indicated to approach the pulmonary hilus for a lobectomy. The left approach is also used in the surgical exposure of a patent ductus arteriosis and vascular ring anomalies and for a pulmonary arteriotomy.

Anesthesia

Anesthetic considerations frequently include the fact that thoracotomy patients may have preoperative cardiac and/or pulmonary disease. Intermittent positive pressure ventilation is required during the thoracotomy and should be initiated immediately after intubation in the pulmonary-diseased patient. Standard methods are to ventilate the patient 12 to 20 breaths per minute with a peak inspiratory pressure of 15 to 20 cm water pressure and an inspiratory phase comprising one third of the total respiratory cycle. The tidal volume should be 8 to 12 ml/lb. Ideally, ventilation should be to effect, as determined by either the arterial or end-tidal carbon dioxide partial pressure. Following thoracotomy closure and pleural drainage, the artificial ventilation is gradually discontinued as the animal attempts to initiate ventilatory drive. Atelectasis with decreased compliance often develops and may be reduced by frequently "sighing" the lungs with a high tidal volume.

Positive pressure ventilation and the lack of a negative intrapleural pressure during a thoracotomy can reduce venous return and cardiac output. Heart rate and arterial blood pressure should be monitored. Intravenous fluids should be administered, preferably according to urine output and central venous pressure. Cardiac trauma induced by the surgeon can produce arrhythmias, and these can best be evaluated with an electrocardiogram.

Some anesthetic agents (thiamylal sodium and halothane) potentiate ventricular arrhythmias. Anesthesia may be with (1) thiobarbiturate induction and inhalant maintenance; (2) balanced anesthesia with narcotics, nitrous oxide, and muscle relaxants; or (3) inhalant induction and maintenance. Rapid recovery of alertness and ventilatory drive is desirable.

Patient Positioning

The patient should be placed in right lateral recumbency for a left-side thoracotomy. The left forelimb should be extended cranially.

Operative Preparation

Specialized Instruments. A self-retaining chest retractor (e.g., a Harken or Finochietto) is necessary to maintain exposure.

46

SOFT TISSUE SURGERY

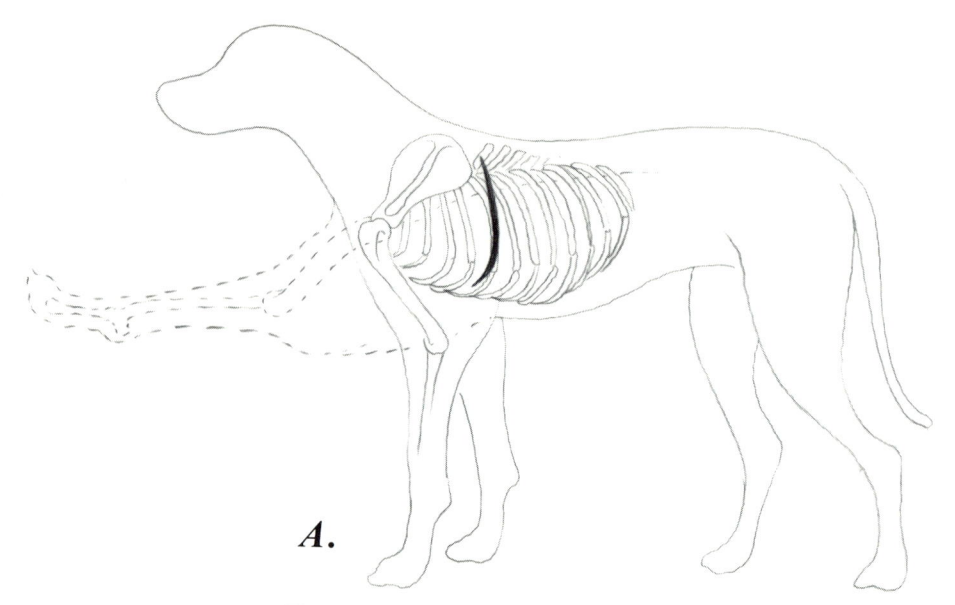

A.

Figure 7–1
Illustration continued on following page.

Details of Procedure

Figure 7–1A. An incision corresponding to the reversed "C" of the left fourth intercostal space is started approximately one space caudal to the caudal portion of the scapula.

Figure 7–1B. The skin and cutaneous trunci are incised. The exact intercostal space is identified by perforating the fascia ventral to the latissimus dorsi and extending a finger medial to this fascial plane to the thoracic inlet. Incise the latissimus dorsi, whose fibers run caudodorsally in the dorsal half of the incision. The intercostal spaces are counted. The latissimus dorsi is incised over the fourth intercostal space. The incision is extended ventrally to incise the scalenus but not the pectoral muscles.

NOTES:

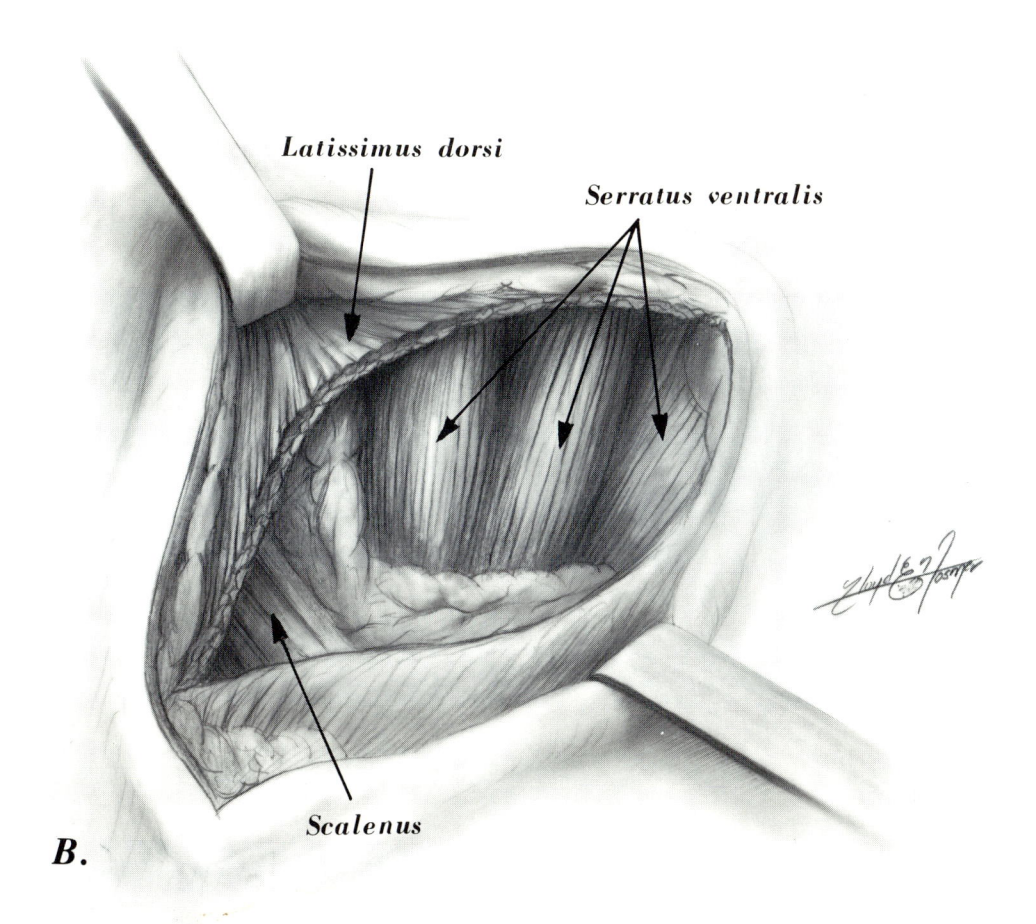

Figure 7–1 Continued
Illustration continued on following page.

48 SOFT TISSUE SURGERY

Serratus ventralis
4th rib
5th rib
C.
4th intercostal muscle
4th rib
Serratus ventralis
D.
8th intercostal space

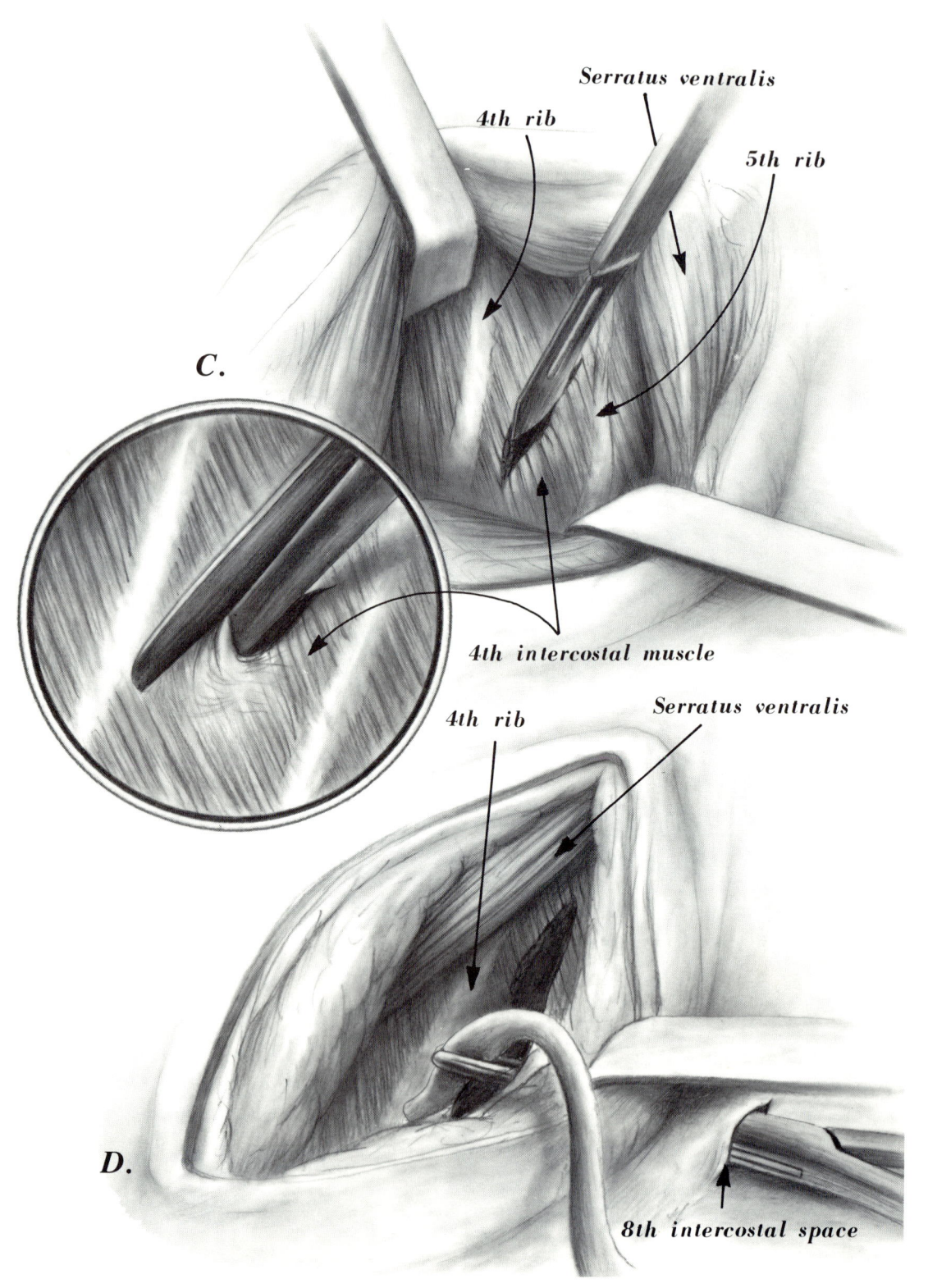

Figure 7–1 Continued

SOFT TISSUE SURGERY

Figure 7–1C. The serratus ventralis muscle is divided in the direction of the muscle bundles over the fourth intercostal space. The intercostal muscles are initially incised by successive strokes with a surgical knife or by perforation with the closed tips of dissecting scissors. The incision is then extended with the scissors. Care should be taken to avoid damage to the lung.

Figure 7–1D. Following the intrathoracic procedure, the mediastinum is perforated, and the chest cavity is lavaged. A chest drain should be placed to enter the thorax one or two spaces caudal to the incision. The chest drain should have a similar position as in Figure 7–8C. The ribs are approximated with three or four paracostal sutures of heavy, absorbable suture material. The serratus ventralis, latissimus dorsi and its fascial plane, subcutaneous tissue, and skin are closed individually.

Postoperative Consideration

The thoracic tube should be left in place for at least 24 hours. During this time, it should be aspirated frequently while the animal is placed in different positions, e.g., ventral recumbency, right lateral recumbency, dorsal recumbency, and left lateral recumbency. The amount and the packed cell volume of the chest-tube aspirate should be recorded on a flow chart. When the tube is removed, the pursestring is tightened to prevent inflow of air into the thorax. This pursestring should be removed after four to five days.

NOTES: *(Continued)*

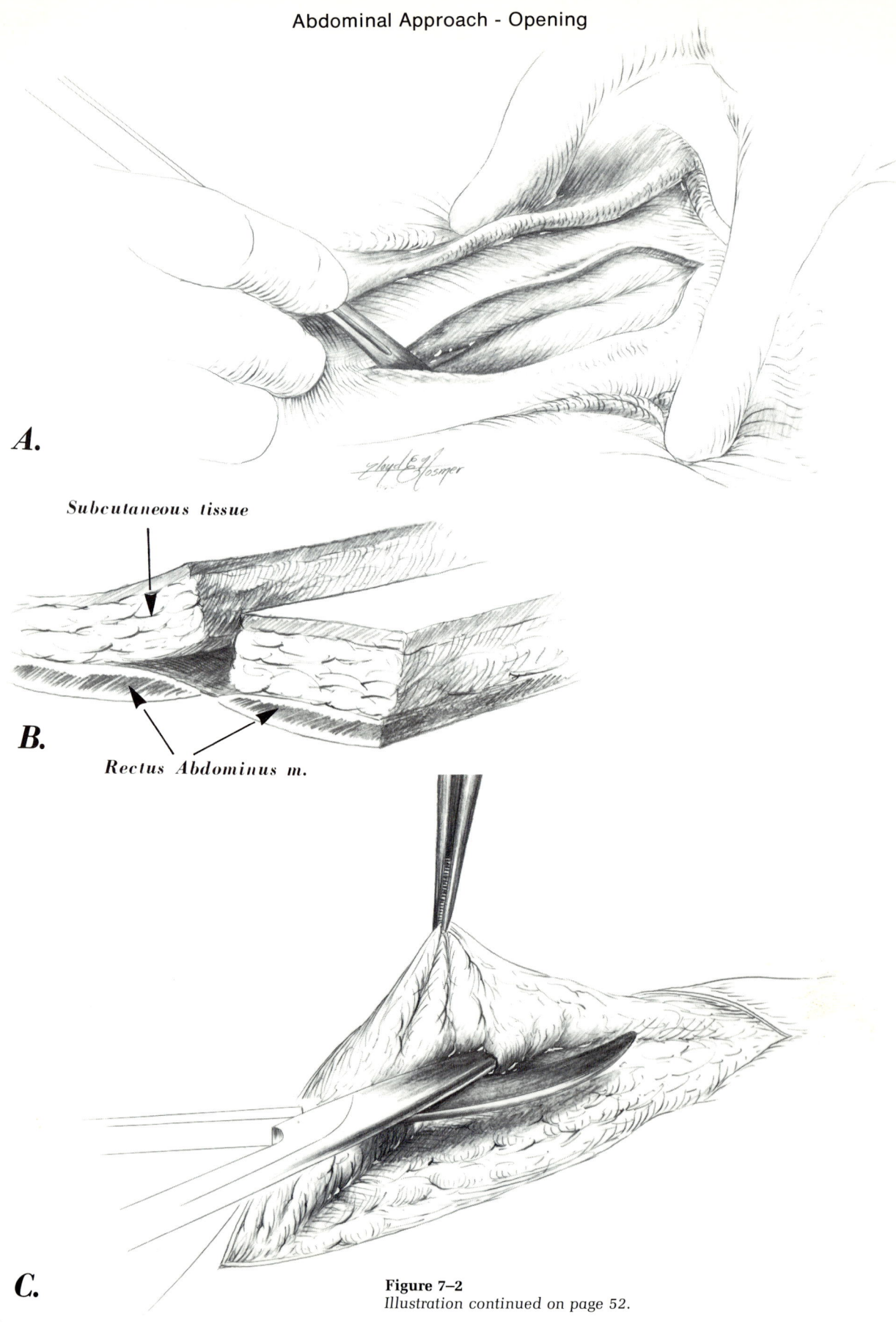

Abdominal Approach - Opening

A.

Subcutaneous tissue

B.

Rectus Abdominus m.

C.

Figure 7–2
Illustration continued on page 52.

7–2 ABDOMINAL APPROACH AND CLOSURE

JONATHAN N. CHAMBERS

Indications

The ventral midline is the most commonly used approach to the abdominal cavity.

Anesthesia

General anesthesia is utilized in an approach to the abdominal organs.

Patient Positioning

The patient is positioned in dorsal recumbency.

Incision and Exposure

Figure 7–2A. Using the umbilicus as a landmark, the dermis and subcutaneous tissue are incised with one stroke. Slight finger tension applied perpendicular to the incision will prevent the skin from sliding with the blade.

Figure 7–2B. The depth of the initial incision is to the linea alba fascia.

Figure 7–2C. The subcutaneous fascia adheres to the deep fascia at the midline. Dissection of this tissue with scissors will facilitate exposure and closure of the linea alba. Excessive undermining of the subcutaneous layer should be avoided.

Figure 7–2D. The surface of the linea alba is grasped with thumb forceps and elevated from the abdominal contents. A stab incision is made in the linea alba, using an inverted knife blade.

Figure 7–2E. The thumb forceps are introduced through the stab incision and elevate the abdominal wall. The linea alba incision is continued by placing the blade between the arms of the forceps and sliding both instruments as one unit. (Note the proper position and angle of the knife blade.)

Figure 7–2F. The incision is completed by reversing the direction of the forceps and knife.

Figure 7–2G. If the incision is on the midline, the falciform ligament remains intact and must be incised to expose the abdominal organs.

Figures 7–2H and 7–2I. The fascia of the rectus abdominus muscle is the strongest and most important tissue layer in the closure. This layer is apposed with simple interrupted sutures. Neither the falciform ligament nor the subcutaneous tissue should be interposed or included in the sutures.

Figure 7–2J. The subcutaneous tissue is sutured to remove dead space and to relieve tension on the dermis. The stitches may include a tacking bite in the rectus fascia to help obliterate the dead space.

Figure 7–2K. The subcutaneous stitches should not include the deep dermal layer, as this will prevent apposition of the dermis and delay wound healing.

Figure 7–2L. The dermis is closed as a single layer, using an appositional suture pattern.

Abdominal Approach-Opening

D.

Subcutaneous tissue

E.

Subcutaneous tissue

F.

Subcutaneous tissue

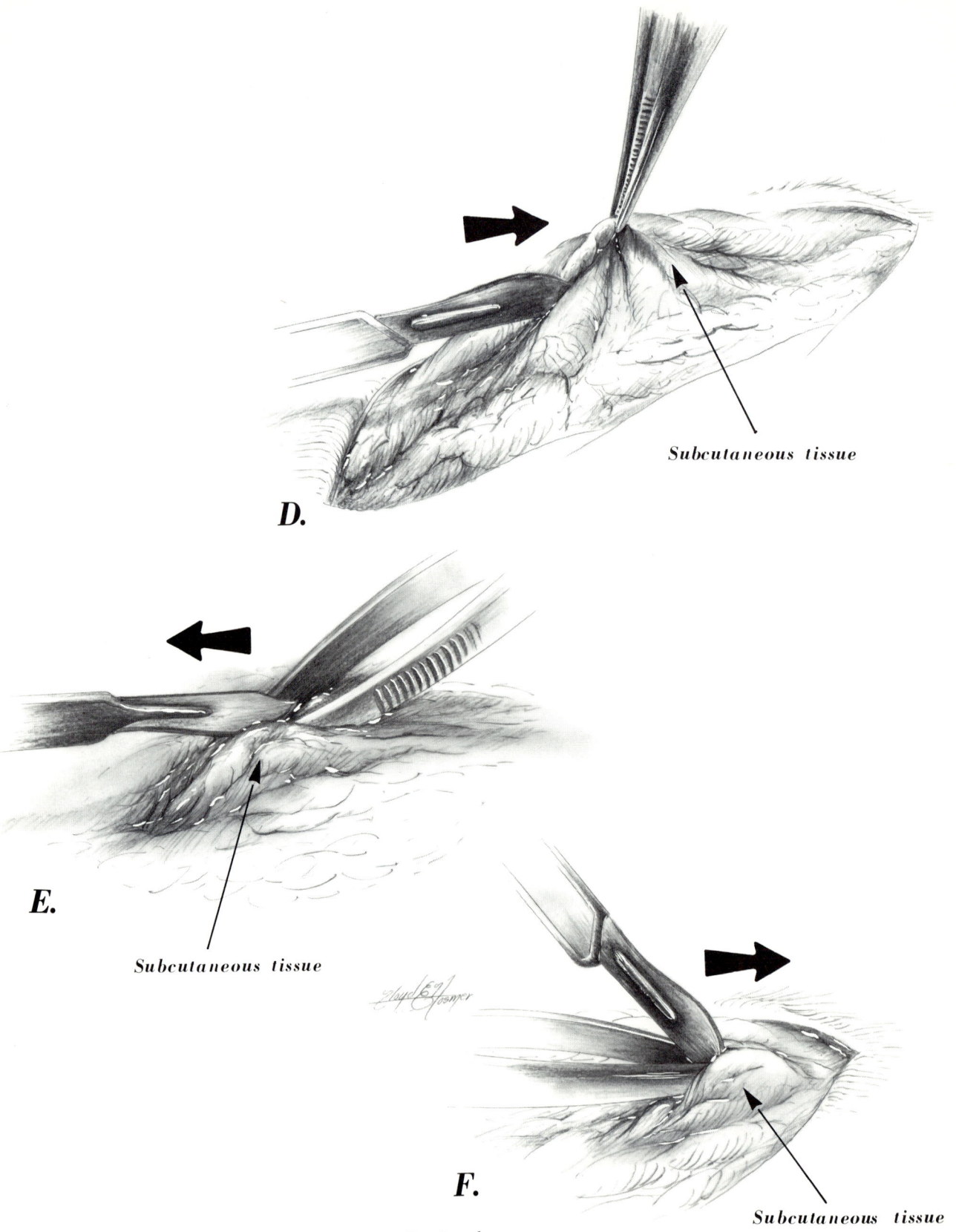

Figure 7–2 Continued.
Illustration continued on opposite page.

Abdominal Approach-Closure

Subcutaneous tissue

G.

Rectus Abdominus m.

Falciform ligament

H.

Rectus Abdominus m.

Subcutaneous

Falciform Ligament

I.

Rectus Abdominus m.

Correct

Incorrect

Falciform Ligament

J.

Rectus Abdominus m.

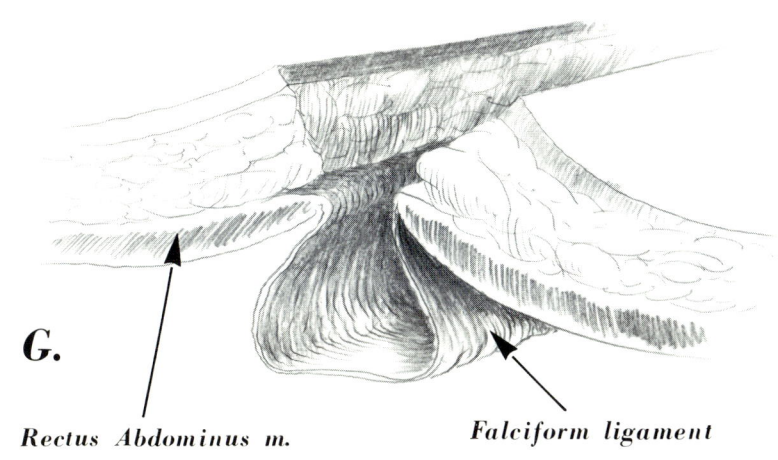

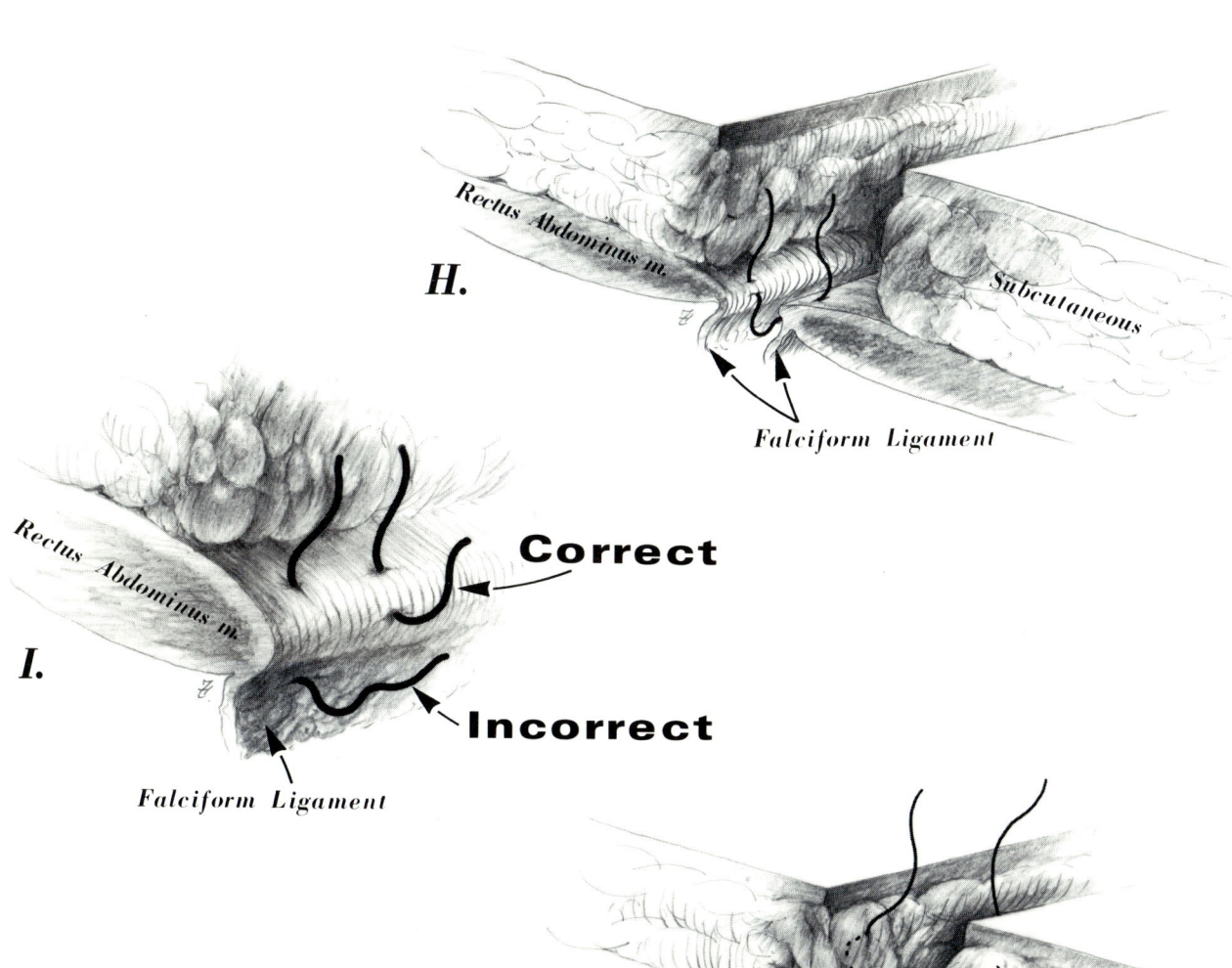

Figure 7–2 Continued.
Illustration continued on following page.

Abdominal Approach-Closure

Correct

Incorrect

Subcutaneous

K.

Subcutaneous

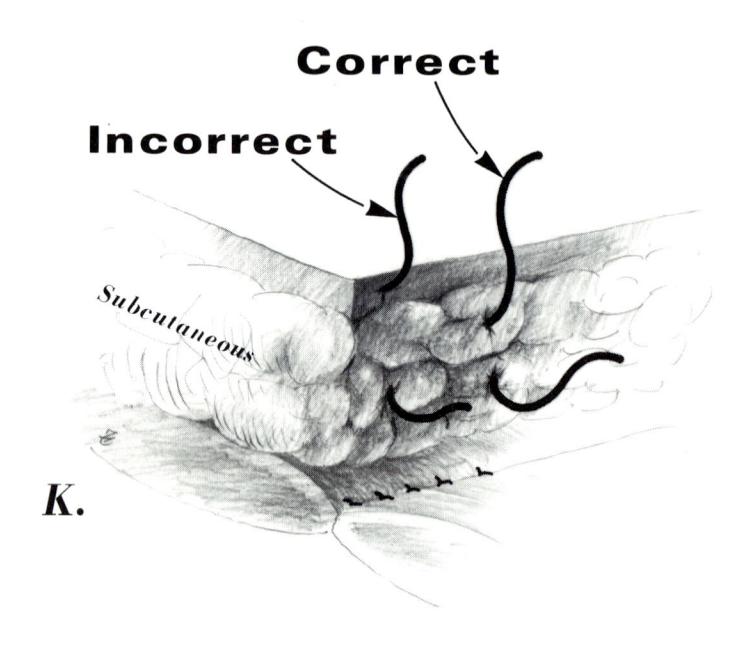

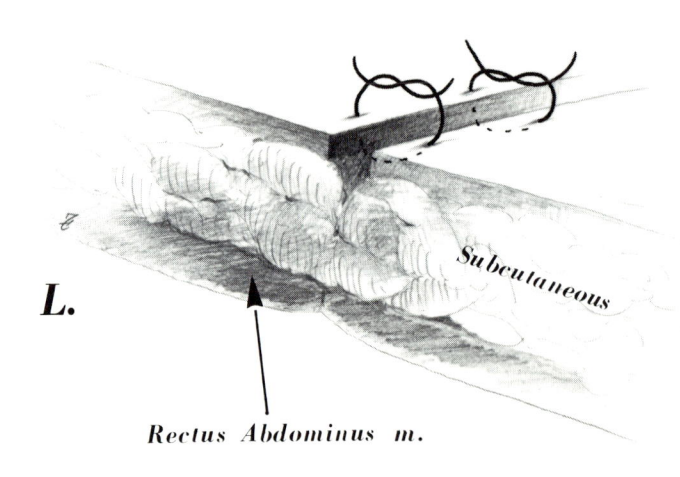

L.

Rectus Abdominus m.

Figure 7–2 Continued

54

NOTES:

7–3 AND 7–4 ESOPHAGOTOMY AND ESOPHAGEAL ANASTOMOSIS

EBERHARD ROSIN

Indications

Surgery of the esophagus is indicated in such conditions as bite or gunshot wounds, foreign objects that cannot be removed *per orum*, granulomas caused by *Spirocerca lupi*, and neoplasms.

Anesthesia

Anesthetic considerations for a thoracotomy (Procedure 7–1) also apply to intrathoracic esophageal surgery. During cervical esophageal surgery, care must be taken to position the endotracheal tube so that neither the retractor nor the surgeon compresses the trachea. Some animals with esophageal disease are either anorectic, depressed, and dehydrated or are victims of aspiration pneumonia. The dehydrated animal needs to be partially rehydrated, and anesthetic considerations applied to the pulmonary patient (Chapter 2) may be required.

Patient Positioning

For exposure of the esophagus in the cervical and thoracic inlet, the patient is positioned in dorsal recumbency. For exposure of the mid-thoracic and caudal thoracic sections of the esophagus, the patient is positioned in left lateral and right lateral recumbency, respectively.

Operative Preparation

Specialized Instruments. Use of a self-retaining retractor, such as the Frazier for the cervical region and the Finochietto for the thoracic cavity, will facilitate good exposure. Mobilization, handling, and isolation of the esophagus is aided by the use of Penrose rubber drains as traction devices and laparotomy sponges for "packing off." The use of clamps is avoided whenever possible. When performing an end-to-end anastomosis of the esophagus, the ends are held with noncrushing forceps, such as pediatric Doyen or Pearlman bulldog intestinal forceps.

Suture Material. Meticulous technique in suturing the esophagus is more important than the type of suture material employed; however, preference is given to 4-0 synthetic absorbable (Dexon, Vicryl) or non-absorbable monofilamentous (nylon, Prolene) suture materials combined with high-quality, tapered needles.

Esophagotomy

Esophagotomy

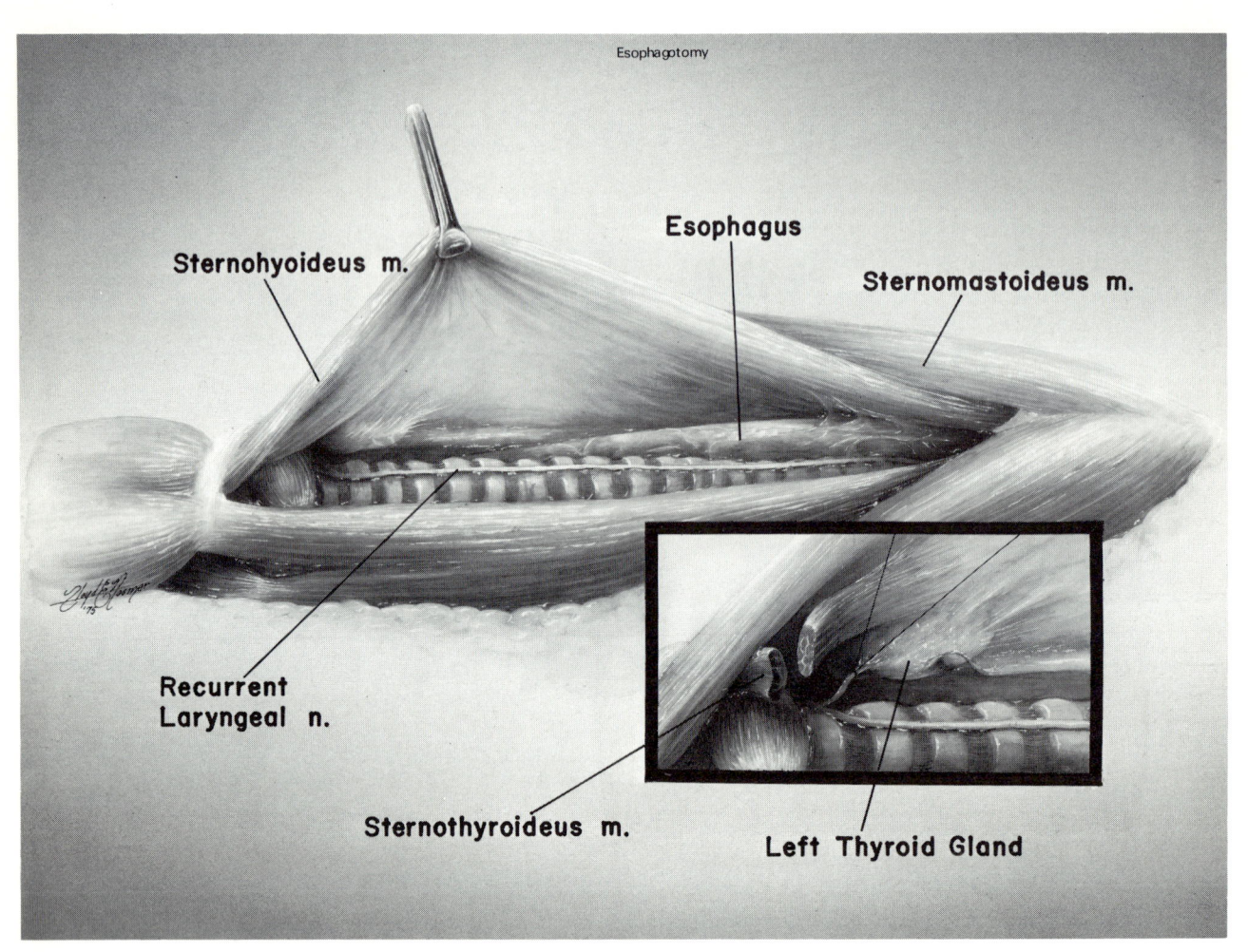

Sternohyoideus m.
Esophagus
Sternomastoideus m.
Recurrent Laryngeal n.
Sternothyroideus m.
Left Thyroid Gland

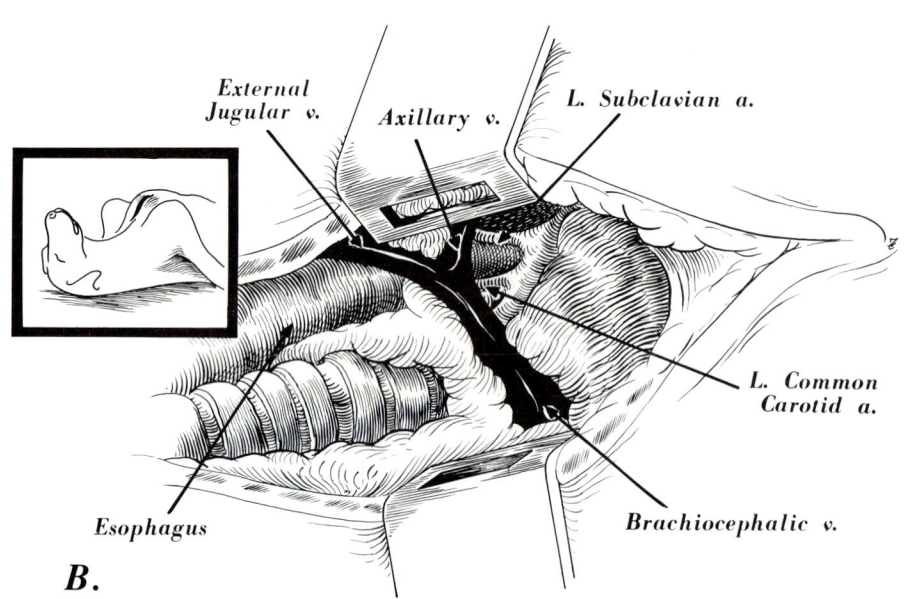

A.

External Jugular v.
Axillary v.
L. Subclavian a.
L. Common Carotid a.
Brachiocephalic v.
Esophagus

B.

Figure 7–3
Illustration continued on opposite page.

SOFT TISSUE SURGERY

Incision and Exposure

Figure 7–3A. Exposure of the cervical section of the esophagus (pharynx to C-7) is initiated by ventral midline incision and dissection between the median raphe of the sternomastoid and sternohyoid muscles. The incision may extend from the larynx to the manubrium. The esophagus is approached to the left of the trachea. Care must be taken to avoid injury to the left recurrent laryngeal nerve that lies adjacent to the trachea, to the left carotid sheath that lies between the esophagus and the sternothyroideus muscle, and to the left thyroid gland that lies in a fascial compartment adjacent to the sternothyroideus muscle and the carotid sheath.

Figure 7–3B. The thoracic inlet section of the esophagus (C-6 to T-2) is difficult to expose satisfactorily. This segment may be partially exposed by retraction after caudal or cranial mobilization following a cervical or cranial right thoracic approach, respectively. Alternatively, the ventral cervical incision is continued into the manubrium. Care is taken to stay on the midline as the scalpel is used to divide subcutaneous tissues and fascia overlying the sternum. The sternum is scored, and the first four sternebrae are split. A chisel, power saw, or scalpel is used to split the sternum, using the scored midline as a guide. Severance of the internal thoracic vessels is avoided by not deviating from the midline. Retraction of the incision will expose mediastinal pleura and, in the young dog, the thymus gland. Reflection of the cranial mediastinal pleura will expose the "Y" junction of the jugular and axillary veins, which forms the brachiocephalic vein. Continued dorsal dissection will expose the common carotid arteries branching from the brachiocephalic artery. The esophagus can be visualized to the left and dorsal to the left common carotid artery. Retraction of these vessels will permit exposure of a limited segment of the esophagus.

Figure 7–3C. The mid-thoracic portion of the esophagus (T-2 to T-7) is exposed by right lateral thoracotomy at the fourth intercostal space. The cranial and middle lung lobes are retracted caudally. The azygos vein is ligated and divided as it obliquely crosses the lateral surface of the esophagus. The middle mediastinal pleura is incised to expose the esophagus. Care must be taken to avoid injury to the vagal trunks.

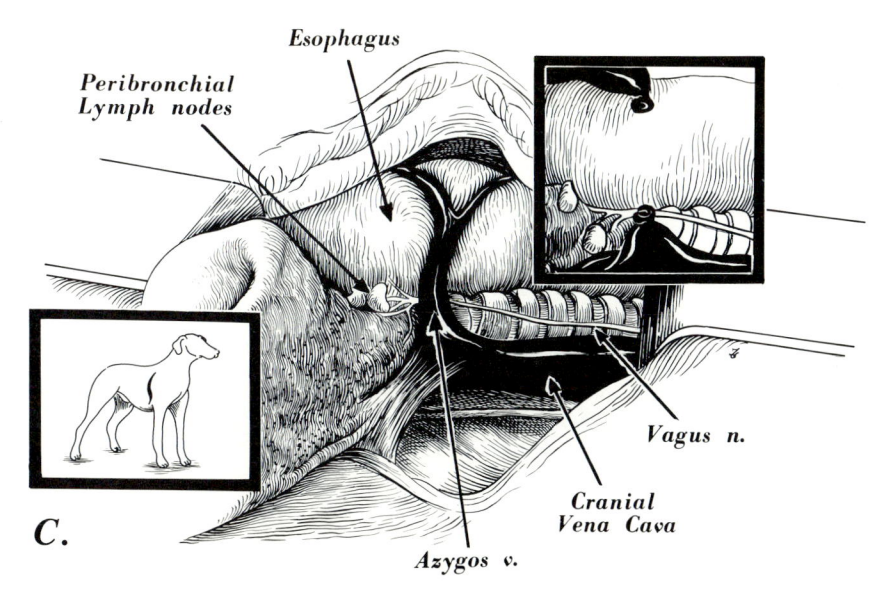

Figure 7–3 Continued
Illustration continued on following page.

Esophagotomy

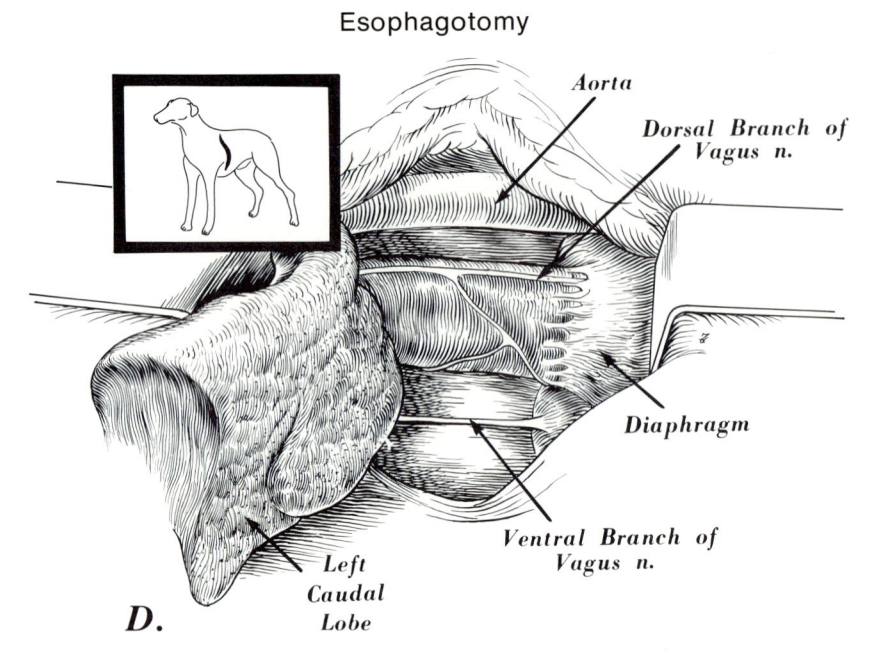

D.

Labels: Aorta, Dorsal Branch of Vagus n., Diaphragm, Ventral Branch of Vagus n., Left Caudal Lobe

Figure 7–3 Continued.

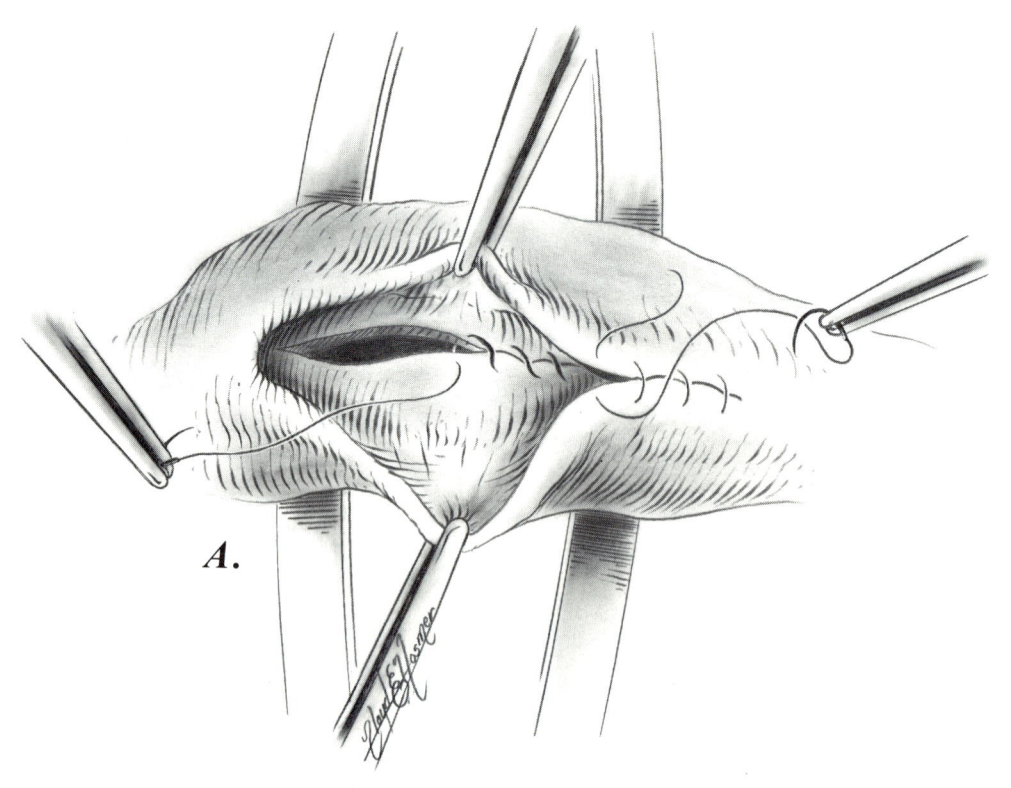

A.

Figure 7–4
Illustration continued on page 60.

Figure 7–3D. Exposure of the caudal thoracic section of the esophagus (T-6 to diaphragm) is initiated by left lateral thoracotomy at the appropriate intercostal space. The avascular left pulmonary ligament is transected, and the left caudal lobe of the lung is retracted cranially. Care is taken to avoid injury to the dorsal and ventral vagal trunk as the caudal mediastinal pleura is incised to expose the esophagus.

Details of Procedure

Following exposure, the esophagus is mobilized with regard for segmental blood supply. Mobilization, however, can be adequate for thorough "packing off" with either gauze sponges or laparotomy sponges without significant interference with vascularity to the proposed surgical site.

Incision and closure of the esophagus are performed with minimal trauma to the esophageal wall. The use of clamps and forceps is avoided when possible. Suction and adequate packing will often suffice to control contamination.

Figure 7–4A. A two-layer closure is used in the esophagotomy. The mucosa-submucosa is sutured in a simple continuous pattern. The muscularis-adventitia is closed with a second row of simple interrupted stitches. Stitches are placed approximately 2 mm from the cut edge and from 2 to 3 mm apart and tied with sufficient tension for a tight seal without interference with the blood supply.

NOTES:

Esophagotomy

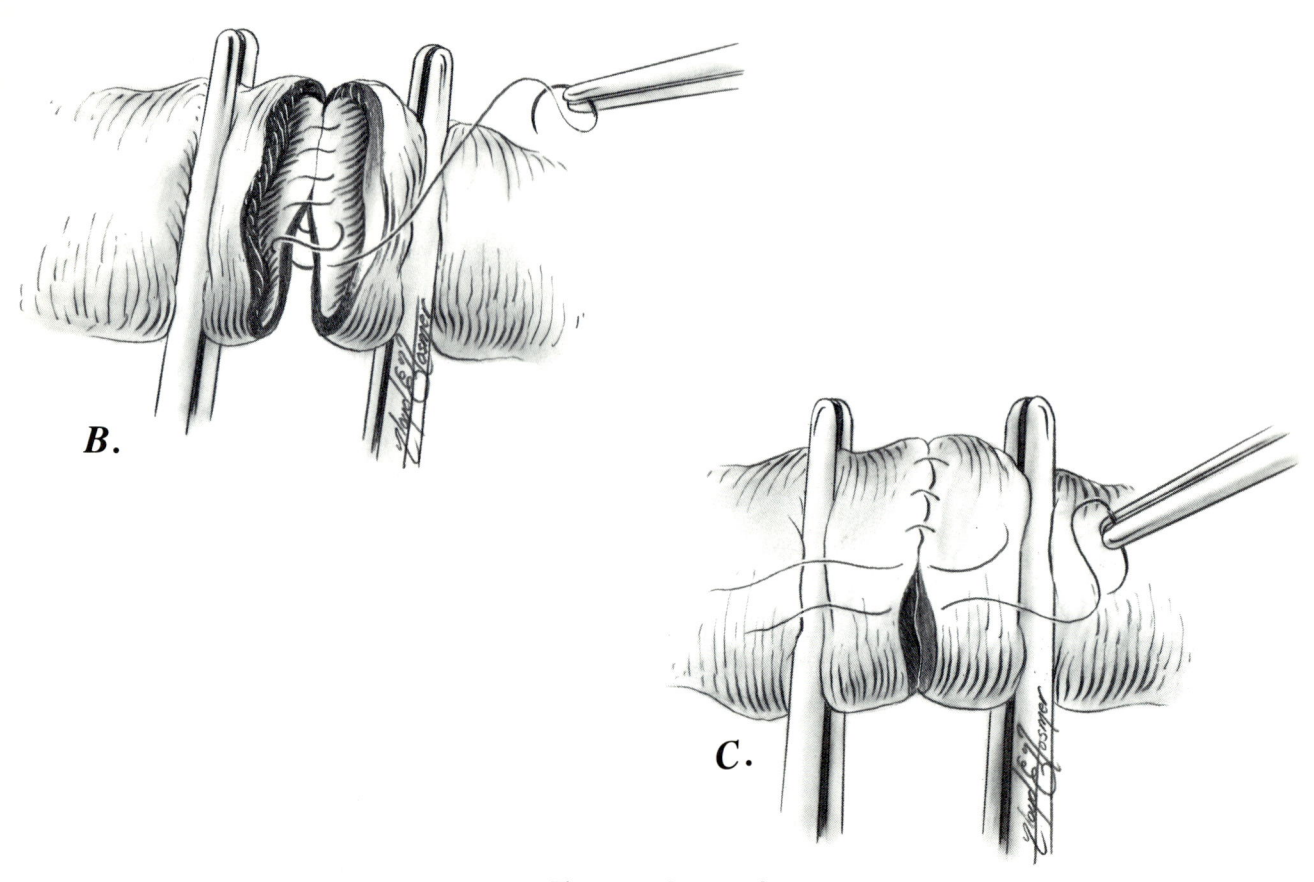

Figure 7–4 Continued

Figure 7–4B. When performing an end-to-end anastomosis, the ends of the esophagus are occluded and manipulated, using noncrushing intestinal forceps. Sutures are placed similarly to those in the esophagotomy, except that they include the circumference of the esophagus.

Figure 7–4C. A second suture layer, using simple interrupted stitches, is placed to unite the muscularis-adventitia.

Closure of the approach incision is performed in the standard manner. Because of contamination with esophageal contents, the operative site should be irrigated copiously with warm, sterile, isotonic fluids. Consideration should be given to placing a Penrose rubber drain into the cervical incision. A chest drain should be inserted prior to closure of the thoracotomy incision. (See Procedure 7–8.)

NOTES: *(Continued)*

Postoperative Considerations

Broad-spectrum antibiotics are administered. *Per orum* food and water are restricted for six to eight days. Insertion of a pharyngostomy tube (Procedure 7–6) will facilitate adequate caloric and water intake. Requirements are determined and provided in the form of food homogenized with tap water and administered in divided feedings.

7–5 SALIVARY GLAND EXCISION

WAYNE E. WINGFIELD

Indications

Excision of the mandibular or sublingual salivary glands is most commonly encountered in the treatment and prevention of recurrence of salivary mucoceles. A neoplasm involving these glands that might require removal of the glands is occasionally encountered.

Anesthesia

Intubation of the trachea and inhalation anesthesia are indicated prior to excising the salivary glands.

Patient Positioning

The animal is placed in dorsal recumbency, with a sandbag placed under the neck, the forelimbs tied caudally, and tape placed over the tip of the mandible to secure the patient with its neck extended over the sandbag.

Operative Preparation

Special Draping. Quadrant draping is utilized after preparation of the surgical site. The external jugular, linguofacial, and maxillary veins should be available for visualization. Cranially, the intermandibular area to the level of the frenulum of the tongue provides access to the duct systems of the salivary glands.

Specialized Instruments. A standard surgical pack is required for this operative procedure. Penrose drains measuring 3/8 to 1/2 inch in diameter are used prior to closure of the incision.

Incision and Exposure

The skin incision extends from the external jugular vein, between the linguofacial and maxillary veins, and proceeds to the medial side of the mandibular body.

Salivary Gland Excision

A.

Labels: Lingual facial v.; Lingual v.; Facial v.; Maxillary v.; Cranial retropharyngeal lymph node; Mandibular salivary gland

B.

Labels: Maxillary v.; Mandibular salivary gland

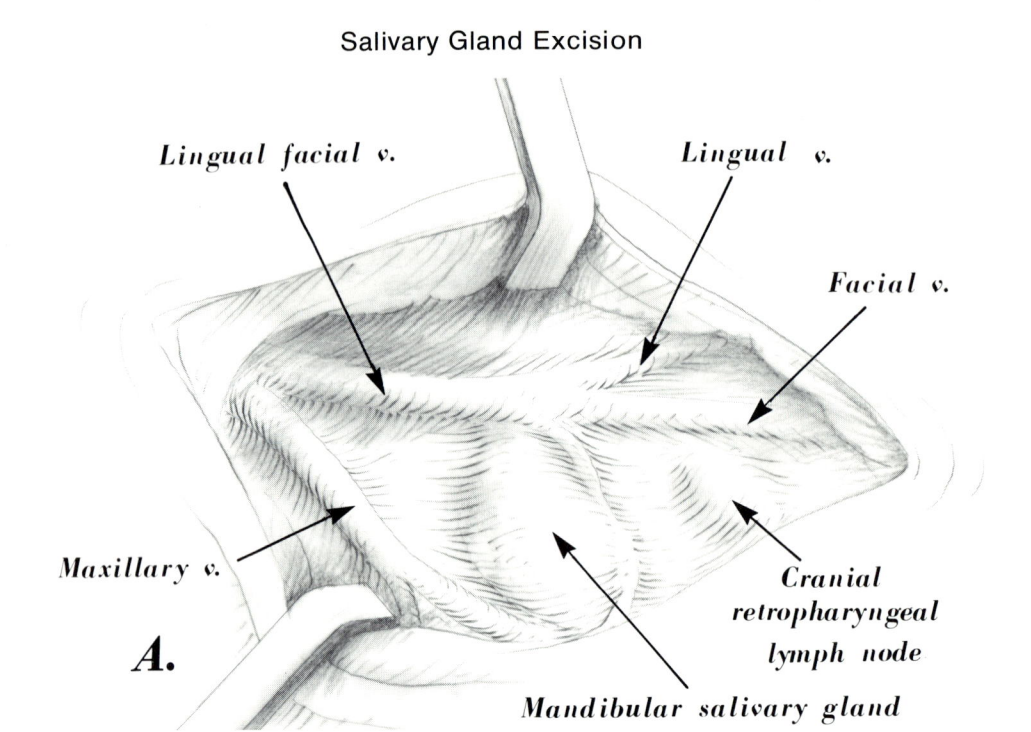

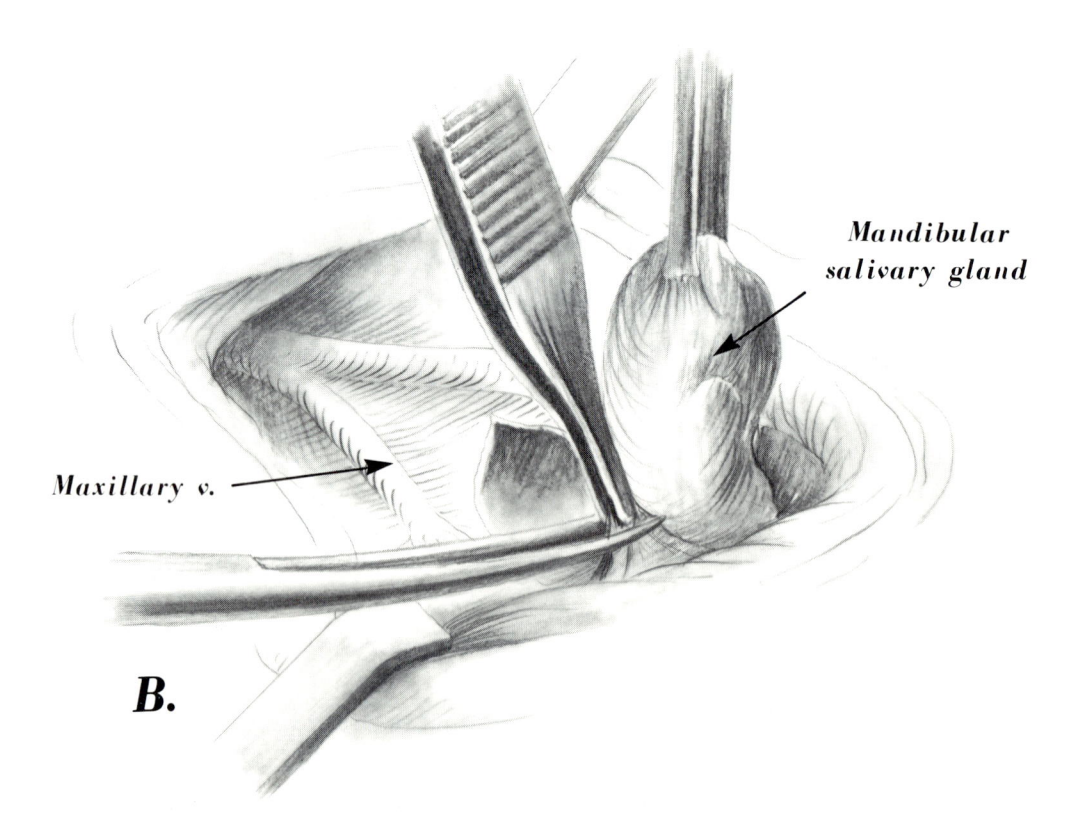

Figure 7–5
Illustration continued on opposite page.

SOFT TISSUE SURGERY

Details of Procedure

NOTES:

Figure 7–5A. Continue the incision through the subcutaneous tissues and platysma muscle until the linguofacial and maxillary veins are noted to form the external jugular vein. Where these two veins come together, the mandibular salivary gland will be seen.

Because the mandibular salivary gland and the caudal sublingual salivary gland share a common capsule, separation is difficult. Generally, the two glands are surgically excised as a unit because they frequently also share a common duct system.

Figure 7–5B. Incise the capsule overlying the mandibular salivary gland and utilize Allis forceps to provide traction while dissecting the glands free. Continue careful dissection until the glands and their ducts disappear beneath the digastricus muscle.

Figure 7–5C. Metzenbaum scissors are used to dissect on the medial side of the digastricus muscle. Separation of the styloglossus muscle from the digastricus muscle will expose the large hypoglossal nerve. Avoid deep dissection in this area, as the carotid and the lingual arteries may be easily damaged.

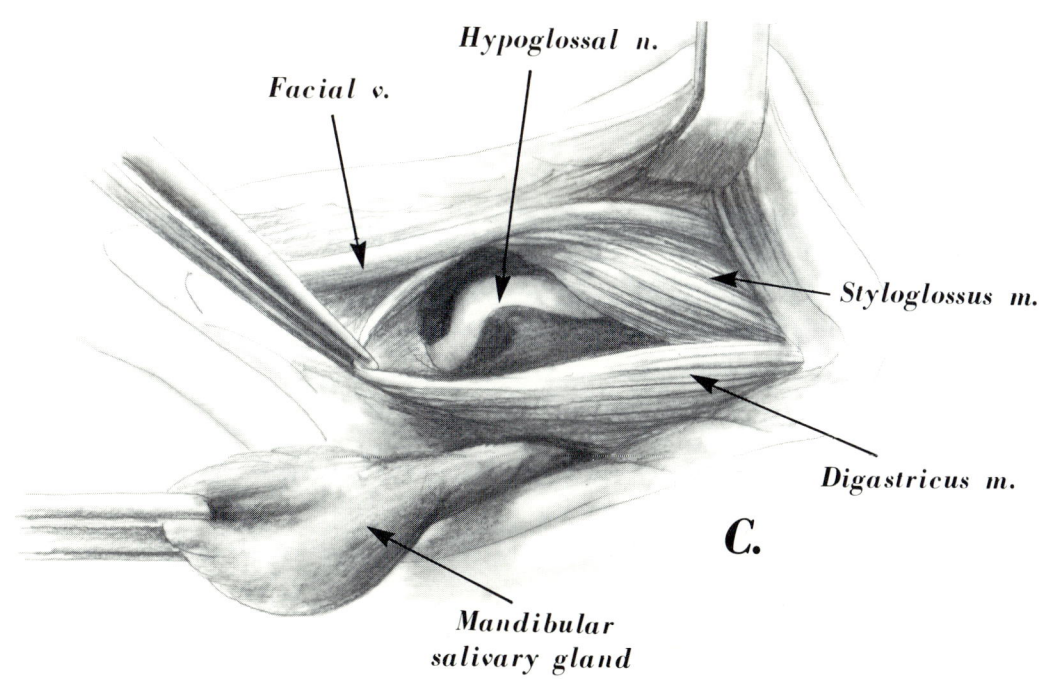

Figure 7–5 Continued
Illustration continued on following page.

64   SOFT TISSUE SURGERY

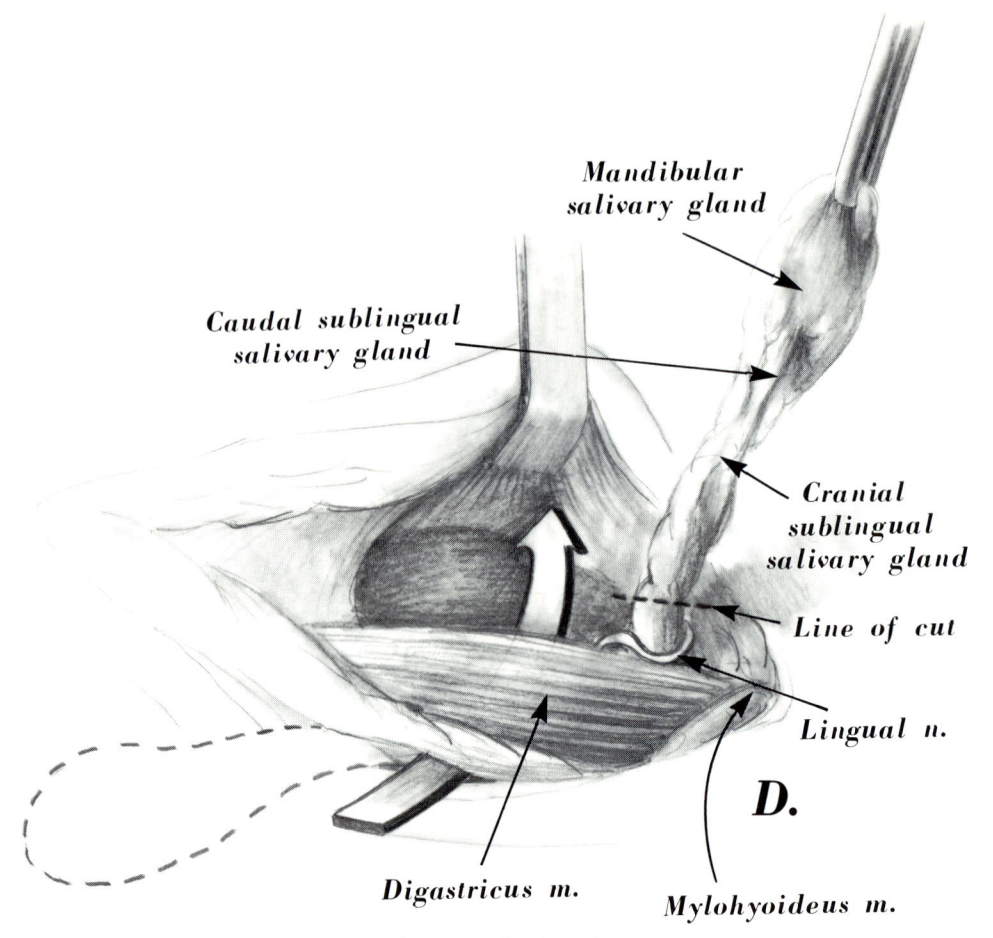

Figure 7–5 Continued.

Figure 7–5D. To remove the cranial sublingual salivary tissue surrounding the duct system, pass the dissected mandibular and caudal sublingual glands beneath the digastricus muscle. This is most easily accomplished by first excising the bulk of the salivary tissue. Note the mylohyoideus muscle overlying the salivary ducts. This muscle must be incised to continue the rostral dissection of the salivary tissue. Continue the dissection until the lingual branch of the trigeminal nerve is seen to pass around the salivary ducts. At this point, place a ligature around the duct systems and excise proximal to the ligature.

NOTES:

Closure of the operative site is initiated by placement of a Penrose drain beneath the digastricus muscle and into the space vacated by the ducts of the salivary tissue just removed. The drain should exit just lateral to the initial skin incision over the external jugular vein. Reappose the mylohyoideus muscle with simple interrupted sutures. Closure of the remainder of the incision involves closing dead space cavities to avoid leaving areas in which tissue fluids may accumulate postoperatively.

Postoperative Considerations

The Penrose drain can usually be removed after three days. Allow the exit hole for the drain to heal by secondary intention. Surgical drains are kept clean and are removed after three to five days.

NOTES: *(Continued)*

7–6 PHARYNGOSTOMY

Clarence A. Rawlings

Indications

A pharyngostomy tube is indicated for animals that have difficulties in normal alimentation because of pharyngeal and esophageal disease and for animals that require gastric gavage for a prolonged period of fluid and nutrient administration.

Anesthesia

Either general anesthesia or heavy sedation is required to permit the animal's mouth to stay open with an oral speculum and to reduce pharyngeal and laryngeal reflexes.

Patient Positioning

The patient is placed in lateral recumbency.

Operative Preparation

<u>Specialized Instruments.</u> An oral speculum is required. Pharyngostomy tubing should be long enough to reach from the pharynx to the thirteenth rib.

Incision and Exposure

The oral speculum is placed on the lower canine teeth to provide exposure.

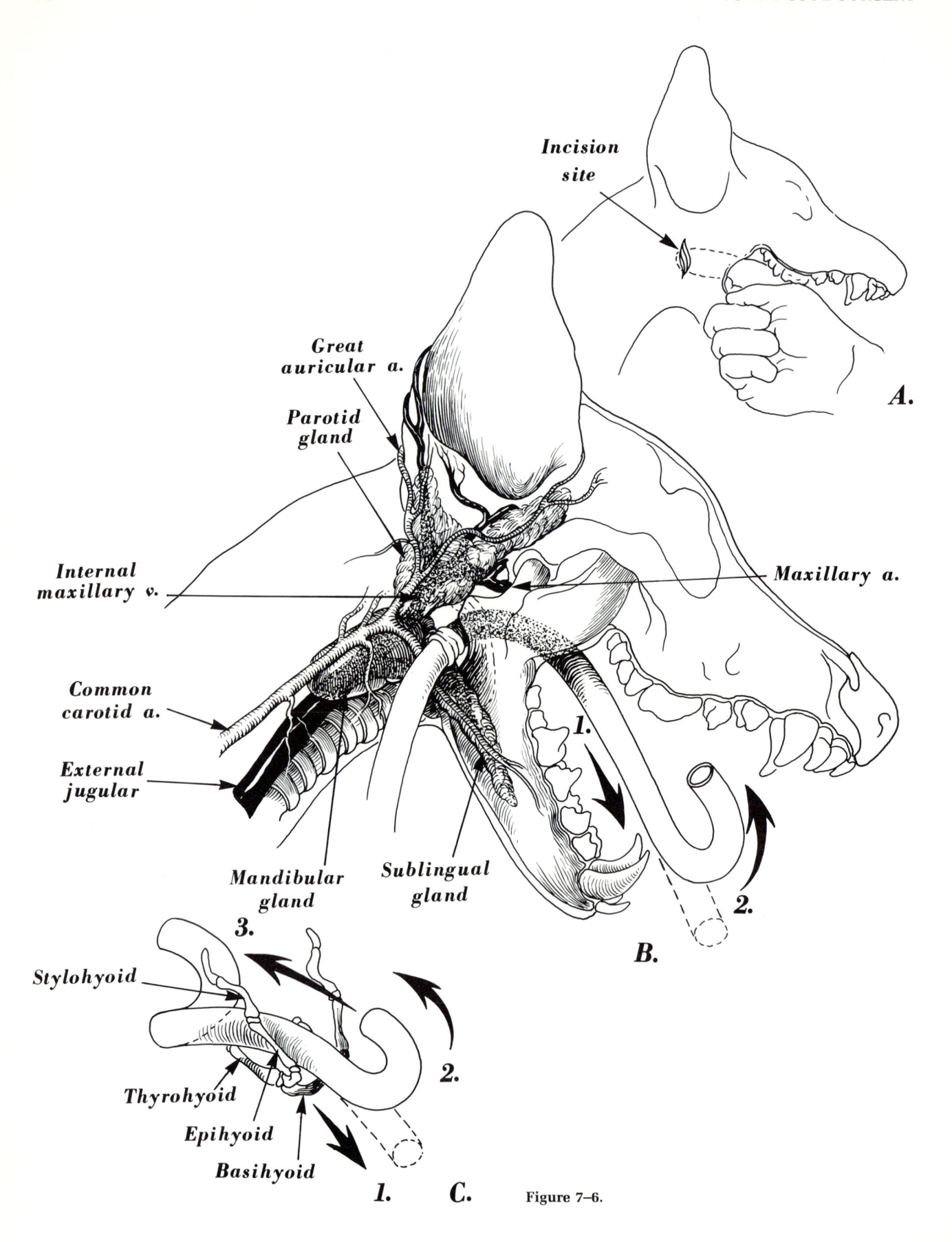

66 SOFT TISSUE SURGERY

Incision site

Great auricular a.
Parotid gland
Internal maxillary v.
Maxillary a.
Common carotid a.
External jugular
Mandibular gland
Sublingual gland

Stylohyoid
Thyrohyoid
Epihyoid
Basihyoid

A.

B.

C.

Figure 7–6.

Details of Procedure

Figure 7–6A. The index finger is placed into the oral pharynx and is passed caudal to the stylohyoid, epihyoid, and basihyoid bones. The tip of the finger should be forced laterally. To determine the position of the external jugular vein and its tributaries, the jugular vein should be obstructed at the thoracic inlet. Avoiding the structures in Figure 7–6B, the skin is incised over the finger.

Figure 7–6B. The position of the pharyngostomy tube is demonstrated. The tract for this tube is created by thrusting Halsted forceps through the skin incision and into the pharynx. The pharyngeal mucosa may need to be incised over the tips of the Halsted forceps to permit perforation. The tube end is grasped with the forceps and is withdrawn from inside the pharynx to outside the skin. Prior to placement, the tube should be marked so that placement of the tube will result in its end being at the level of the thirteenth rib. The illustration demonstrates structures (jugular vein with its tributaries, common carotid artery, salivary glands, and lymph nodes) that should not be damaged.

Figure 7–6C. Following withdrawal of the tube to its position in Figure 7–6B, the end within the pharynx is turned around and passed into the esophagus. The tube is properly positioned with relationship to the hyoid apparatus and is secured to the skin in a manner similar to that in which the chest tube is secured. It should be further stabilized with an encircling neck bandage.

Postoperative Considerations

Tube feedings are prepared by making a gruel of canned food and water in a food blender. These feedings are administered at least three times a day. The amount of food should be determined by nomogram requirements for calories, water, and protein. Supplementation with other nutrients should be considered, especially in the diseased animal that is undergoing catabolic changes. When alimentation by pharyngostomy tube is completed, the tube is withdrawn. The incision should not be closed, because it will close by granulation.

NOTES:

Figure 7–7
Illustration continued on page 70.

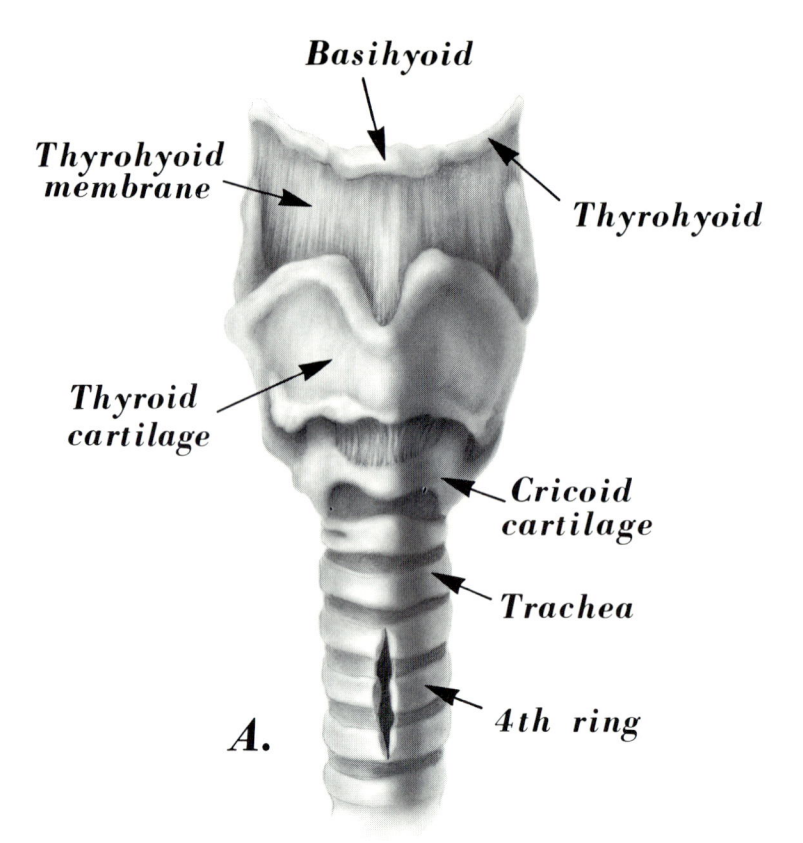

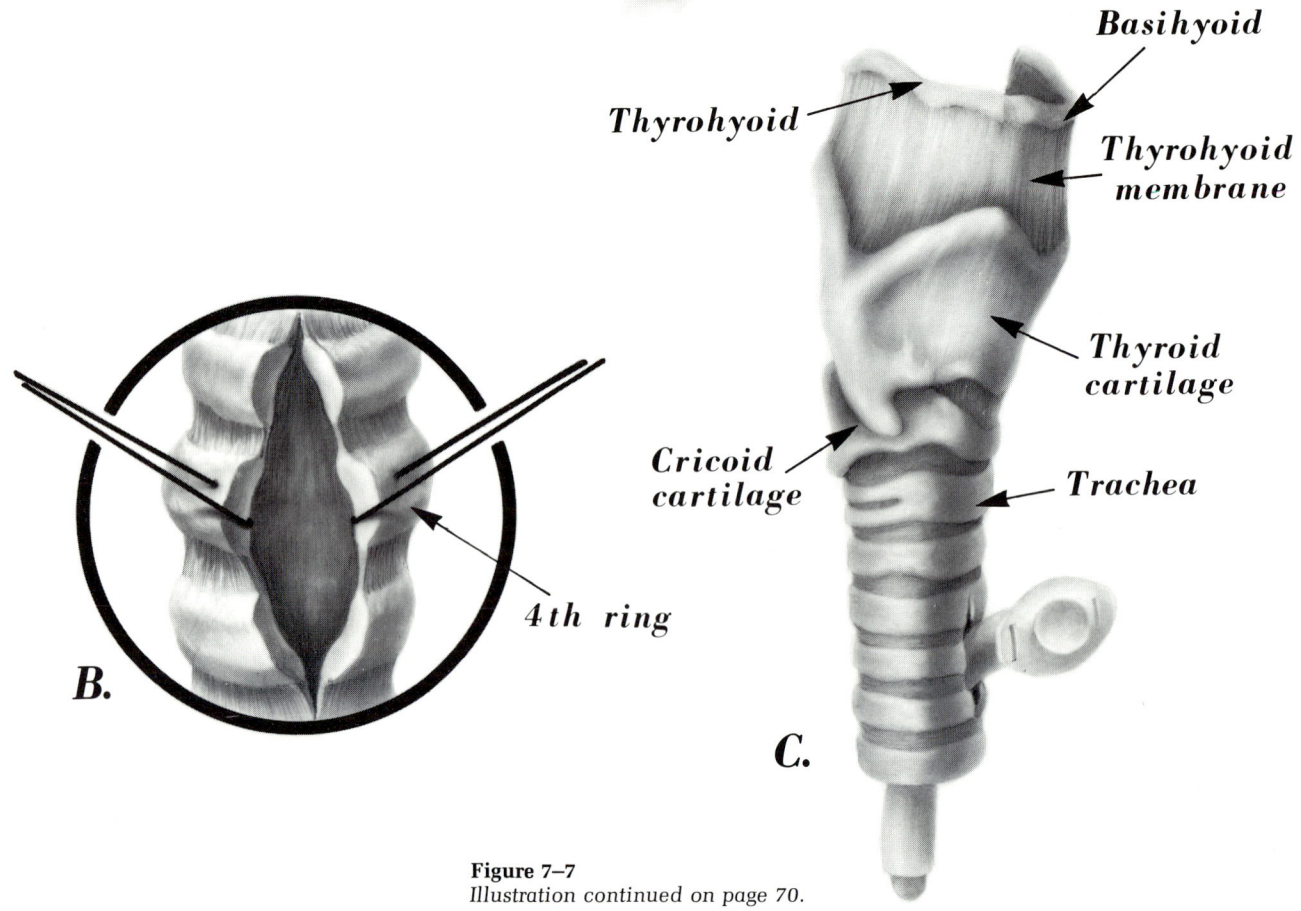

7–7 TRACHEOTOMY

Clarence A. Rawlings

Indications

A tracheotomy is indicated in many animals with upper airway obstruction and/or disease, and in many animals that require surgery.

Anesthesia

Many animals with upper airway problems require prebreathing with 100 per cent oxygen. Induction is rapid to permit intubation soon after initial depression. Patients must be monitored closely, because they frequently develop hypoxemia, respiratory acidosis, and ventricular arrhythmias. Drugs such as the thiobarbiturates and halothane potentiate these ventricular arrhythmias and must be used with caution.

Patient Positioning

The patient is positioned in dorsal recumbency, with the neck extended over a sandbag.

Operative Preparation

Specialized Instruments. A tracheotomy airway may be temporarily supplied by an endotracheal tube or, preferably, by a commercially available tracheotomy tube.

Incision and Exposure

A midline, cranial, cervical incision is performed to approach the trachea. The most cranial tracheotomy site should be the second tracheal cartilage ring.

Details of Procedure

Figure 7–7A. The tracheal rings are incised on their ventral side. The incision should be just large enough to permit passage of the tracheotomy cannula.

Figure 7–7B. Traction sutures are placed through cartilage rings on either side of the incision. Tension on these sutures will expose the tracheal lumen.

Figure 7–7C. The tracheotomy outer cannula and an obturator are passed through the tracheotomy incision. The obturator is withdrawn, and the inner cannula is inserted. A small endotracheal tube can be used for short-term tracheotomies.

NOTES:

opening for retention sutures

Outer canula

Obturator

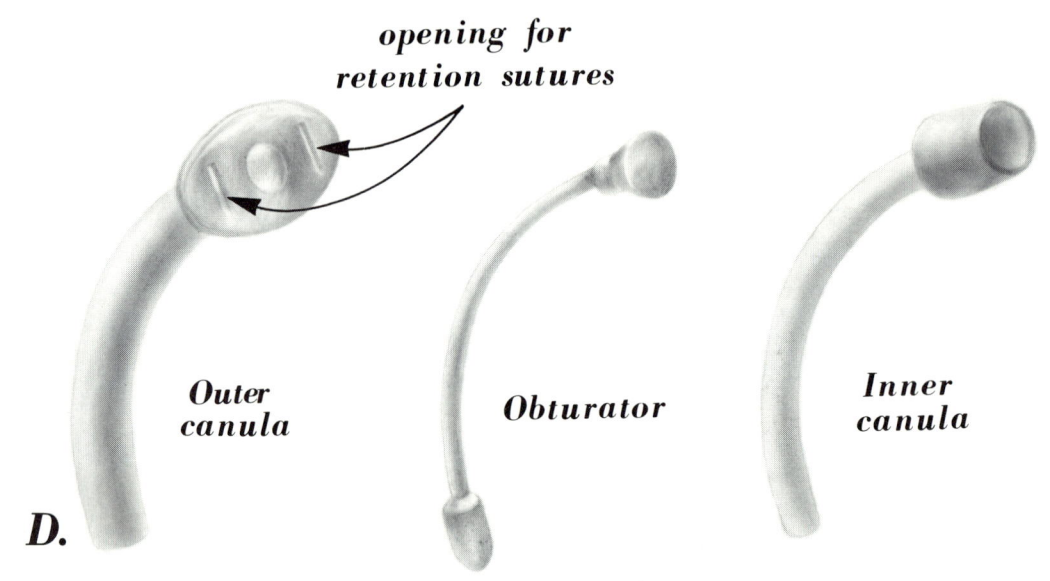

Inner canula

D.

Figure 7–7 Continued.

Figure 7–7D. The complete tracheotomy assembly is illustrated. The outer cannula should remain within the trachea throughout the tracheotomy. Retention sutures are attached between the skin and openings on the outer cannula. The remainder of the tracheotomy incision is closed with skin sutures up to the outer cannula. The obturator is used only during insertion.

a day. The tracheotomy tube is left in place until ventilatory support is no longer required. Constant technical attention is required, and the tracheotomy site and tube should be frequently cleaned. At extubation, the tube is removed, with surgical intervention generally not required.

NOTES: (Continued)

Postoperative Considerations

The inner cannula should be maintained within the outer cannula at all times except for cleansing. The inner cannula should be withdrawn, and the trachea should be lavaged with saline several times

7-8 CHEST DRAINS

Clarence A. Rawlings

Indications

Drainage of the chest by tubes is indicated to remove fluid and air from the pleural space. The chest tube is placed into the most severely affected side or both sides of the chest in animals requiring thoracic lavage.

Anesthesia

General anesthesia is seldom required and is frequently contraindicated. Sedation may be required, whereas only physical restraint is needed for depressed patients. Local anesthesia should be injected at the chest tube placement site.

Patient Positioning

The patient should be placed in lateral recumbency, with the recumbent side having the less affected hemithorax.

Operative Preparation

Specialized Instruments. The chest tube can be fashioned as described in Figure 7–8A or may be obtained commercially (Argyle).

Details of Procedure

Figure 7–8A. A 10 or 12 French sterile, disposable urethral catheter (Sherwood Medical Industries, Inc., St. Louis, MO 63103) is used as the drain tube. The flared end should be fashioned to accept either a three-way stopcock or a Heimlich valve, and multiple side holes are cut into the tip. A metal stylet with handle is passed the entire length of the catheter and makes the catheter rigid enough for the forceful thrust through the chest wall.

NOTES:

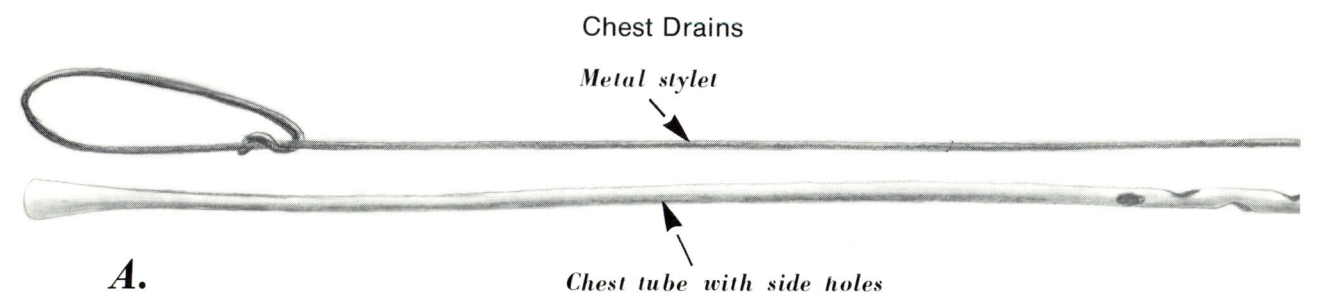

Figure 7–8
Illustration continued on following page.

Chest Drains

B.

9th intercostal space

7th intercostal space

C.

9th intercostal space

7th intercostal space

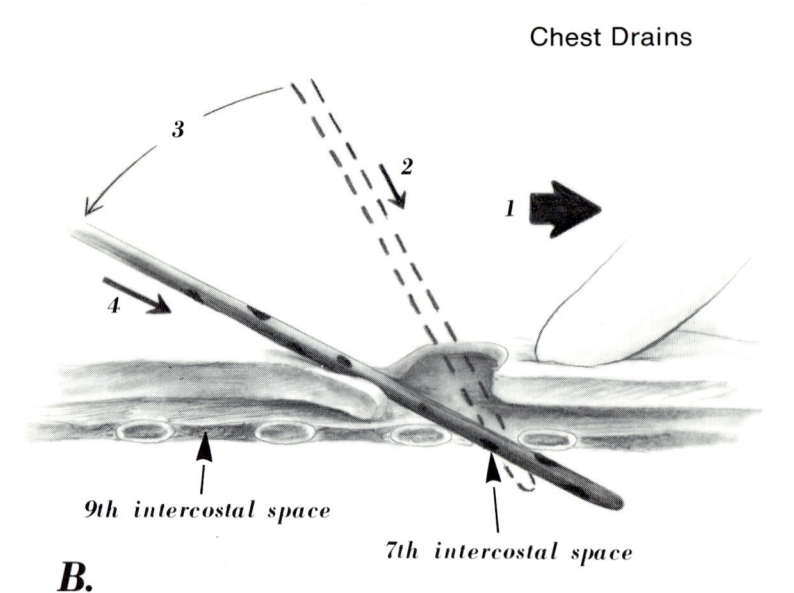

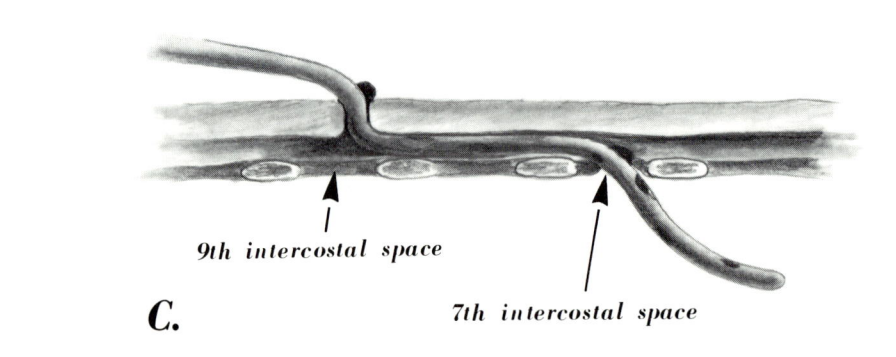

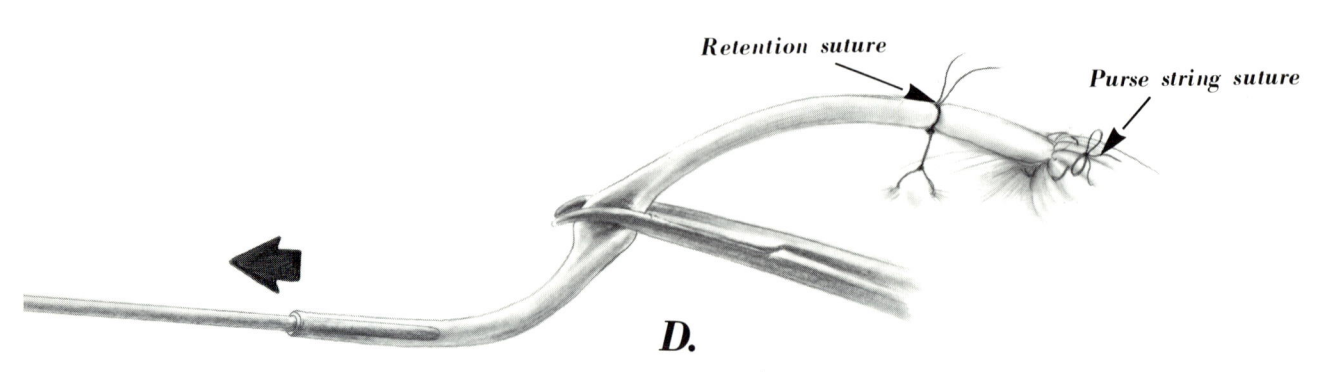

D.

Retention suture

Purse string suture

Figure 7–8 Continued.

SOFT TISSUE SURGERY

Figure 7–8B. An incision just large enough for the tube is made over the ninth intercostal space. The skin is pulled forward two spaces (motion 1). The drain tube with stylet is passed through the incision and superficial muscles (motion 2); the outside end of the catheter is lowered caudally (motion 3); and the catheter is thrust forward through the seventh intercostal space (motion 4). During the thrust through the intercostal space, care should be taken to prevent penetration of thoracic structures, such as the heart and great vessels. All side holes must be inside the thorax.

Figure 7–8C. The desired entry through the chest wall creates a flap-type valve that prevents fluid and air passage. Intrathoracic tube position can be determined radiographically, and the cranial end should be positioned ventrally at the first or second intercostal space.

Figure 7–8D. After penetration of the chest wall, the stylet is withdrawn. Prior to complete withdrawal of the stylet, a heavy clamp is placed across the tube. A three-way stopcock or Heimlich valve is attached to the tube. A pursestring suture is placed around the entry site and tied in a shoestring bow. A retention suture is placed near the tube exit from the skin. The suture is placed and tied to the skin. The ends are passed around the tube twice and tied snugly enough to slightly indent the tube. A chest bandage should be used as a protective wrap around the chest tube. Fatal pneumothorax can be produced by the animal's laceration of the tube. To withdraw the tube, the bow is undone, the chest tube is withdrawn, and the pursestring suture is retightened and tied.

Postoperative Considerations

Following placement of the chest tube, culture and cytology of the thoracic fluid are performed. The tube is frequently aspirated. The packed cell volume and the condition of the buffy coat are periodically determined, evaluated, and recorded on a flow chart.

NOTES: *(Continued)*

7–9 PATENT DUCTUS ARTERIOSUS

Clarence A. Rawlings

Indications

A patent ductus arteriosus should be ligated when it is diagnosed, when there is a left to right shunting of blood, and when congestive heart failure is not present or is medically managed.

Anesthesia

Dogs with congestive heart failure should be treated with diuretics and digitalization. Anesthetic considerations discussed for the thoracotomy (Procedure 7–1) also apply to ligation of the patent ductus arteriosus. Drugs that reduce cardiac force of contraction and potentiate ventricular arrhythmias, such as halothane and the barbiturates, should not be used or should be used with caution. Drugs that have limited cardiovascular effects (e.g., the narcotics and nitrous oxide) are preferred. Muscle relaxants are useful adjuncts to balanced anesthesia, but positive pressure ventilation must be performed during muscle paralysis.

Patient Positioning

The patient is placed in right lateral recumbency, with the left forelimb extended cranially.

Operative Preparation

Special Draping. The lungs are reflected with moist laparotomy pads.

Specialized Instruments. A self-retaining thoracic retractor, such as a Finochietto or Harken retractor, is needed to maintain good exposure. Dissection instruments required are DeBakey tissue forceps, Metzenbaum scissors, and right-angle forceps. Cardiovascular arterial clamps and needle holders would be required to oversew a severed ductus.

Suture Material. The ductus is ligated with 2-0 or larger nonabsorbable suture material. Cardiovascular suture of 6-0 monofilamentous strands (nylon or polypropylene) would be necessary to oversew severed or transected arteries and ductus.

Incision and Exposure

The patent ductus arterious is approached through a left side thoracotomy at the fourth intercostal space (See Procedure 7–1.)

Details of Procedure

Figure 7–9A. Initial exposure of the region of the patent ductus arteriosus (PDA) reveals a connection between the pulmonary artery (PA) and the aorta. Turbulence within the vessels can be detected by digital palpation. The left phrenic and left vagus nerves should be identified and avoided.

Figure 7–9B. Dissection around the PDA can be improved by traction with sutures or umbilical tapes placed around the aorta. One traction suture should be placed around the aorta proximal to the PDA and

SOFT TISSUE SURGERY

another distal to the PDA. Traction on these sutures presents the aorta for dissection, and these sutures can be used to initiate hemostasis in case of a lacerated vessel. A dissection plane is established between the aorta and the PA on the cranial and caudal sides of the PDA. Dissection instruments should include DeBakey tissue forceps, right-angle forceps, and Metzenbaum scissors.

NOTES:

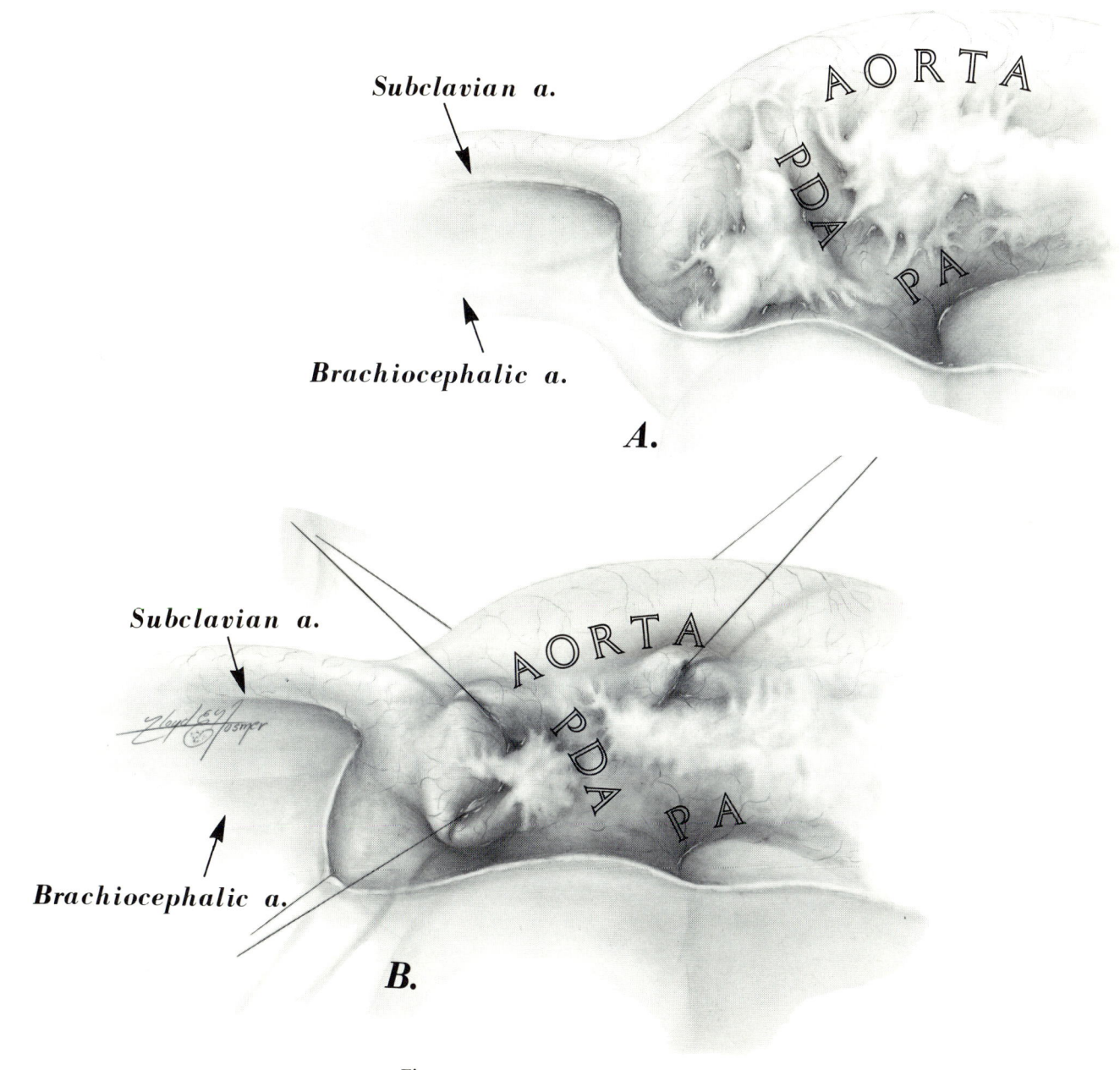

Subclavian a.

Brachiocephalic a.

AORTA
PDA
PA

A.

Subclavian a.

Brachiocephalic a.

AORTA
PDA
PA

B.

Figure 7–9
Illustration continued on following page.

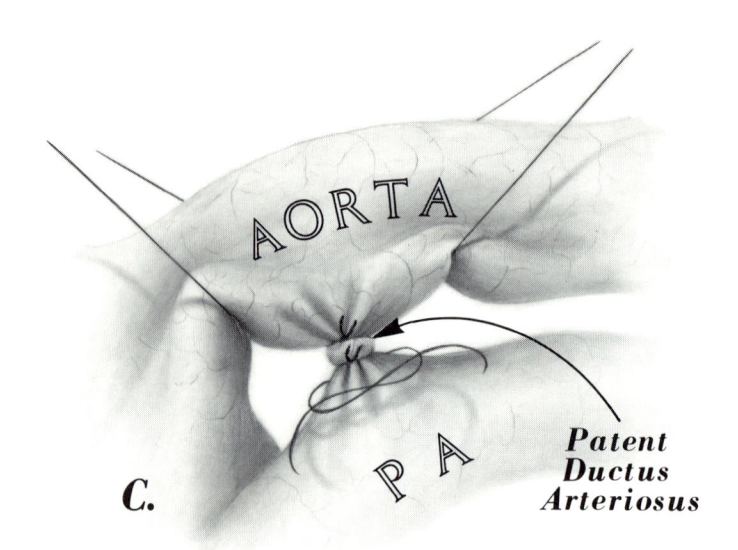

Figure 7–9 Continued

Figure 7–9C. Ligatures of 2-0 or larger nonabsorbable suture material are passed around the PDA by using right-angle forceps. During passage of a ligature medial to the PDA, care must be taken to avoid puncturing the right pulmonary artery, which divides to the right from the main pulmonary artery just ventral to the PDA. At least two ligatures should be positioned, and the ligature closest to the aorta should be tied first. A chest tube should be positioned prior to routine closure of the thoracotomy.

findings should be determined frequently and logged on a flow chart. The chest-tube aspirate should also be obtained frequently and recorded.

NOTES: *(Continued)*

Postoperative Considerations

The electrocardiogram, venous pressure, systemic artery pressure, and auscultatory

7–10 PULMONARY LOBECTOMY

Clarence A. Rawlings

Indications

Amputation of a lung lobe is indicated when that lobe is nonfunctional because of neoplasia, lobar pneumonia, or torsion of the pulmonary lobe.

Anesthesia

The patient should be anesthetized according to the suggestions for the thoracotomy and the pulmonary disease patient (Procedure 7–1; Chapter 2).

Patient Positioning

The patient should be placed in lateral recumbency.

Operative Preparation

Special Draping. To reduce the spread of bacteria from a pneumonic lung lobe and the spread of neoplastic cells from pulmonary neoplasms, the lung should be isolated by moist laparotomy pads.

Specialized Instruments. A self-retaining thoracic retractor (Harken or Finochietto) is needed to provide thoracic exposure. Dissection instruments, such as Metzenbaum scissors and DeBakey forceps, and noncrushing cardiovascular clamps (atrial clamps or right-angle forceps) are required.

Suture Material. Swaged cardiovascular suture material of 5-0 polypropylene is used to close the bronchus.

Incision and Exposure

A lateral thoracotomy through the fifth intercostal space provides access to the hilus of the lung (Procedure 7–1).

78 SOFT TISSUE SURGERY

Ventral view

Cranial lobe
Middle lobe
Bronchus
Pulmonary veins
Aorta
P.A.
L. Auricle

A.

Caudal lobe
L. Bronchus
Bronchus
Middle lobe
Pulmonary arteries
Pulmonary a.
Aorta
Bronchus
L. Auricle
P.A.
Cranial lobe

B.

Dorsal view

Distal

Transfixation suture

C.

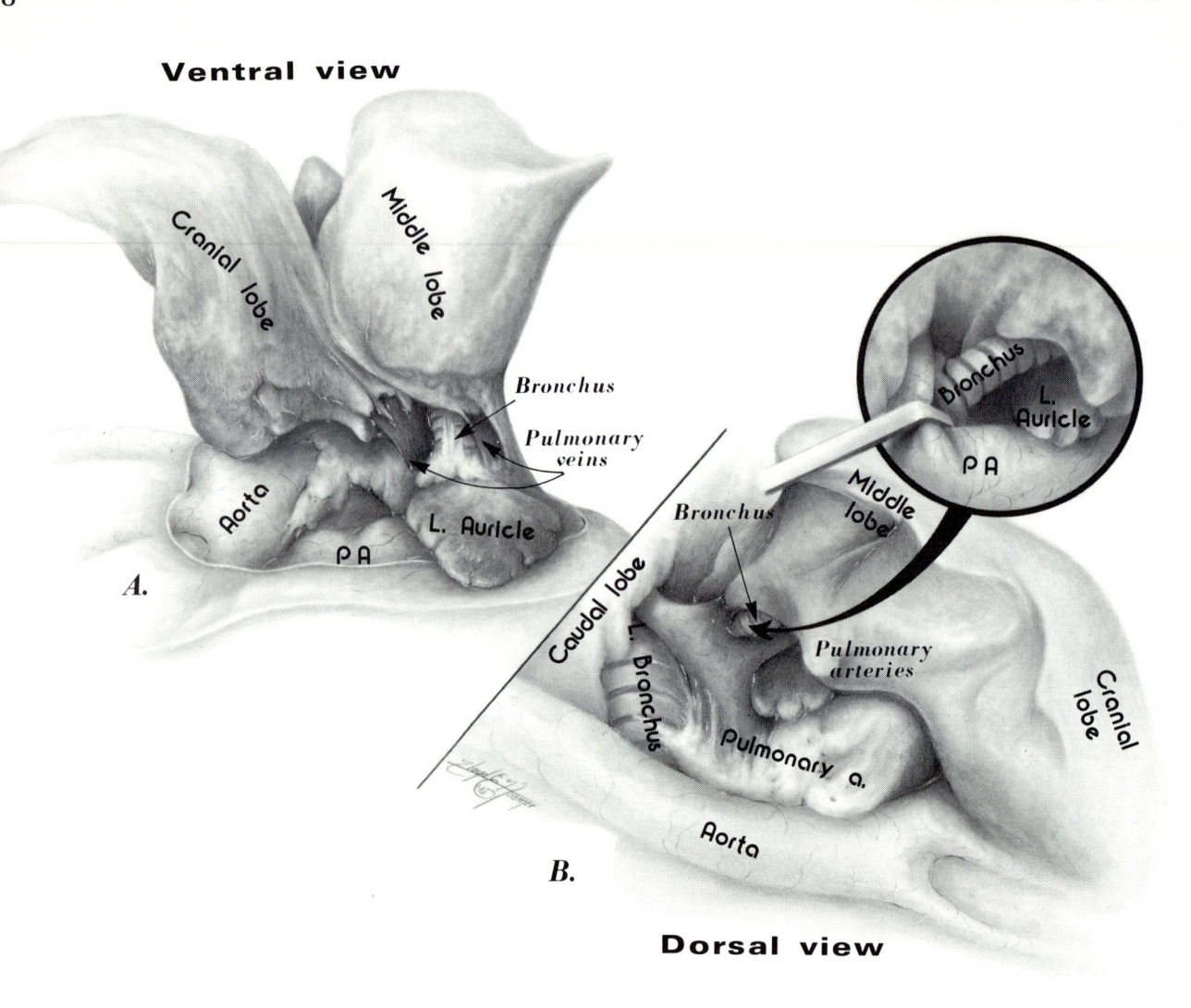

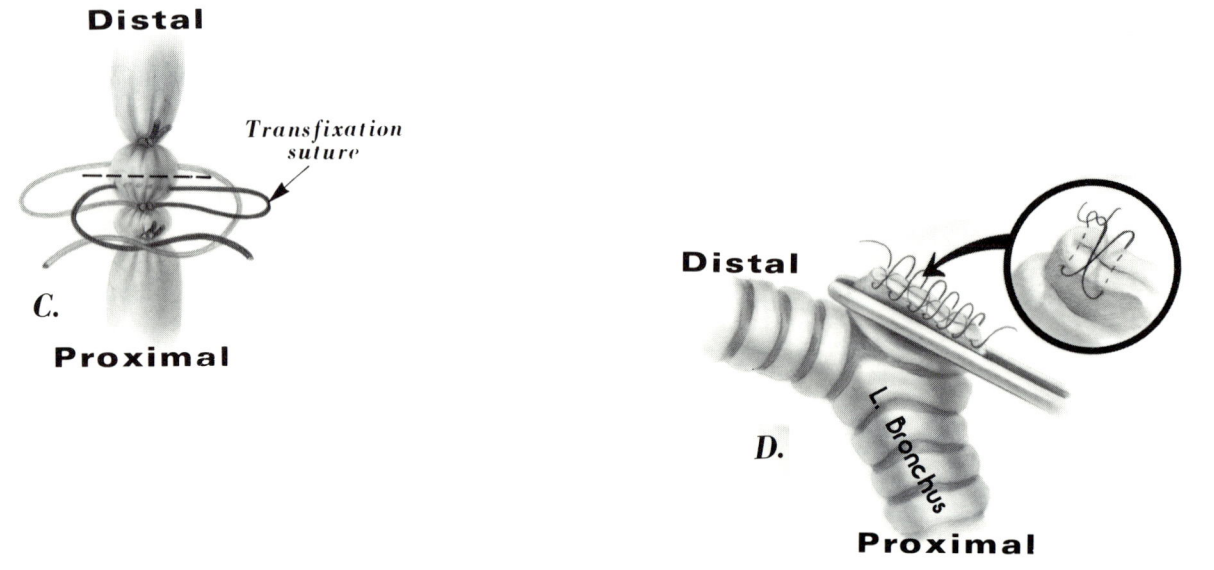

Proximal

Distal

D.

L. Bronchus

Proximal

Figure 7–10.

Details of Procedure

Figure 7–10A. The structures around the hilus of the left cranial and middle lung lobes are viewed from the ventral aspect of the thoracotomy. The bronchus can be readily palpated and exposed by dissection. The pulmonary veins course toward the left atrium and are ventral and caudal to the bronchus. Note the pulmonary artery (PA).

Figure 7–10B. When the hilus of the left cranial and middle lung lobes is viewed from a dorsal direction, the pulmonary arteries are dorsal and cranial to the bronchi. The bronchi, arteries, and veins should be dissected by sharp dissection using DeBakey forceps and Metzenbaum scissors.

Figure 7–10C. The pulmonary arteries are ligated close to their origin from the left pulmonary arteries. Two ligatures, a simple ligature and a second ligature as a transfixing suture, are placed proximal to the intended incision. Either a third ligature or a hemostat can be placed distal to the intended incision. The pulmonary veins are then ligated and incised in a similar manner.

Figure 7–10D. After the vessels have been ligated and incised, they can be reflected to expose the bronchus. The bronchial cartilage is flattened, and the noncrushing cardiovascular clamp is applied. The clamp should be adjacent to the origin of the bronchus from the left bronchus. The bronchus on the pulmonary lobe side is occluded with another clamp, and the bronchus is incised parallel and 5 mm distal to the noncrushing clamp. Two rows of sutures of a 5-0 cardiovascular suture material are used to close the bronchus. The first suture line is composed of interrupted figure eight sutures (see inset). The second suture line is a simple continuous pattern. Patency of the suture line should be checked by positive pressure inflation of the lung while the bronchus is submerged in saline. Mediastinal tissue can be sutured over the vessels and bronchus. A chest tube is positioned, and the chest is closed in the routine manner.

Postoperative Considerations

Amputated lung lobes should be cultured, and appropriate antibiotic therapy should be initiated. Histopathology should be obtained on the excised tissue. A chest tube should be left in place for 24 hours and aspirated frequently.

NOTES:

7–11 DIAPHRAGMATIC RUPTURE

Wayne E. Wingfield

Indications

A ventral abdominal approach provides ready access to repair a ruptured diaphragm. This approach is more familiar than a thoracic approach and is useful for all but the chronic hernia, which may have multiple areas of adhesion between abdominal and thoracic organs.

Anesthesia

Positive pressure ventilation is required when repairing a diaphragmatic rupture. The considerations applied to the thoracotomy and pulmonary patients (Procedure 7–1; Chapter 2) are applicable. Rapid induction and intubation and early initiation of positive pressure ventilation are critical. With the open thorax, a chest drain coupled to underwater seals, Heimlich valves, or intermittent suction via a three-way stopcock will be required postoperatively.

Patient Positioning

The patient is positioned in dorsal recumbency, with support on either side by sandbags or a V-trough to facilitate the abdominal approach through the linea alba.

Operative Preparation

Patient stabilization is important prior to the administration of an anesthetic agent. Treatment for shock and temporary immobilization of existing fractures should precede anesthesia. Incarceration of the liver may result in fluid accumulation within the thorax and/or abdomen. Likewise, the stomach may dilate with air while in the thorax and impair respiration more severely. In general, a timed surgical intervention following patient stabilization is important.

Specialized Instruments. Use of a Balfour retractor will provide ready access to the diaphragm. Postoperatively, the surgeon should be prepared to manage a thoracic drain for removal of air and/or fluid.

Suture Material. Nonabsorbable suture materials are preferred for their tensile strength and longer-lasting characteristic.

Incision and Exposure

A midventral abdominal incision is made from the xiphoid process to the umbilicus. For additional exposure, the incision may be enlarged by either splitting the xiphoid or extending the incision in a paracostal direction.

Details of Procedure

Figure 7–11A. The size and location of the diaphragmatic tears determine which abdominal viscera will enter the thorax. With incarceration of abdominal organs, the tears should be surgically enlarged rather than risk tears in the organ in attempting to replace the normal anatomy.

Use of moistened laparotomy towels to

SOFT TISSUE SURGERY 81

pack the abdominal organs away from the diaphragm will provide better visualization. Coordination between the anesthetist and the surgeon is mandatory in order to avoid laceration of organs during surgical suturing. The adequacy of lung expansion can be evaluated through the diaphragmatic tear.

Prior to closing the diaphragm, the abdominal and thoracic walls should be carefully examined to assure that there are no unforeseen traumatic injuries. Abnormal fluid accumulations in the thorax and abdomen are aspirated with suction, and the mediastinum is fenestrated to assure good drainage of air and fluids postoperatively. Following mediastinal fenestration, the thoracic drain is positioned in the ventral floor of the thorax.

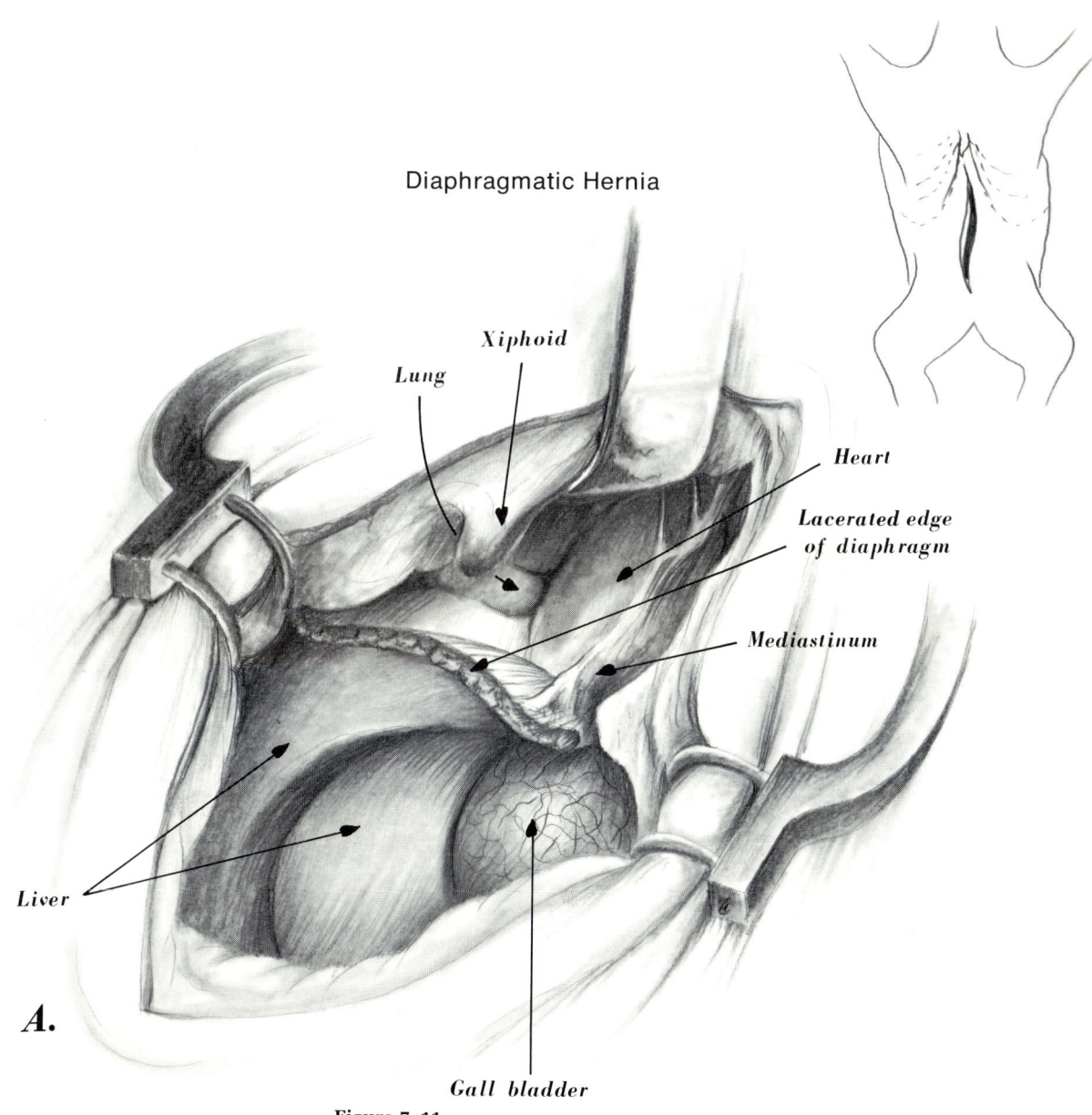

Figure 7–11
Illustration continued on following page.

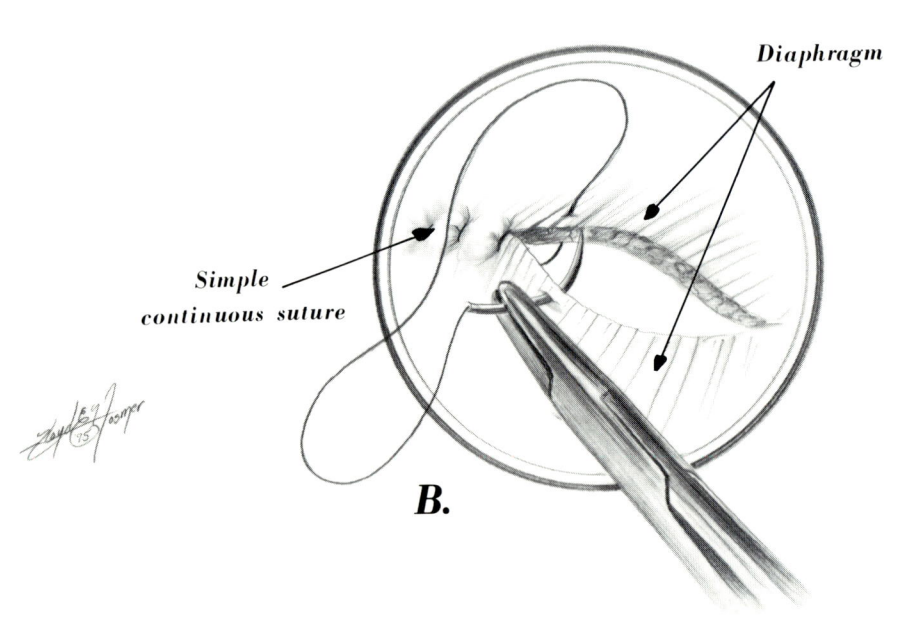

Figure 7–11 Continued

Figure 7–11B. The diaphragm is closed with suture patterns of the surgeon's preference. The suturing of a tear should begin at the most remote site and progress to the most accessible site. Preplacement of sutures will allow visualization of the diaphragm and may help to avoid stricturing areas around the esophagus or caudal vena cava. A simple continuous suture is illustrated and provides a good closure with a rapid serosal seal. This pattern requires passage of the suture needle 3 to 4 mm from the cut edge of the diaphragm to assure good holding strength by the diaphragmatic muscle.

Following closure of the diaphragmatic tear, the adequacy of the suture line may be checked by inflating the lungs while simultaneously dripping saline. The presence of air bubbles would suggest an inadequate seal and simple interrupted or horizontal mattress sutures should be utilized to close the area of leakage more firmly.

The abdominal incision is closed in a routine three-layer closure.

Postoperative Considerations

The chest drain is used to remove fluid and air from the thorax. Through the use of a flow chart delineating the time of aspiration and the quantities of air and fluid, when to pull the chest drain can be determined. The drain is usually required for less than 24 hours.

NOTES:

7–12 GASTROTOMY

Wayne E. Wingfield

Indications

Gastrotomy is utilized most frequently in small animal surgery for the removal of foreign bodies. Additional indications for gastrotomy include uncontrolled hematemesis, chronic gastric ulcers, removal of nonviable tissue in acute gastric dilation-volvulus, excision of small gastric neoplasms, and for biopsy in the diagnosis of food allergy or chronic gastritis.

Anesthesia

Consideration should be given to improving the anesthetic risk status prior to gastrotomy. Dehydration, acid-base imbalance, and electrolyte losses are encountered in vomiting patients. These derangements increase anesthetic risk and should be at least partially corrected prior to induction of a general anesthetic.

Patient Positioning

A V-trough or sandbags are used to maintain dorsal recumbency in preparation for gastrotomy.

Operative Preparation

Special Draping. Prior to gastrotomy, the stomach should be packed away from other abdominal organs through the use of laparotomy towels. After completion of the gastrotomy, soiled instruments should be discarded, and the surgeon should be prepared to exchange contaminated gloves for sterile gloves.

Incision and Exposure

A cranial midventral abdominal incision is used to expose the stomach. Frequently a large, fat-filled falciform ligament is encountered as the linea alba is incised. This structure will hamper accurate apposition of tissue layers during surgical closure of the abdomen. Total excision of this structure at its junction with the peritoneum will facilitate closure as well as visualization in the cranial abdomen. Because the falciform ligament extends ventral to the xiphoid process, the cranial deep epigastric vessels will be encountered. These vessels should be ligated.

SOFT TISSUE SURGERY

Details of Procedure

Figure 7–12A. Retention sutures are placed in the stomach and are used to retract the stomach from the abdominal cavity. Moistened laparotomy towels are used to protect the abdominal cavity from potential contamination from accidental spills of gastric contents.

Because the epiploic vessels extend from the greater curvature and the gastric vessels extend from the lesser curvature, there will be a relatively avascular area where these two groups of vessels approach each other. This avascular area will be the site of the gastrotomy incision.

NOTES:

Gastrotomy

Retention suture

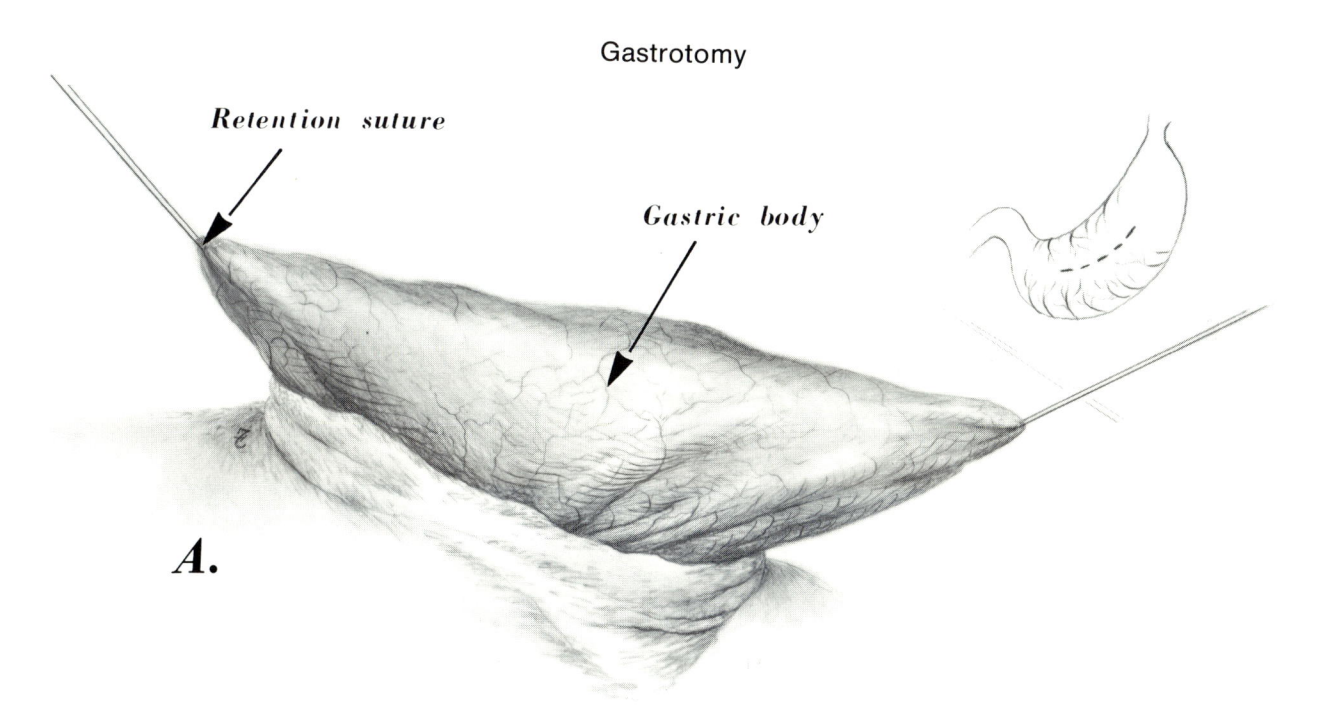

Gastric body

A.

Figure 7–12
Illustration continued on following page.

Figure 7–12B. A No. 10 surgical blade is used to make the stab incision into the gastric lumen. Considerable resistance can be expected as the blade is thrust through the submucosa and the mucosa.

Figure 7–12C. Next, Metzenbaum scissors are inserted into the gastric lumen through the stab incision, and the incision is enlarged to the appropriate size. While enlarging the incision, maintain a line parallel to the retention sutures and within the least vascular area of the stomach.

Figure 7–12D. Gastric mucosa will bulge from the incision. Adequate exploration of the lumen should include an assessment of the cardia, fundus, pyloric antrum, and pylorus.

NOTES: *(Continued)*

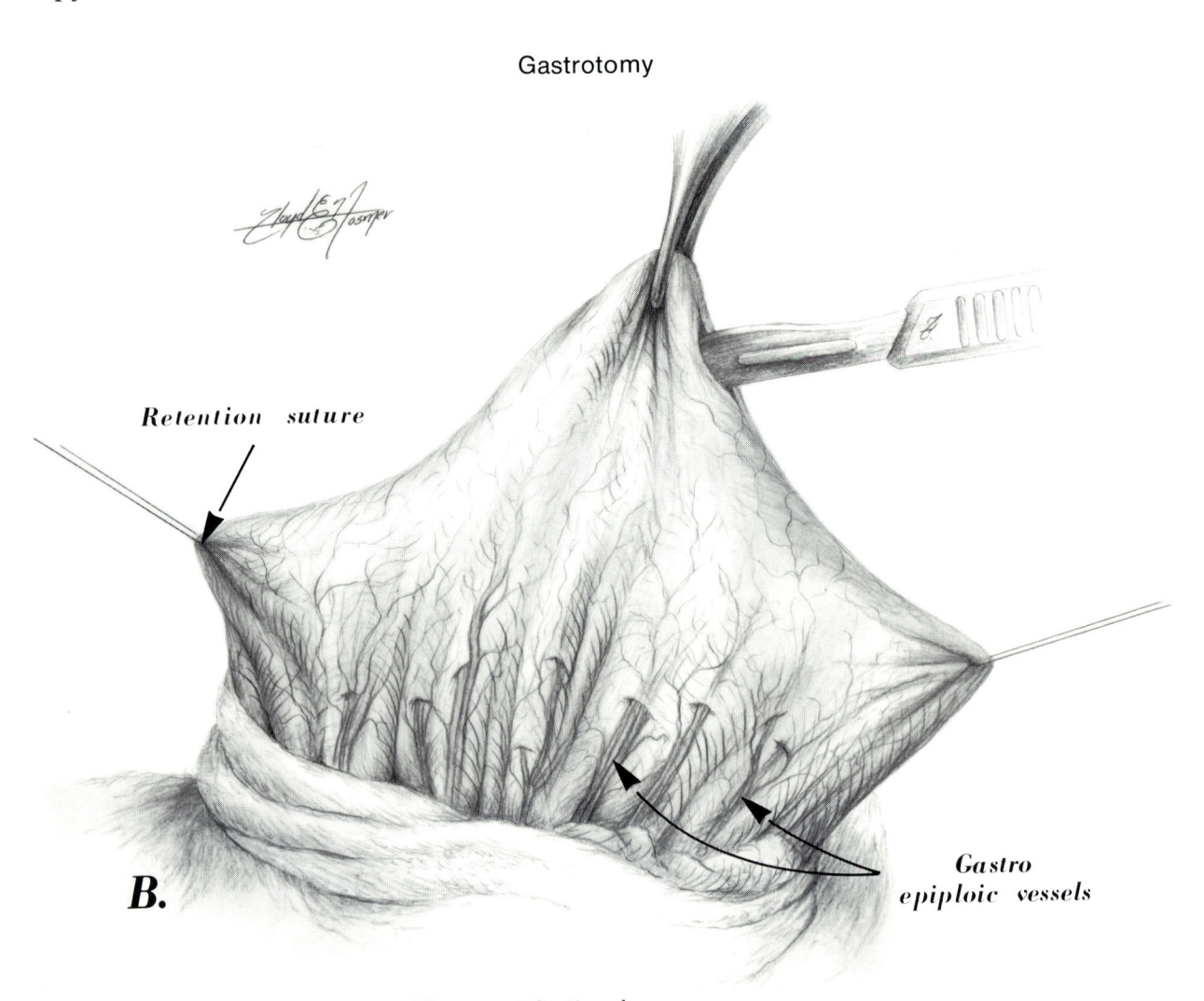

Figure 7–12 Continued
Illustration continued on opposite page.

SOFT TISSUE SURGERY

Gastrotomy

C.

Gastro epiploic vessels

Retention suture

D.

Gastric lumen

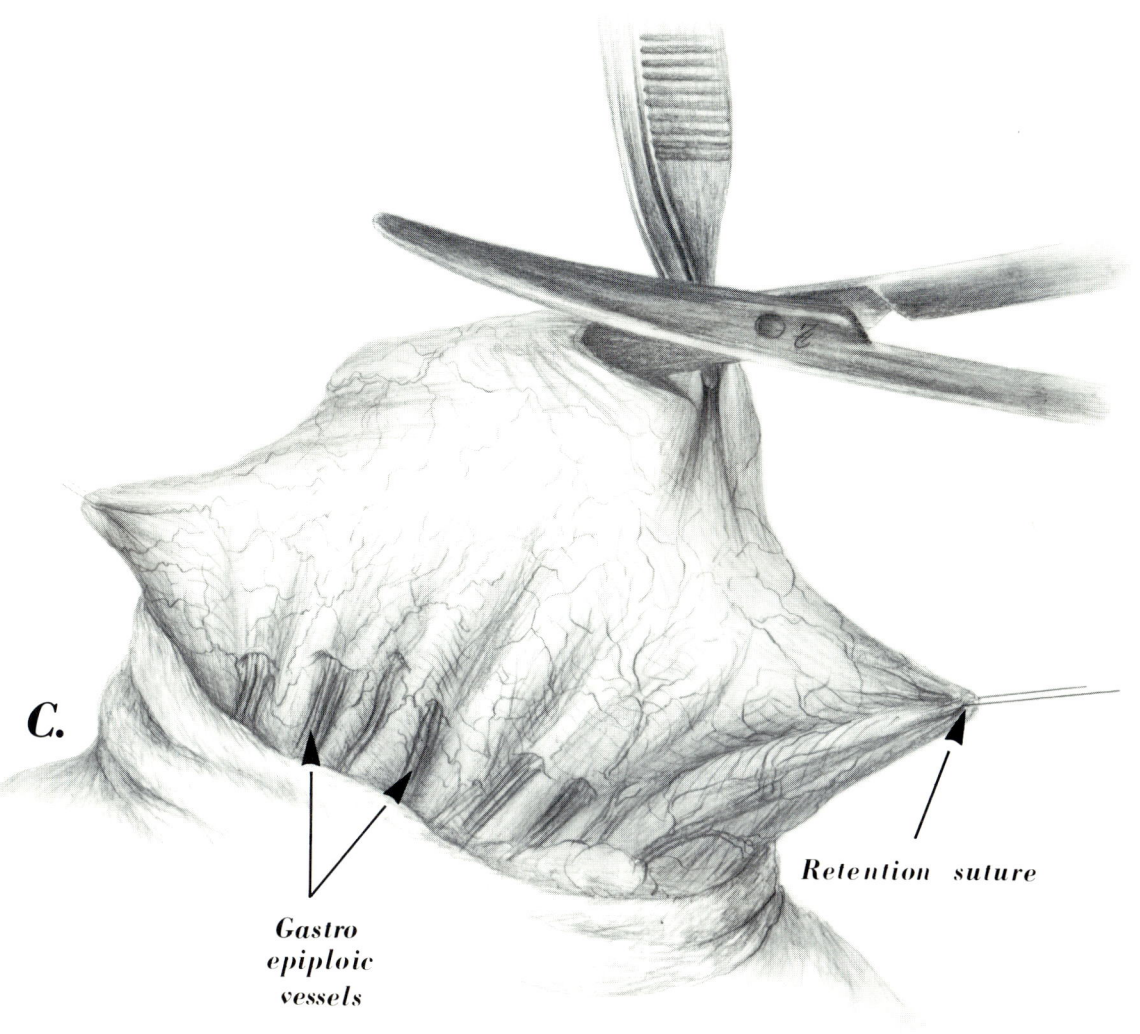

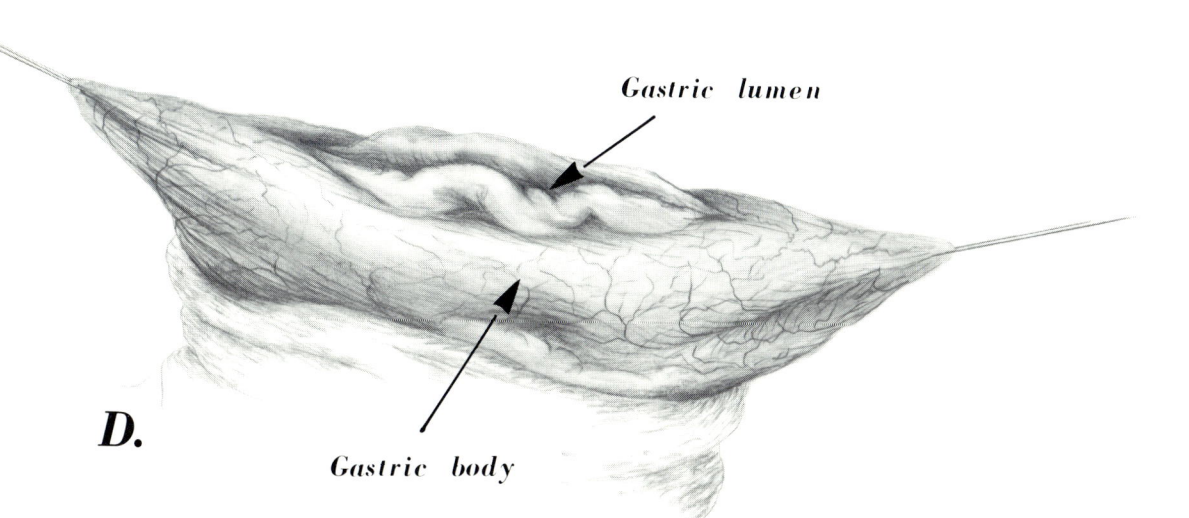

Gastric body

Figure 7–12 Continued
Illustration continued on following page.

Gastrotomy

E. 1st Layer of Closure

Gastric lumen

Retention suture

Gastro epiploic vessels

F.

Gastric mucosa
Muscularis mucosa
Submucosa
Muscularis
Serosa

Gastric lumen

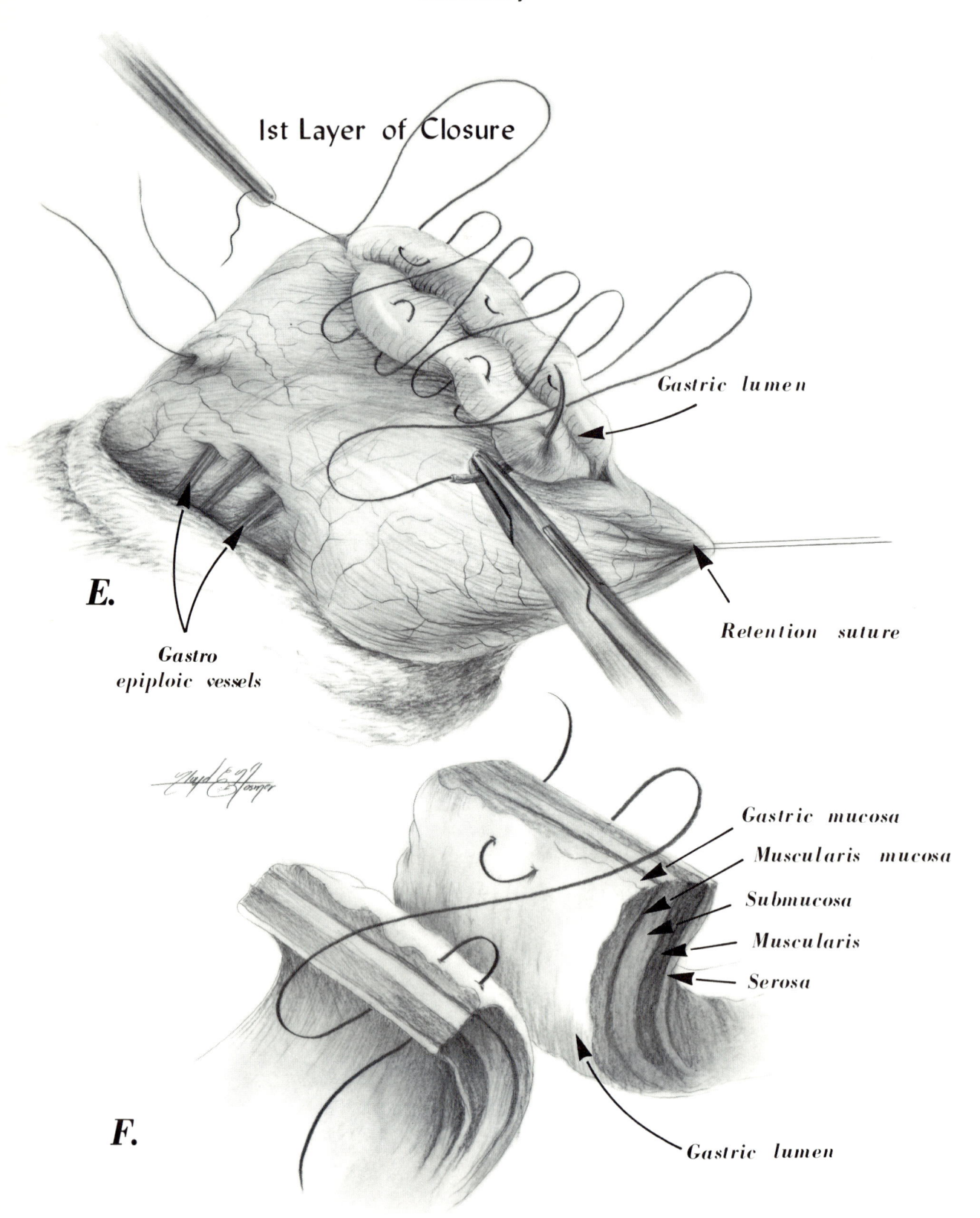

Figure 7–12 Continued
Illustration continued on opposite page

SOFT TISSUE SURGERY

Figure 7–12E. Closure of the gastrotomy incision involves two suture layers. A Connell stitch is used for the first layer of closure. This inverting suture pattern is begun by tying the suture away from the end of the gastric incision. A Connell stitch extends from the serosa through the mucosa and is continuous.

Figure 7–12F. A Connell suture passes through all tissue layers of the stomach and is passed from side to side and parallel to the incision. Each suture is about 3 mm from the incision edge. As each stitch is placed, it is tightened to invert the tissue edges and provide serosa-to-serosa contact. (In Figure 7–12E, the sutures have not been tightened to illustrate the continuous appearance of the Connell pattern.) Continue the Connell suture pattern approximately 5 mm beyond the edge of the incision before tying it off.

Figure 7–12G. A second layer of closure is inserted over the Connell sutures. The Halsted pattern is used for this second layer of closure. Because it is an interrupted pattern, the Halsted pattern will provide good holding strength if the stomach becomes distended postoperatively with gas

NOTES: *(Continued)*

Gastrotomy

G.

1st layer of closure
Retention suture

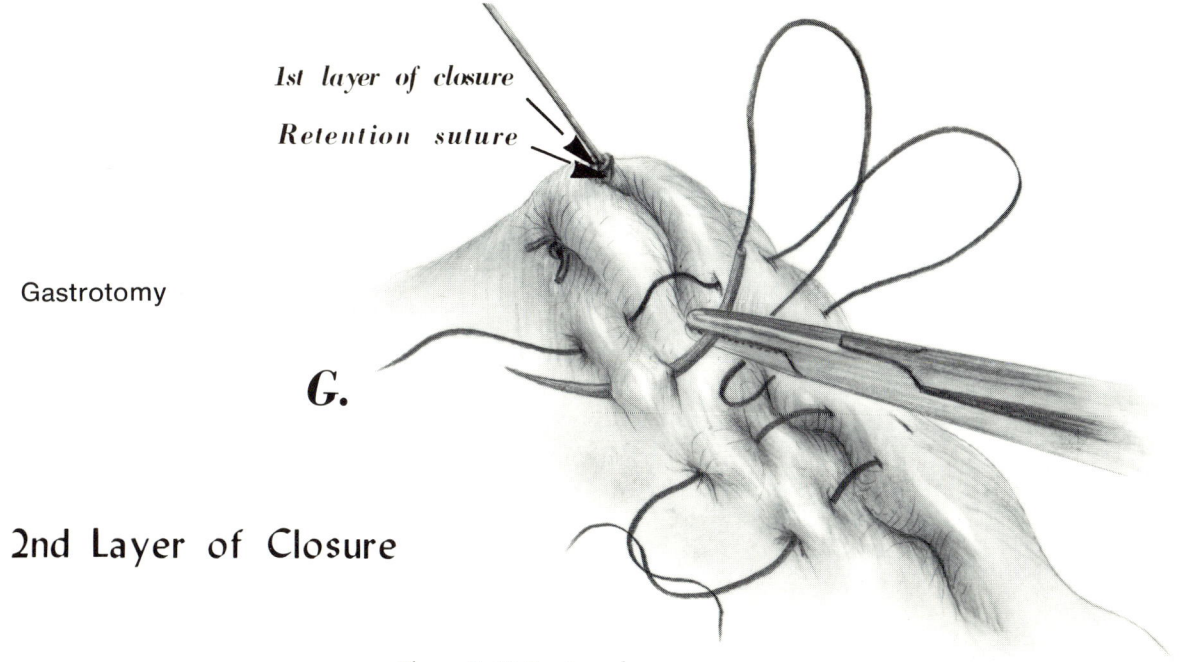

2nd Layer of Closure

Figure 7–12 Continued
Illustration continued on following page.

Gastrotomy

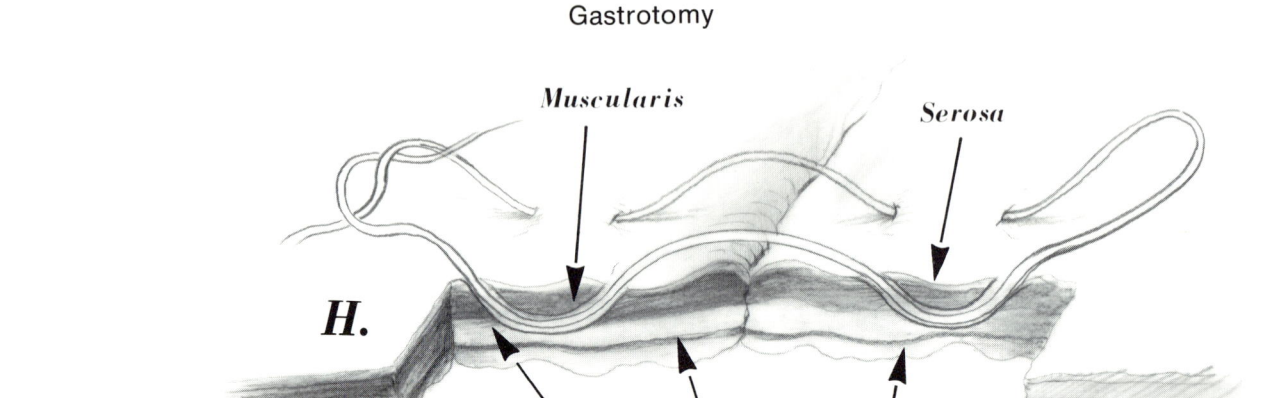

Figure 7–12 Continued

or food. Placement of the Halsted sutures will provide a second inverting pattern to the closure of the gastrotomy incision.

Figure 7–12H. Notice that the Halsted stitch extends only to the depth of the submucosa. Each suture extends 3 to 5 mm apart. Upon completion of the second layer of closure, the retention sutures and laparotomy towels are removed. Warm Ringer's lactate is used to lavage the abdomen. Contaminated instruments and gloves are discarded prior to a routine three-layer closure of the abdominal wall.

NOTES: *(Continued)*

Postoperative Considerations

Small amounts of a bland diet and water are offered to the animal after 12 to 24 hours. Small volumes of food should be continued for 10 days to prevent disruption of the suture line by overdistention of the stomach.

7–13 PERMANENT GASTROPEXY

CHARLES WILLIAM BETTS

Indications

Recurrence of gastric volvulus in dogs is not unusual. To prevent the stomach from rotating into a volvulus, a permanent gastropexy has been shown to be effective preventive surgery.

Anesthesia

General anesthesia is required.

Preoperative Preparation

The dog should be clipped from the dorsal midline to the ventral midline, from the caudal half of the thorax to the flank.

Patient Positioning

The patient is positioned in right lateral recumbency.

Operative Preparation

Special Draping. Four corner draping is used.

Specialized Instruments. Babcock intestinal forceps are useful for gentle grasping of the stomach.

NOTES:

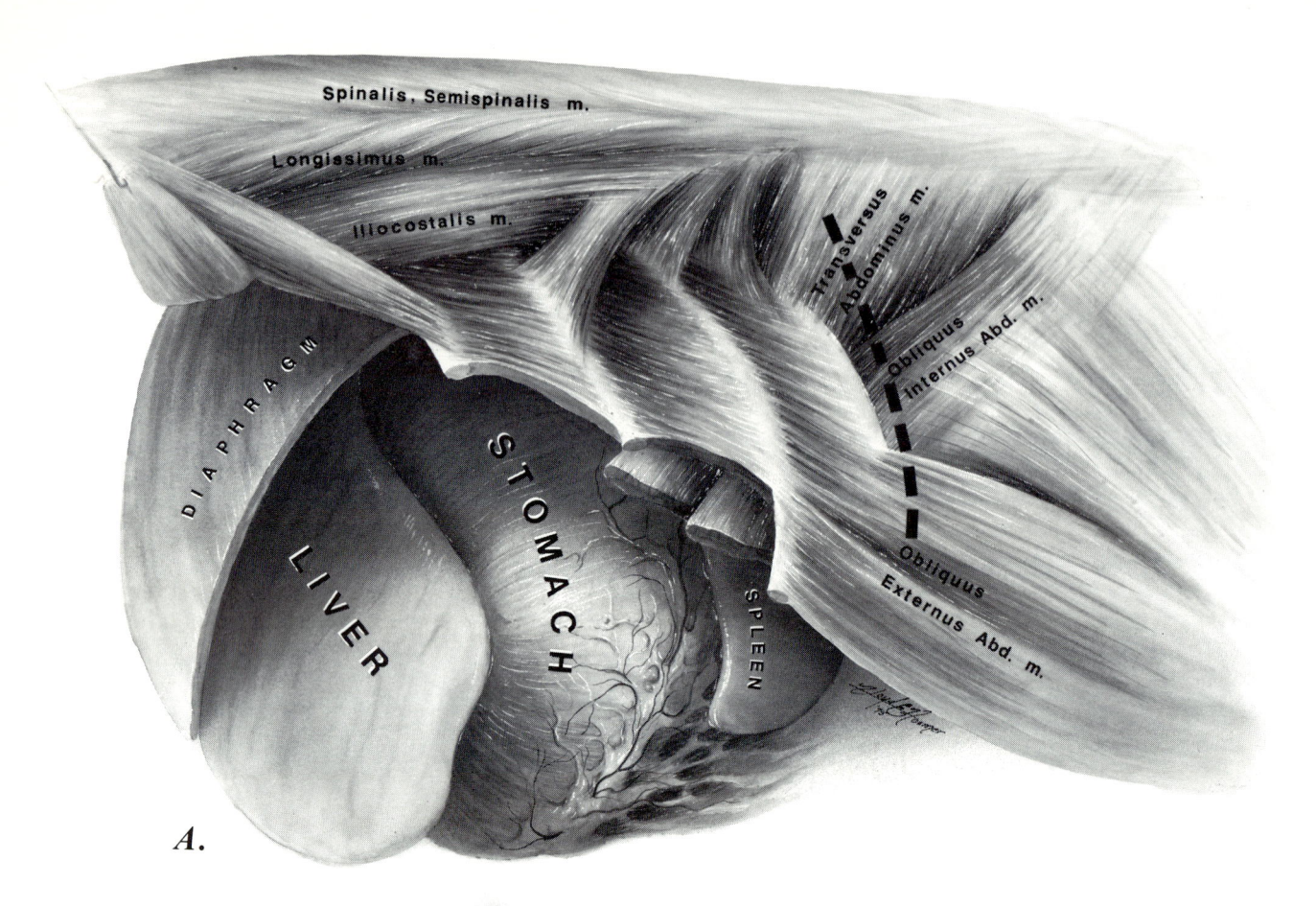

92 SOFT TISSUE SURGERY

A.

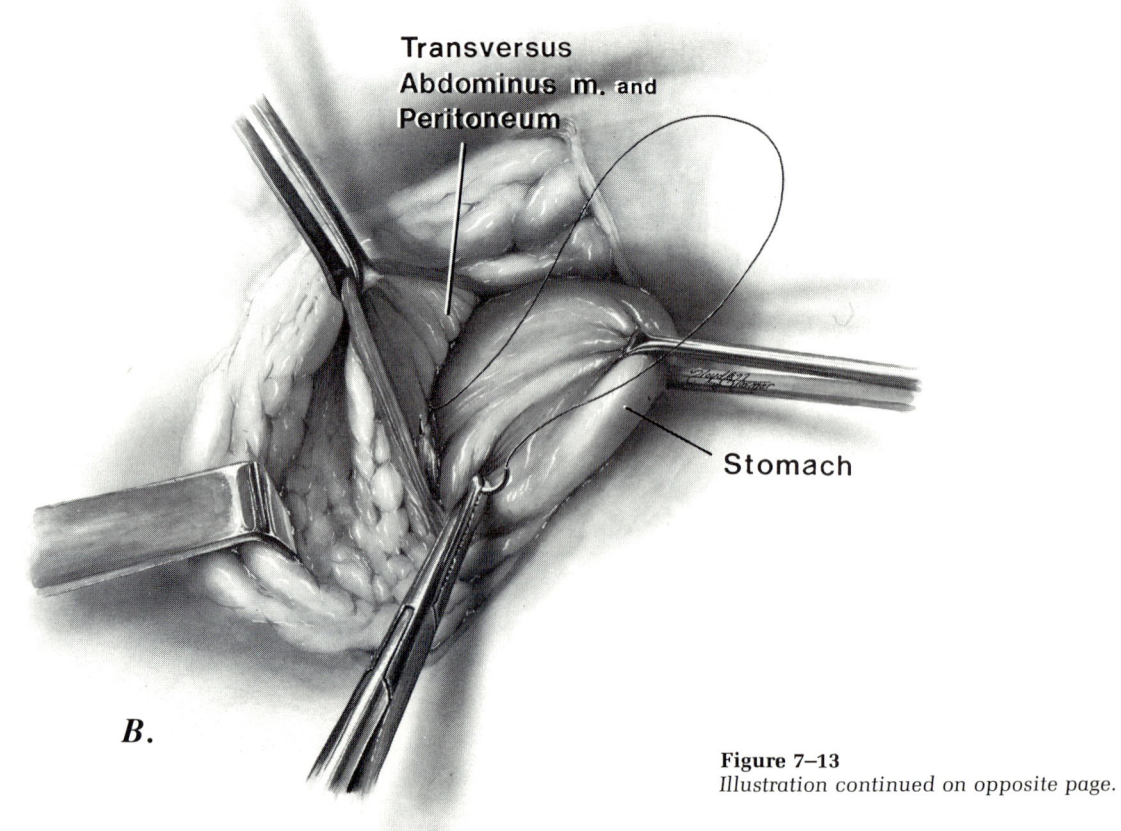

B.

Figure 7–13
Illustration continued on opposite page.

SOFT TISSUE SURGERY

Transversus Abdominus m.

Obliquus Internus m.

Stomach

Obliquus Externus m.

C.

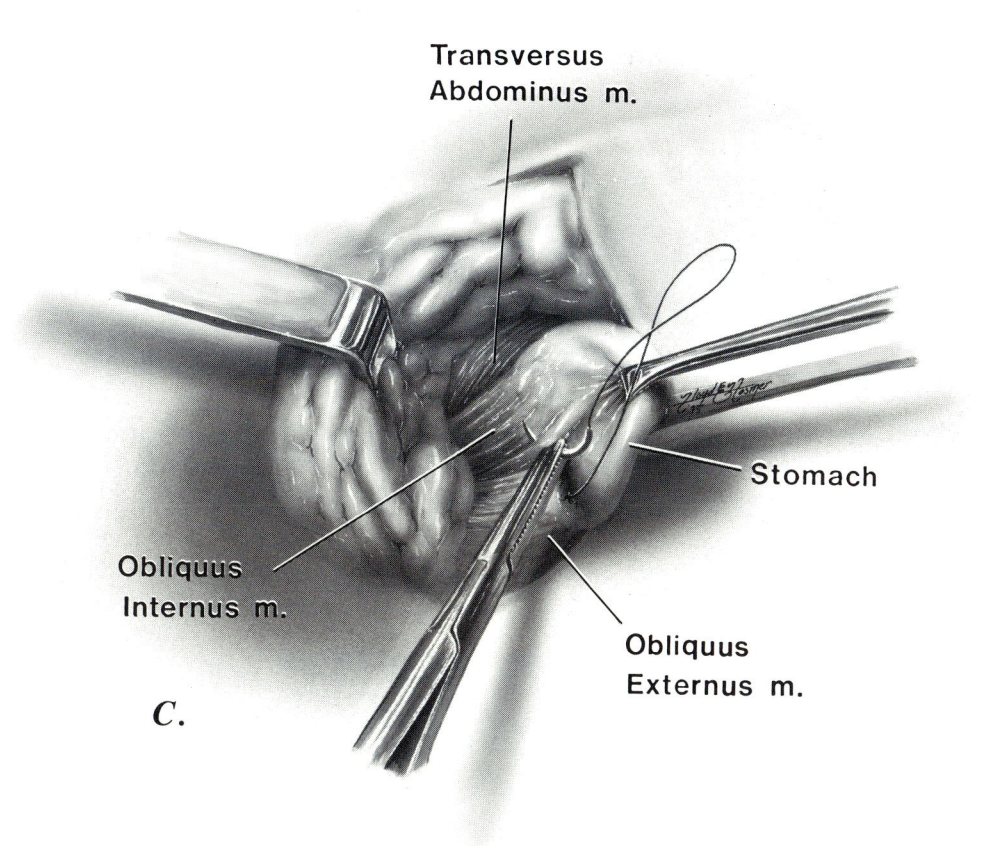

Figure 7–13 Continued

Details of Procedure

Figure 7–13A. The operative site for a permanent gastropexy is in the left paracostal region (dotted line).

Figure 7–13B. The avascular fundic portion of the stomach is grasped, and 2-0 chromic catgut is sutured in a simple continuous pattern to the peritoneum and transversus abdominis muscle. In suturing, be sure the submucosal layer of the stomach is sutured with each passage of the suture needle. The entire circumference of the incision is traversed, leaving adequate stomach to suture the next muscle group (internal abdominal oblique muscle).

Figure 7–13C. A simple continuous suture pattern using 2-0 chromic catgut is used to suture the submucosal layer of the stomach to the external abdominal oblique muscle. Next the subcutaneous tissues and skin are closed in the routine manner.

Postoperative Considerations

The dog should be given small amounts of gruel for 4 to 6 days, starting 12 to 24 hours after surgery. Water should be given frequently in small amounts until the dog's thirst is satisfied; then water is given *ad libitum*. Exercise should be limited to several short, daily sessions of leash walks for 7 to 10 days. Any precautions necessary to prevent vomiting should be taken. A light protective bandage may be necessary to prevent the dog from licking or scratching the area.

NOTES:

7–14 PYLOROMYOTOMY

Charles William Betts

Indications

This procedure is indicated to relieve pylorospasm refractory to medical management and pyloric stenosis and to assist emptying of the stomach as part of the management of the gastric dilatation-volvulus syndrome.

Preoperative Preparation

The abdomen should be clipped from slightly cranial to the xiphoid cartilage and costal arch to the pubic rim if exploratory surgery is contemplated.

Pyloromyotomy

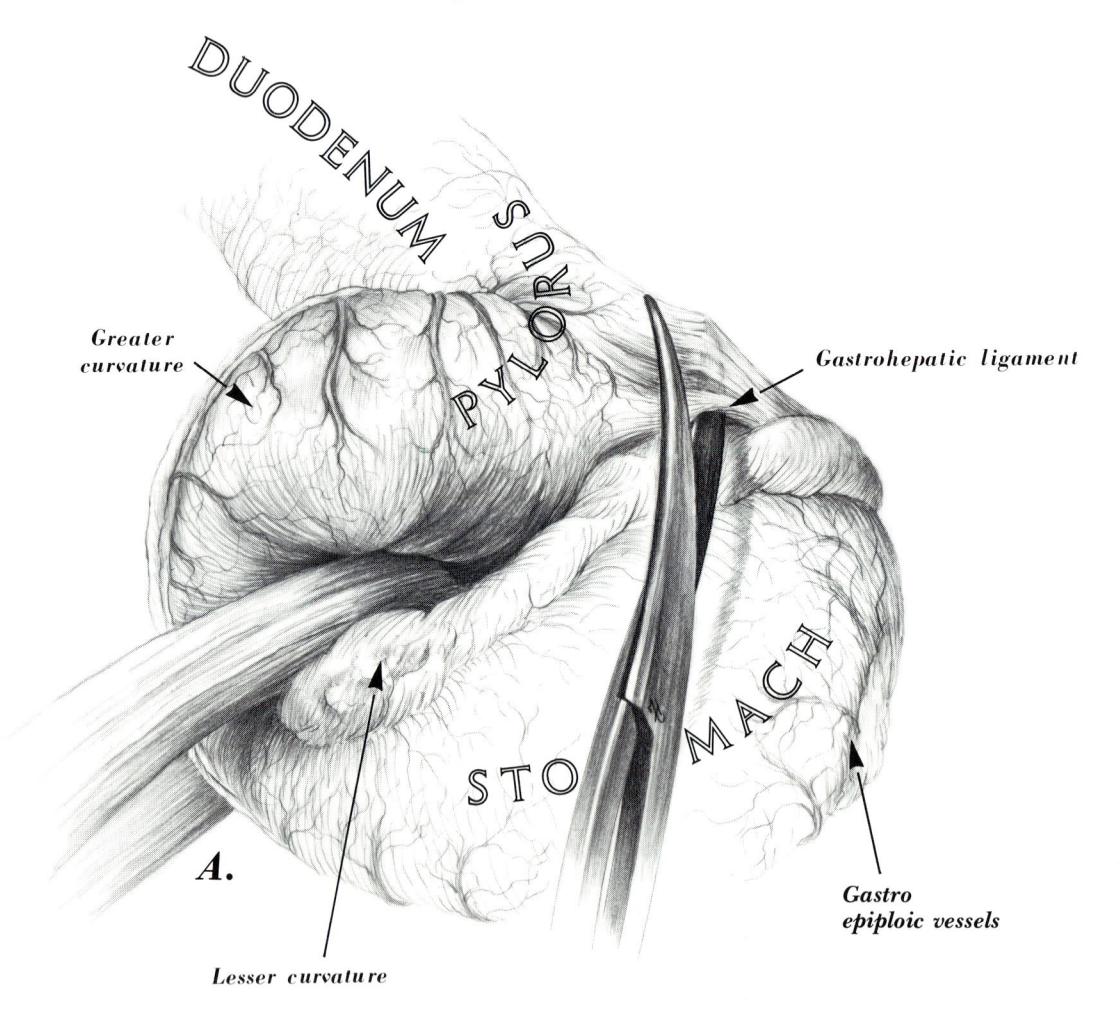

Figure 7–14
Illustration continued on page 96.

Anesthesia

General anesthesia is required.

Patient Positioning

The animal is placed in dorsal recumbency.

Operative Preparation

Special Draping. Four corner draping is utilized. Laparotomy pads should be used to line the sides of the incision and to pack off the intestines.

Specialized Instruments. A Balfour self-retaining abdominal retractor is of considerable benefit.

Suture Material. The suture material used is the same as that for any abdominal closure.

Incision and Exposure

A cranial midventral abdominal incision is made to expose the stomach for a pyloromyotomy. Moist laparotomy pads should be placed laterally against the inner abdominal wall prior to placement of the Balfour self-retaining abdominal retractor. Be cognizant of the pancreas, the liver, and the common bile duct and handle them gently.

Details of Procedure

Figure 7–14A. Identify the greater and lesser curvatures of the stomach, the pylorus, the gastrohepatic ligament, and the common bile duct. Mobilize the stomach by caudal and left lateral retraction at the lesser curvature — use umbilical tape, a Penrose drain, or the left index finger (if right-handed). Carefully incise the gastrohepatic ligament and adjacent connective tissue. Never incise craniodorsally toward the common bile duct.

NOTES:

Pyloromyotomy

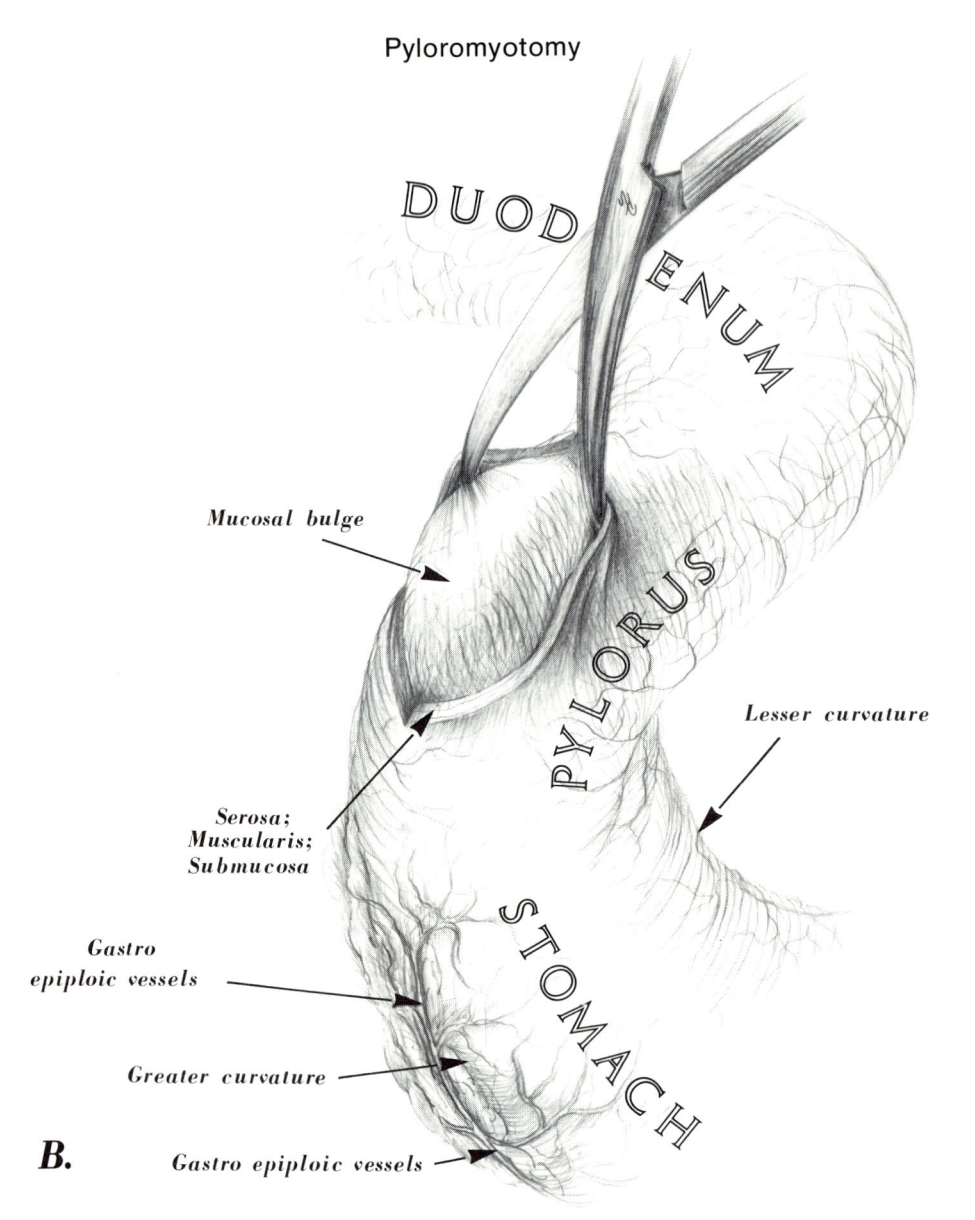

Figure 7–14 Continued

Figure 7–14B. Make a liberal, linear incision over the pyloric antrum, the pylorus, and the proximal duodenum. The incision should be carried carefully to the level of the mucosa by incising the serosal, longitudinal, and circular muscle layers. The submucosa is not a distinguishable layer. Dissection is facilitated by the caudal and left lateral retraction of the stomach and the right lateral retraction of the proximal duodenum. A tissue-dissection plane should be established between the mucosa and the superficial tissue layers with a mosquito hemostat or Metzenbaum scissors. This plane should be established as far laterally as possible to allow the mucosa to bulge. All circular muscle fibers must be incised to create a smooth, even mucosal bulge. This can be done with Metzenbaum scissors or a No. 10 surgical blade. Small mucosal perforations can be sutured with a simple interrupted pattern. If a large perforation occurs, convert the pyloromyotomy to a pyloroplasty (Heineke-Mikulicz) by suturing the longitudinal incision in a transverse direction. Closure of the abdomen is performed in the routine manner.

Postoperative Considerations

In the absence of electrolyte imbalances and/or vomiting, no special feeding regimen is required. Smaller amounts of food than normally eaten given two to three times a day for 24 to 48 hours will suffice. Feeding may be resumed a few hours after surgery if the dog is hungry. Routine wound management and supervision of exercise are necessary.

7–15 ENTEROTOMY

Clarence A. Rawlings

Indications

Enterotomies of healthy intestines are required to remove foreign bodies and to obtain biopsies. If the intestine containing the foreign body appears devitalized, this area should be resected and anastomosed (Procedure 7–16).

Anesthesia

Preanesthetic preparation should partially correct fluid and electrolyte disturbances in the patient that is vomiting and dehydrated because of the foreign body. General anesthesia is required, with preference given to halothane and narcotic agents. These agents produce minimal depression of splanchnic blood flow, can be given to effect, and are readily reversible. If anesthesia is induced by inhalation, nitrous oxide should probably not be used, as this distends gas pockets.

Patient Positioning

The patient is placed in dorsal recumbency.

Operative Preparation

Special Draping. In addition to routine laparotomy draping, moist laparotomy pads are required to reduce peritoneal contamination by intestinal contents.

Specialized Instruments. A self-retaining abdominal retractor, e.g., a Balfour retractor, is needed to provide abdominal exposure. Occluding but noncrushing intestinal forceps, e.g., Doyen or Pearlman bulldog clamps, are optimal and may be used for obstructing chyme movement. A second set of instruments for laparotomy is required following completion of the enterotomy and removal of contaminated drapes and instruments. A vacuum pump and sterile suction device are necessary to evacuate the peritoneal cavity following peritoneal lavage.

Suture Material. The intestine is closed with 3-0 or 4-0 synthetic absorbable suture material.

Incision and Exposure

The abdomen is approached through a cranial midline laparotomy.

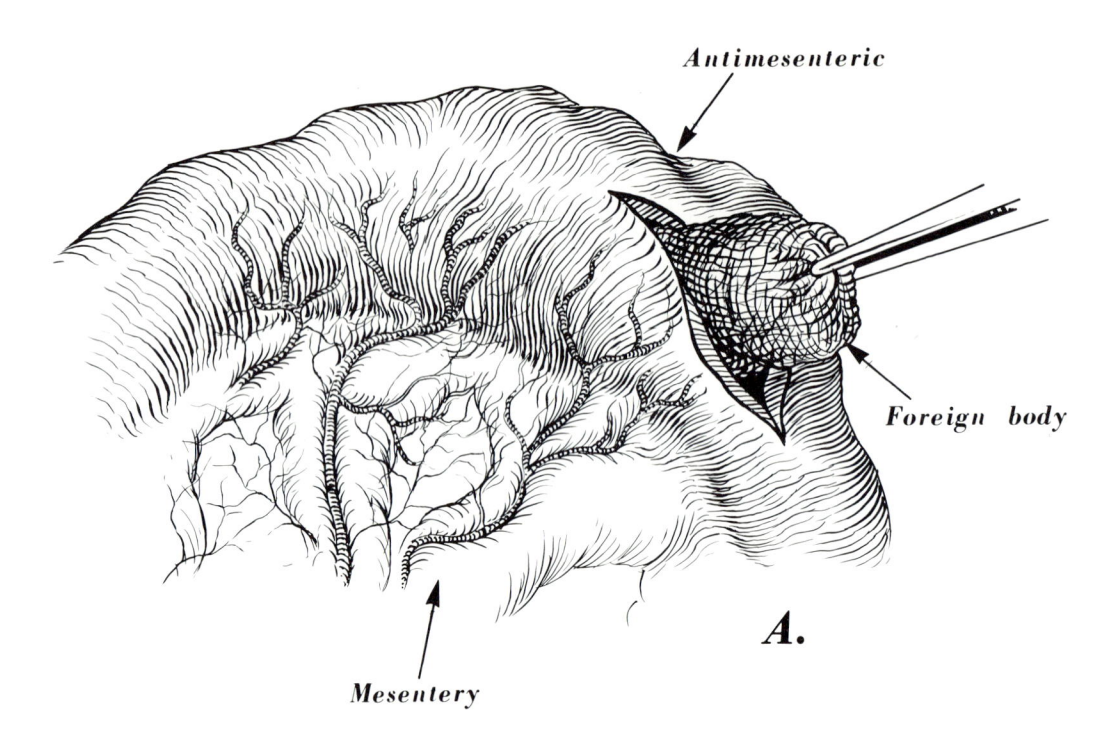

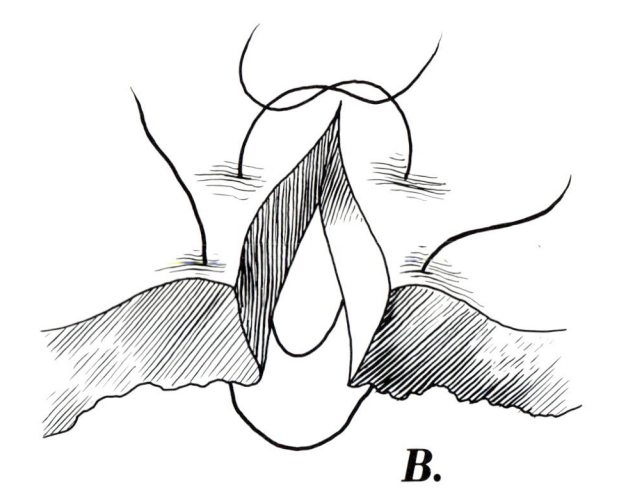

Figure 7–15

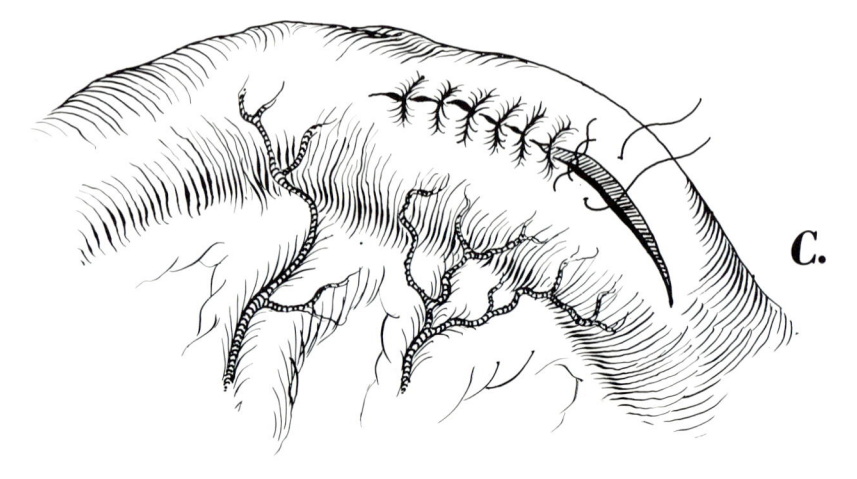

Details of Procedure

Figure 7–15A. A longitudinal incision is made over one end of the foreign body and on the antimesenteric side of the intestine. The foreign body should be gently removed. The intestine should be examined to determine if resection is necessary.

Figure 7–15B. The enterotomy is closed by a single layer of simple interrupted sutures of 3-0 or 4-0 absorbable suture material.

Figure 7–15C. The enterotomy is closed so that there is an effective seal against chyme. The longitudinal incision, in contrast to a transverse incision, permits lengthening of the incision and will reduce the lumen size. Should closure of the enterotomy constrict the diameter of the lumen excessively, this incision may be sutured transversely to avoid stenosis. When intestinal biopsies are performed, they should be full thickness.

Postoperative Considerations

Within 12 hours of surgery, the animal is encouraged to eat small meals of its regular diet and to drink water. The diet should be restricted in the animal with intestinal disease (lymphangiectasia, neoplasia, malabsorption) in which the initiating cause of disease was not removed by surgery. The patient should be observed closely for vomiting and signs of ileus.

NOTES:

100　　　　　　　　　　　　　　　　　　　　　　　　　　　　　　　　　　　　　　SOFT TISSUE SURGERY

Intestinal Anastomosis

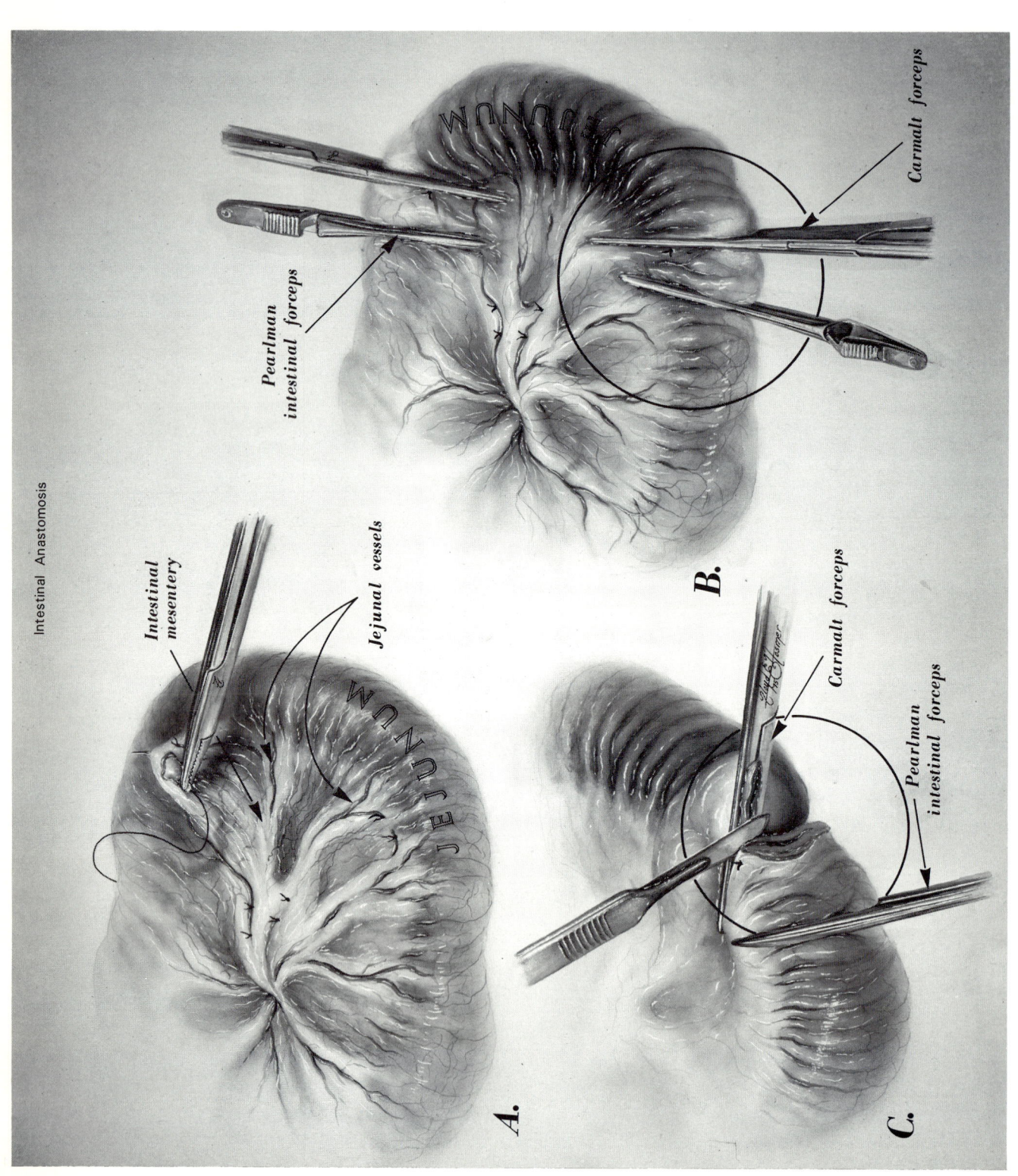

A.
Intestinal mesentery
Jejunal vessels
JEJUNUM

B.
Pearlman intestinal forceps
Carmalt forceps
DUODENUM

C.
Carmalt forceps
Pearlman intestinal forceps

Figure 7–16
Illustration continued on page 102.

7–16 INTESTINAL ANASTOMOSIS

Eberhard Rosin

Indications

Intestinal resection and anastomosis are indicated in such conditions as an intestinal foreign body, intussusception, volvulus, and abdominal trauma.

Anesthesia

Patients with intestinal disease are frequently dehydrated and depressed. Their fluid and electrolyte status must be evaluated and partially corrected prior to surgery. Induction and maintenance may be of the surgeon's choice, with the exception of those for toxic and depressed animals. Induction and maintenance with halothane should be considered. The use of nitrous oxide should be discouraged when the intestinal disease has produced a bowel obstruction and potential gas pocket.

Patient Positioning

The patient is positioned in dorsal recumbency.

Operative Preparation

Specialized Instruments. Use of a Balfour self-retaining retractor will facilitate good exposure of the abdominal cavity. Laparotomy sponges are used to protect exposed tissues and minimize contamination. The ends of the intestine may be held with noncrushing forceps, such as pediatric Doyen or Pearlman bulldog intestinal forceps.

Suture Material. Anastomosis is accomplished using 3-0 or 4-0 synthetic absorbable (Dexon, Vicryl) or nonabsorbable monofilamentous (nylon, polypropylene) suture materials combined with high-quality tapered needles.

Incision and Exposure

Exposure for intestinal resection and anastomosis is through a midventral abdominal incision.

Details of Procedure

Figure 7–16A. A loop of jejunum is withdrawn from the abdomen, and a moistened laparotomy sponge is placed around the intestine. The arcadial blood supply of the portion of the intestine to be resected is identified and doubly ligated. The communicating branches of the vasa recta vessels along the mesenteric borders are ligated.

Figure 7–16B. Crushing forceps are applied across the intestine at the transection sites. These forceps are placed next to the ligation of the vasa recta vessel and at a slight angle to insure good blood supply to the antimesenteric border. The intestinal contents are milked away from the crushing forceps for a distance of 2 to 3 cm, and noncrushing intestinal forceps are applied.

Figure 7–16C. The intestine is transected along the edge of the crushing forceps with a scalpel. The mesentery is transected between the ligatures with scissors.

102　　SOFT TISSUE SURGERY

Intestinal Anastomosis

D. Everted intestinal mucosa

E. Mesenteric border / Direction of suturing / Antimesenteric border

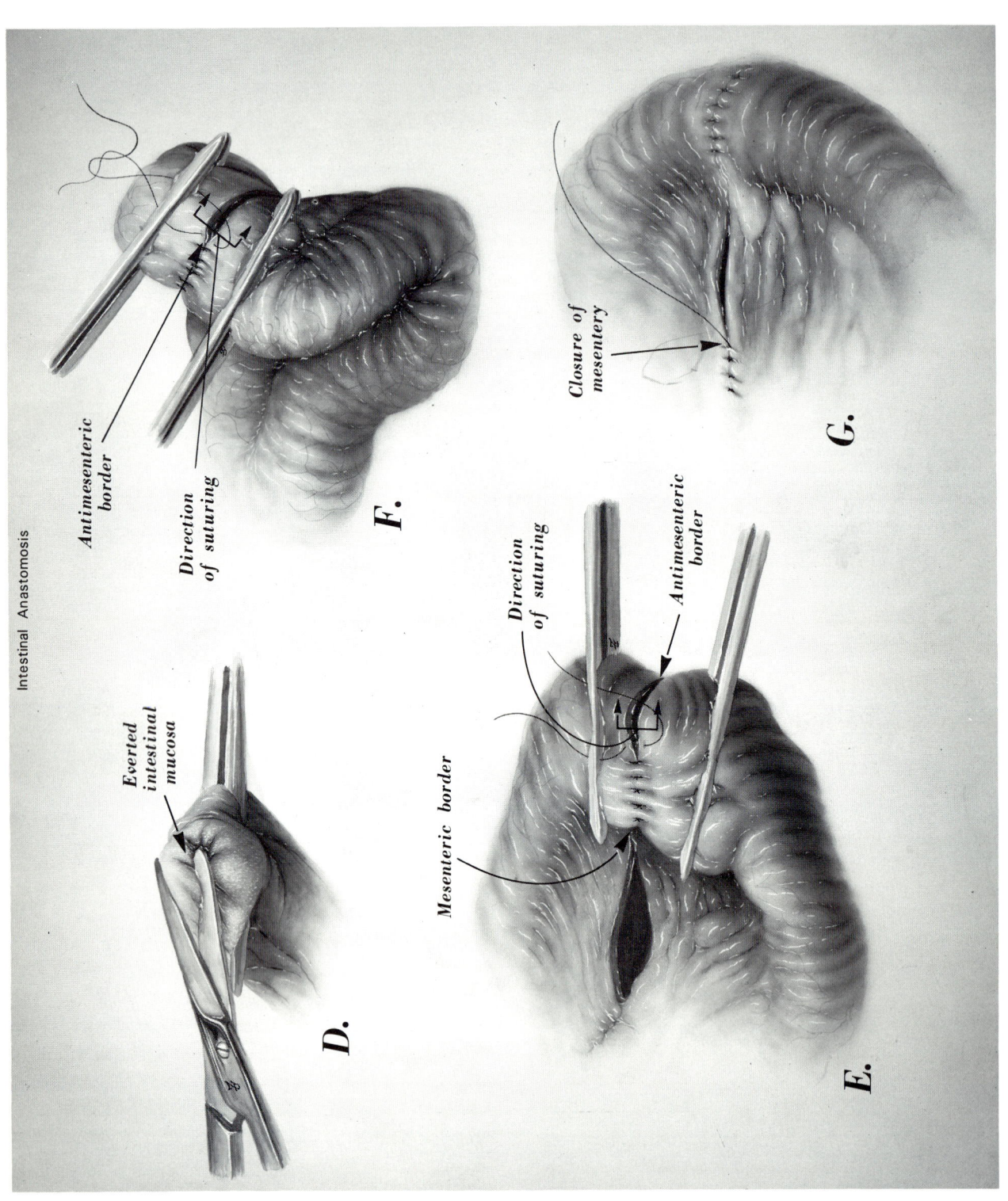

F. Antimesenteric border / Direction of suturing

G. Closure of mesentery

Figure 7–16 Continued

Figure 7–16D. The intestinal mucosa will bulge from the incised edge. This everted mucosa should be trimmed prior to beginning the anastomosis. Half of each circumference is trimmed at one time.

Figure 7–16E. The anastomosis is accomplished with a simple interrupted suture pattern. Starting at the mesenteric border, sutures are inserted approximately 3 mm from the incised edge and pass through all layers of the intestine. The stitch is tied with appositional tension. A series of simple interrupted sutures are placed 3 mm apart and directed toward the antimesenteric border. An attempt is made to invert any bulging mucosa as each knot is secured.

Figure 7–16F. When half of the intestine has been sutured, the intestine is turned for placement of a series of simple interrupted sutures in the open side. The everting mucosa is trimmed prior to beginning the suture pattern. The sutures are again directed from the mesenteric toward the antimesenteric border.

Figure 7–16G. The mesenteric defect is closed with simple interrupted sutures. Care must be taken to avoid the mesenteric vessels. The greater omentum is draped over the anastomosis site. All contaminated instruments, toweling, and gloves are discarded.

The abdominal cavity is lavaged with warm, sterile, isotonic fluids. Drain tubes are inserted if necessary for postoperative peritoneal lavage. Closure of the abdomen is performed in the routine manner.

Postoperative Considerations

Systemic antibiotics are employed, and the patient is monitored for detection of peritonitis. The patient is offered water, and food is given when initial thirst is satisfied.

NOTES:

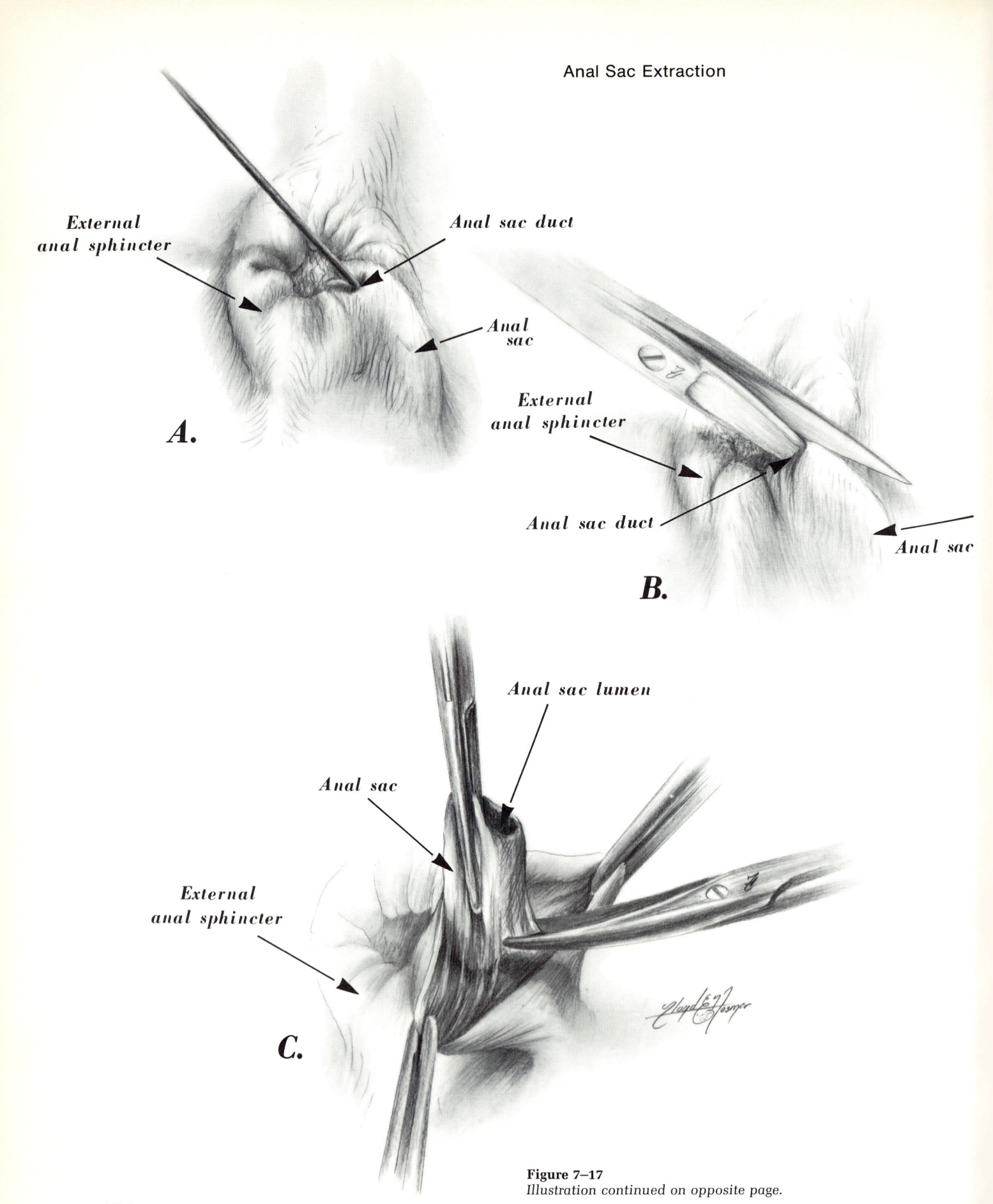

Anal Sac Extraction

A.
External anal sphincter — Anal sac duct — Anal sac

B.
External anal sphincter — Anal sac duct — Anal sac

C.
Anal sac — Anal sac lumen — External anal sphincter

Figure 7–17
Illustration continued on opposite page.

7–17 ANAL SAC EXTRACTION

Clarence A. Rawlings

Indications

Removal of the anal sacs is indicated for chronic anal sac obstipation and infection.

Anesthesia

Either general anesthesia or sedation combined with epidural anesthesia is indicated. The surgeon may request that the rear quarters of the animal be elevated. If the animal's rear quarters are elevated, an epidural block is contraindicated. The pressure of the abdominal viscera on the diaphragm decreases pulmonary compliance. Spontaneous breathing should be supplemented by three to four positive pressure breaths per minute, and the animal should be sighed every 5 to 10 minutes.

Patient Positioning

The patient is placed in ventral recumbency.

Operative Preparation

Prior to anesthesia, an enema is given, and prior to preparation of the surgical site, the rectum is packed with several pieces of sterile gauze.

Details of Procedure

Figure 7–17A. A blunt probe or grooved director is passed via the duct of the anal sac into the sac. The sacs are located at the four and eight o'clock positions.

Figure 7–17B. The duct of the anal sac is incised by placing the point of sharp scissors into the sac.

Figure 7–17C. The sac should be dissected from the fibers of the external anal sphincter within which they lie. The dark inner surface of the sac and the white connective tissue can be easily distinguished from the surrounding tissue.

Figure 7–17D. The sac is dissected until its duct is freed. This is transected. The incision is closed with simple interrupted subcutaneous and skin sutures.

Postoperative Considerations

Fecal incontinence may develop occasionally.

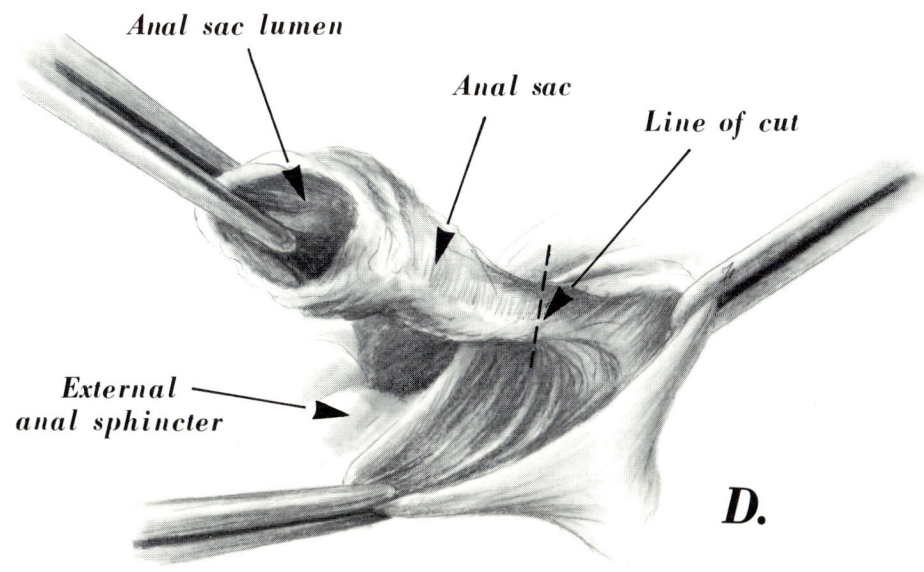

Figure 7–17 Continued

7–18 SPLENECTOMY

Andrew J. Frey

Indications

Splenectomy is indicated for removal of splenic neoplasms, for splenic rupture, splenic torsion, splenic infarcts, hypersplenism, and splenic abscess.

Anesthesia

Choice of anesthetics is based upon the patient's overall condition. Traumatic splenic rupture or rupture of a splenic neoplasm is usually followed by hypovolemic shock. For these patients, whole blood transfusions are preferred.

Patient Positioning

The patient is placed in dorsal recumbency.

Operative Preparation

Specialized Instruments. A Balfour self-retaining retractor is used when the spleen cannot be easily exteriorized through the laparotomy incision. When large amounts of blood or fluid are present in the abdominal cavity, suction is helpful. A minimum of six angiotribes or large hemostatic forceps, as well as several small hemostatic forceps, are necessary. Electrocautery may be used to help control hemorrhage.

Suture Material. Ligation of blood vessels or pedicles of tissue is performed with 3-0 or 4-0 Dexon, nylon, or chromic catgut.

SOFT TISSUE SURGERY 107

Details of Procedure

Figure 7–18A. Either a cranial midventral abdominal incision or a left paramedian incision is made to expose the spleen. Moist laparotomy pads are used to protect the edges of the abdominal incision, and a Balfour self-retaining retractor is positioned to provide exposure of the abdominal viscera.

NOTES:

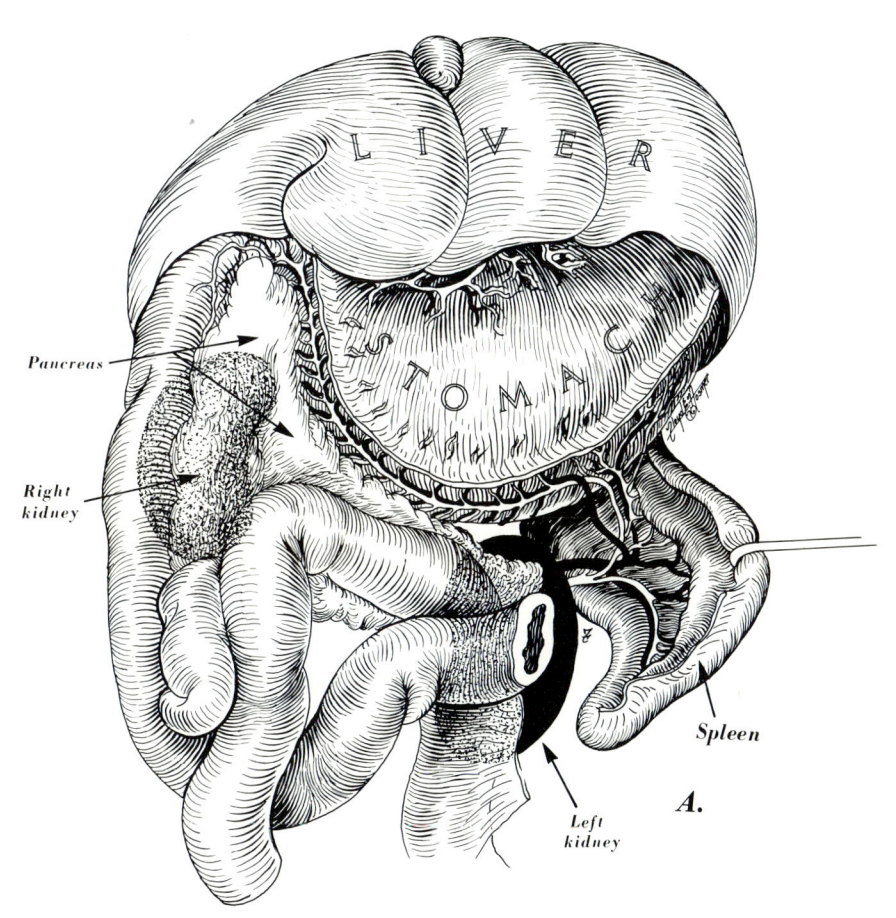

Figure 7–18
Illustration continued on following page.

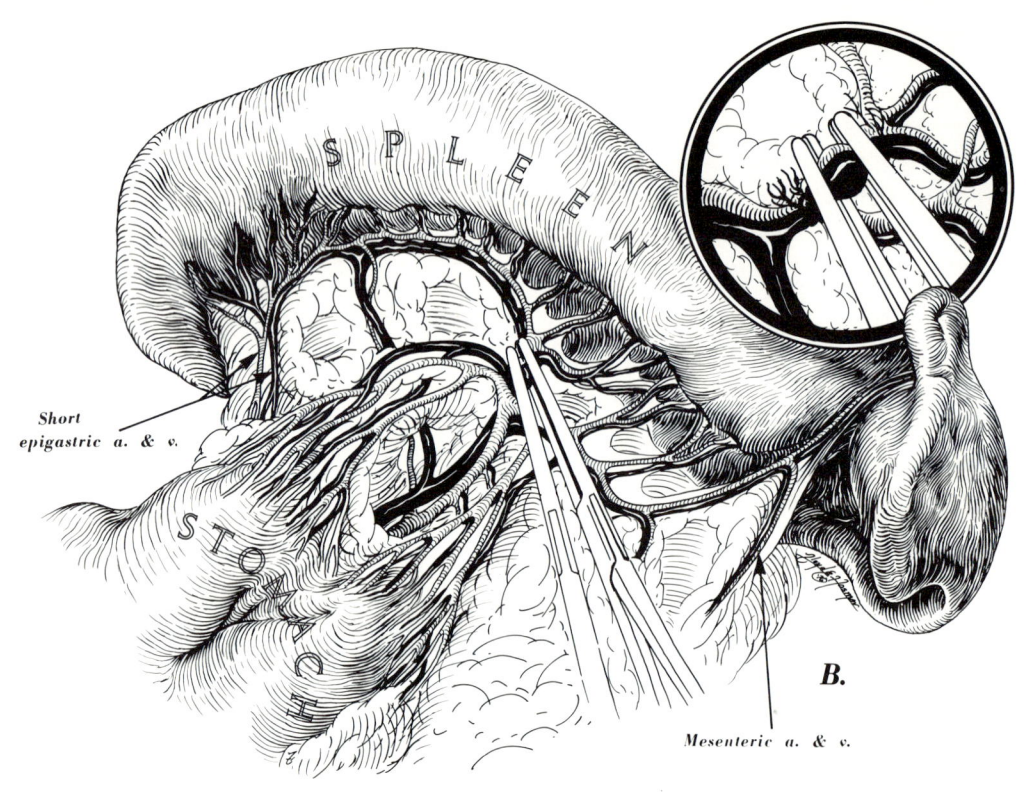

Figure 7–18 Continued

Figure 7–18B. Identify the spleen, the greater curvature of the stomach, the dorsal and ventral layers of the greater omentum, the gastrosplenic ligament, the splenocolic ligament, and the left limb of the pancreas. Trace the splenic artery and vein as they course from the dorsal layer of the greater omentum into the gastrosplenic ligament. Identify the left gastroepiploic artery and vein (there may be more than one), the many splenic arterial and venous branches into the hilus of the spleen, the short gastric vessels, and the vessels continuing into the greater omentum.

A fenestration is made in the gastrosplenic ligament on each side of the splenic artery and vein immediately distal to the bifurcation of the gastroepiploic vessels. Two Crile forceps are then placed across the splenic artery and vein, excluding as much omental tissue as possible.

The vessels are transected between the Crile forceps. After double ligation of the vessels on the gastric side of transection, one pair of forceps is removed. The remaining forceps may be left in place or removed after a single ligature is tied around the vessels leading into the spleen.

The gastrosplenic ligament is then divided into several (five to six) small pedicles by making fenestrations in the ligament and doubly clamping each pedicle. The tissue is transected between each pair of forceps and ligated as described. All ligations are made with 3-0 nonabsorbable suture material (e.g., polypropylene, silk).

During the procedure, several points should be remembered: (1) Handle the pancreas carefully and do not occlude its blood supply. (2) Do not occlude the gastroepiploic blood vessels. (3) Double ligate all major vessels. (4) After removal of the spleen, carefully inspect the ligated tissue for evidence of uncontrolled hemorrhage. (5) The greater omentum is an important abdominal organ and as little as possible should be removed.

The Balfour retractor and laparotomy pads are removed, and the abdominal incision is closed in the routine manner.

Postoperative Considerations

Postoperative care involves monitoring for blood loss encountered should a ligature slip from the ligated vessels.

NOTES: *(Continued)*

7–19 NEPHROTOMY AND NEPHRECTOMY

Clarence A. Rawlings

Indications

Nephrotomy is indicated for removal of renal calculi from functional kidneys. Nephrectomy is indicated to remove an infected and nonfunctional kidney containing renal calculi, a severely traumatized and hemorrhaging kidney, or a renal neoplasm.

Anesthesia

Patients requiring renal surgery generally have renal disease and must be managed according to the considerations discussed for the renal patient (Chapter 2). Diuresis is critical and is initially attempted by volume diuresis.

Patient Positioning

The patient is positioned in dorsal recumbency for a midline laparotomy or in dorsal lateral recumbency for a paramedian laparotomy.

Operative Preparation

Special Draping. In addition to laparotomy draping, the kidney should be isolated by draping with separate laparotomy pads, so that peritoneal contamination by renal bacteria and urine is limited.

Specialized Instruments. Noncrushing cardiovascular clamps for obstruction of

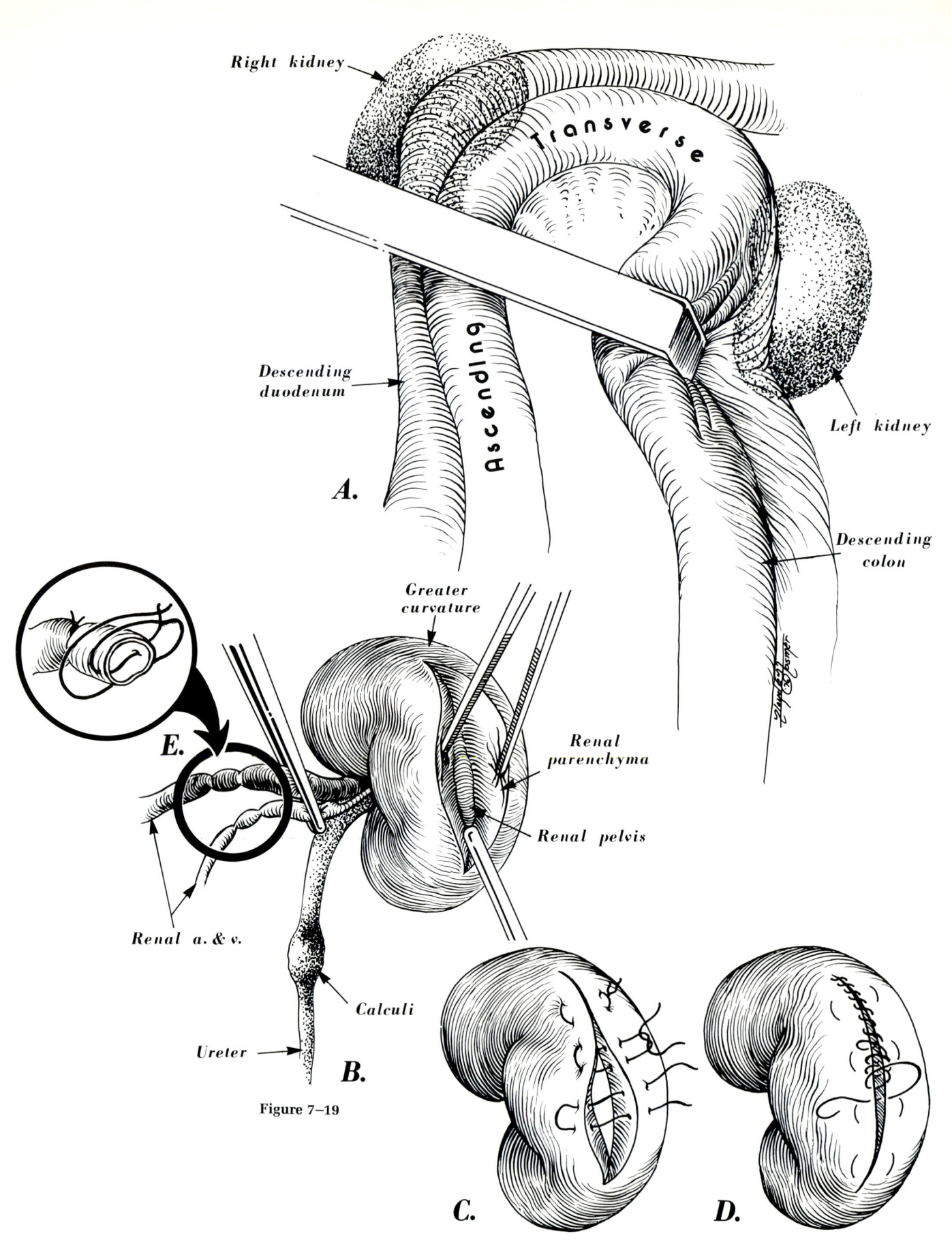

Figure 7-19

flow in the renal arteries and veins are useful. A small (3.5 to 5.0 F) catheter is used to evaluate patency of the ureteral lumen between the kidney and the urinary bladder.

Suture Material. A 2-0 and 4-0 synthetic absorbable suture material is used to close the kidney.

Incision and Exposure

The kidney may be approached through either a caudal midline laparotomy or paramedian laparotomy. The midline laparotomy is preferred if a cystotomy is anticipated.

Details of Procedure

Figure 7–19A. Reflection of abdominal viscera to expose the left kidney is improved by gentle traction of the descending colon and mesocolon. Exposure of the right kidney, which is cranial to the left kidney, is aided by traction on the descending duodenum.

Figure 7–19B. Prior to nephrotomy, either noncrushing cardiovascular clamps or tourniquets should be applied to the renal arteries and veins. An incision is made over the greater curvature of the kidney and into the renal pelvis. Calculi are removed, and the renal pelvis is thoroughly flushed. A catheter is passed through the ureter via the renal pelvis and into the urinary bladder. Ureteral calculi should be flushed into either the urinary bladder or the renal pelvis.

Figure 7–19C. The nephrotomy incision is closed with deeply placed, interruptured horizontal mattress sutures of a 2-0 absorbable suture material.

Figure 7–19D. A second suture line of a simple continuous pattern of 4-0 suture material is placed in the renal capsule. The vascular clamps are removed from the pedicle. Occlusion time should be limited to 30 minutes.

Figure 7–19E. The surgical exposure for nephrectomy is the same as that for nephrotomy. The renal artery should be doubly ligated, with a transfixing ligature being placed distal to the simple ligature. The renal vein and then the ureter are ligated. The kidney is removed, with the ureter detached and ligated at the trigone of the bladder.

Postoperative Considerations

Urine output should be monitored closely, and diuresis should be insured by hydration and possibly by the use of either furosemide (Lasix) or mannitol. Urine and calculi cultures should be performed, and the urinary tract infection should be treated according to antibiotic sensitivity. Management techniques to prevent calculi recurrence should be practiced after biochemical analysis of the stone.

NOTES:

7–20 CYSTOTOMY

Wayne E. Wingfield

Indications

Presence of cystic calculi is the most frequent indication for a cystotomy in small animal surgery. Additionally, the removal of neoplasms or a biopsy of the bladder involves a cystotomy. Following a traumatic rupture of the urinary bladder, the surgical closure is identical to that of cystotomy.

Anesthesia

Preoperative assessment of operative risk should precede anesthetic induction. With evidence of prerenal, renal, or postrenal uremia, every effort should be made to improve the patient's status. With acutely ill patients, preoperative fluid administration and the use of diuretics will help to improve their status. Anesthetic induction with nitrous oxide and halothane provides a safe anesthetic regimen. During anesthesia, the urine output can be readily monitored to measure renal function. Normal urine output in the dog amounts to 0.5 to 2.0 ml/lb/hr, while urine output following diuresis equals 4.0 to 8.0 ml/lb/hr.

Patient Positioning

The patient is placed in dorsal recumbency, with sandbags or V-trough used to maintain this position.

Operative Preparation

Establishment of good renal function and assessment of operative risk should precede a cystotomy. Preoperative placement of a urinary catheter will facilitate monitoring of urine output as well as provide a useful means for flushing calculi from the urethra.

Incision and Exposure

A caudal midventral abdominal incision is made through the linea alba. In the male dog, the prepuce is reflected laterally to allow opening of the linea alba. As the caudal superficial epigastric vessels are encountered near the sheath of the penis, they are ligated and cut to allow lateralization of the prepuce.

SOFT TISSUE SURGERY

Details of Procedure

Figure 7–20A. Once the urinary bladder has been exteriorized, a retention suture is placed in the apex (fundus vesicae) of the bladder to allow caudal retraction in preparation for the cystotomy incision. Moistened laparotomy towels are placed around the urinary bladder to prevent contamination of the peritoneal cavity should urine spill. With a bladder distended with urine, advancement of the urethral catheter or paracentesis with a 22-gauge needle is used to empty the contents.

NOTES:

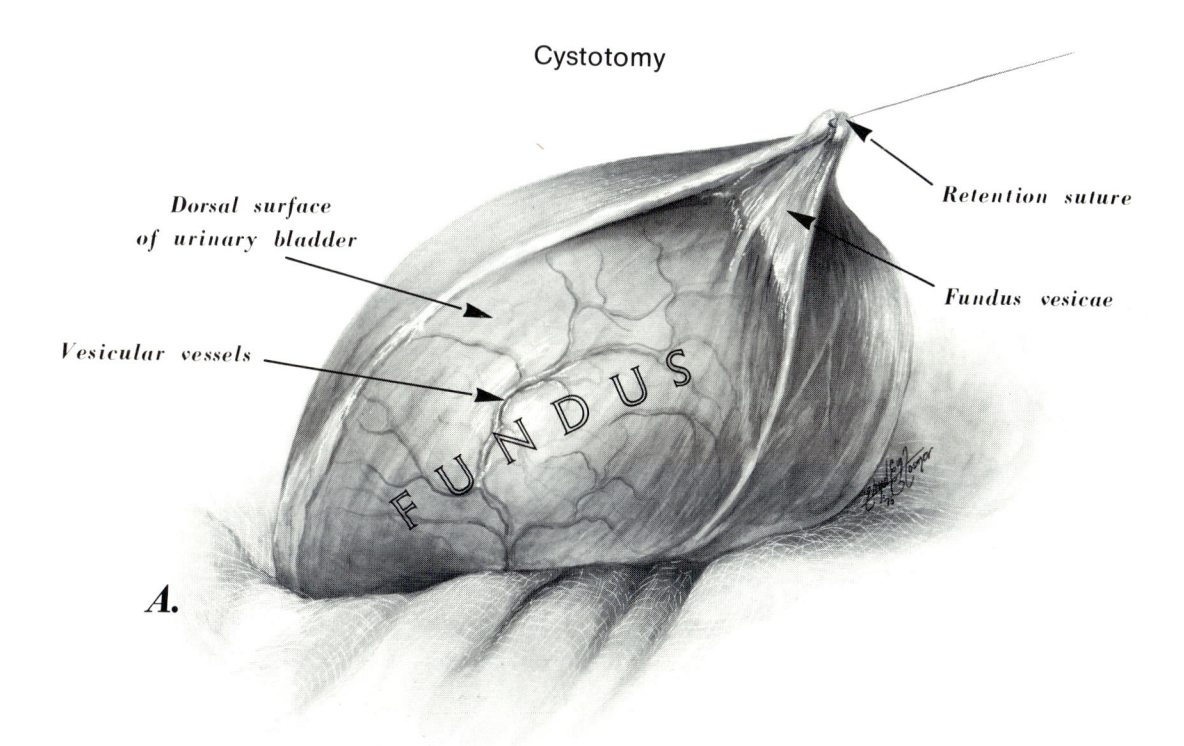

Figure 7–20
Illustration continued on following page.

Cystotomy

B. Retention suture, Fundus vesicae, Vesicular vessels

C. Vesicular lumen, Fundus vesicae

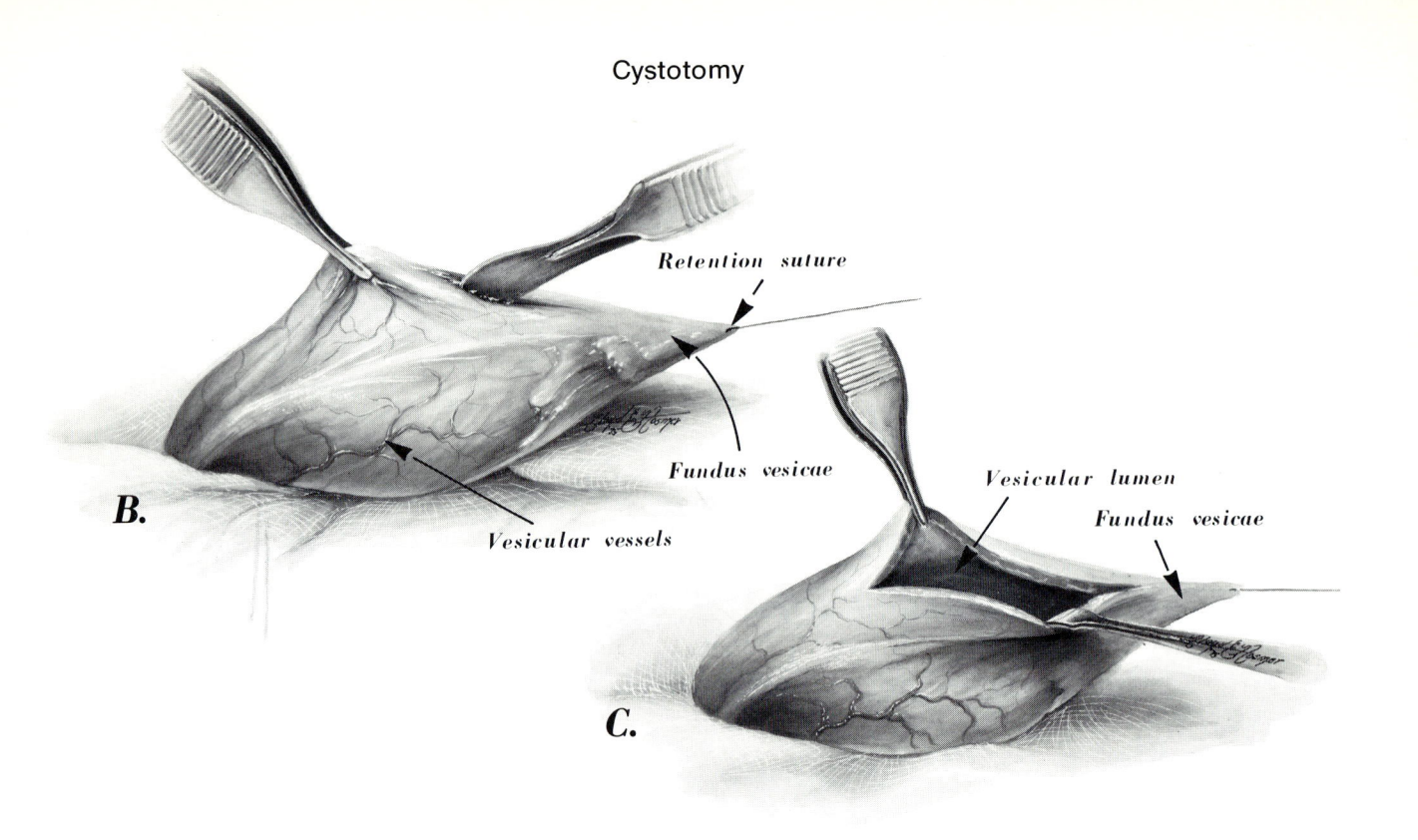

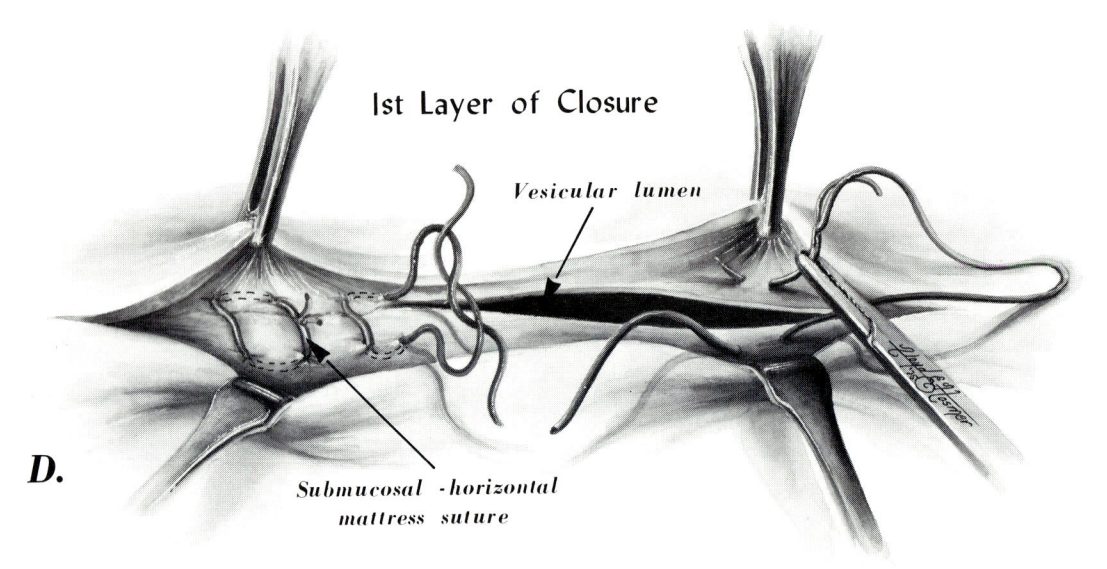

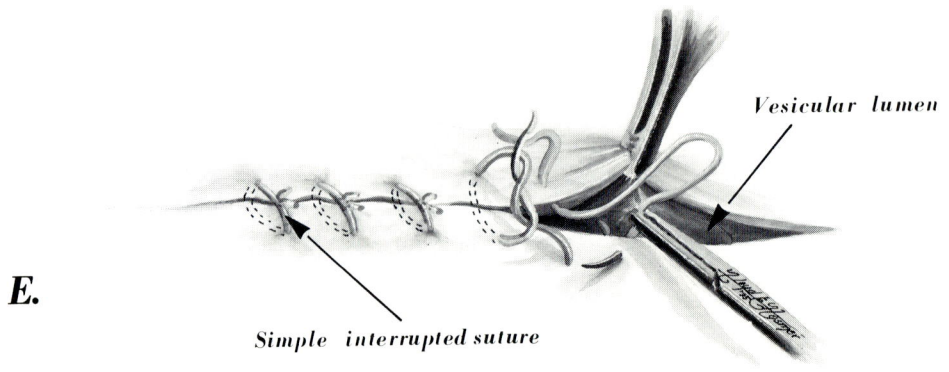

1st Layer of Closure

D. Vesicular lumen, Submucosal-horizontal mattress suture

2nd Layer of Closure

E. Vesicular lumen, Simple interrupted suture

Figure 7–20 Continued.

Figure 7–20B. While maintaining caudal traction, a stab incision is made in the dorsal surface of the urinary bladder. The incision should be made in the least vascular area. Use of the dorsal surface will provide a degree of protection from adhesion formation between the sutured incision and the ventral abdomen. Adhesions in this area could invite disaster should a second operation be required at a later date.

Figure 7–20C. The initial stab incision into the bladder is enlarged for adequate visualization of the vesicular lumen. When removing cystic calculi, the area of the trigone should be thoroughly explored to assure removal of all debris. Retrograde flushing of the proximal urethra and adequate lavage and suction of the bladder will help to eliminate all small calculi, blood clots, and tissue debris that are loose within the lumen.

Figure 7–20D. Closure of the cystotomy incision is initiated with 3-0 to 4-0 suture material. A horizontal mattress pattern within the submucosa is used to accurately appose the incision. Avoid passage of the suture through the mucosa, as this suture may act as a nidus for future cystic calculi. The horizontal mattress pattern is begun at both ends of the incision and is continued to the center.

Figure 7–20E. The second suture layer is a simple interrupted pattern. These sutures are passed through the serosa and muscularis and into the submucosal layer. Remove the retention suture.

Discard the soiled laparotomy towel from around the bladder. Contaminated surgical instruments should be removed and a sterile pair of gloves donned. The abdominal wall is closed with a routine three-layer closure.

Postoperative Considerations

The cystotomy incision must be allowed to heal with minimal tension on the suture line. This is best accomplished by frequent evacuation of the bladder. The removed calculi should be analyzed, and proper therapeutics should be applied. Antibacterial agents are indicated in the presence of infection.

NOTES: *(Continued)*

116   SOFT TISSUE SURGERY

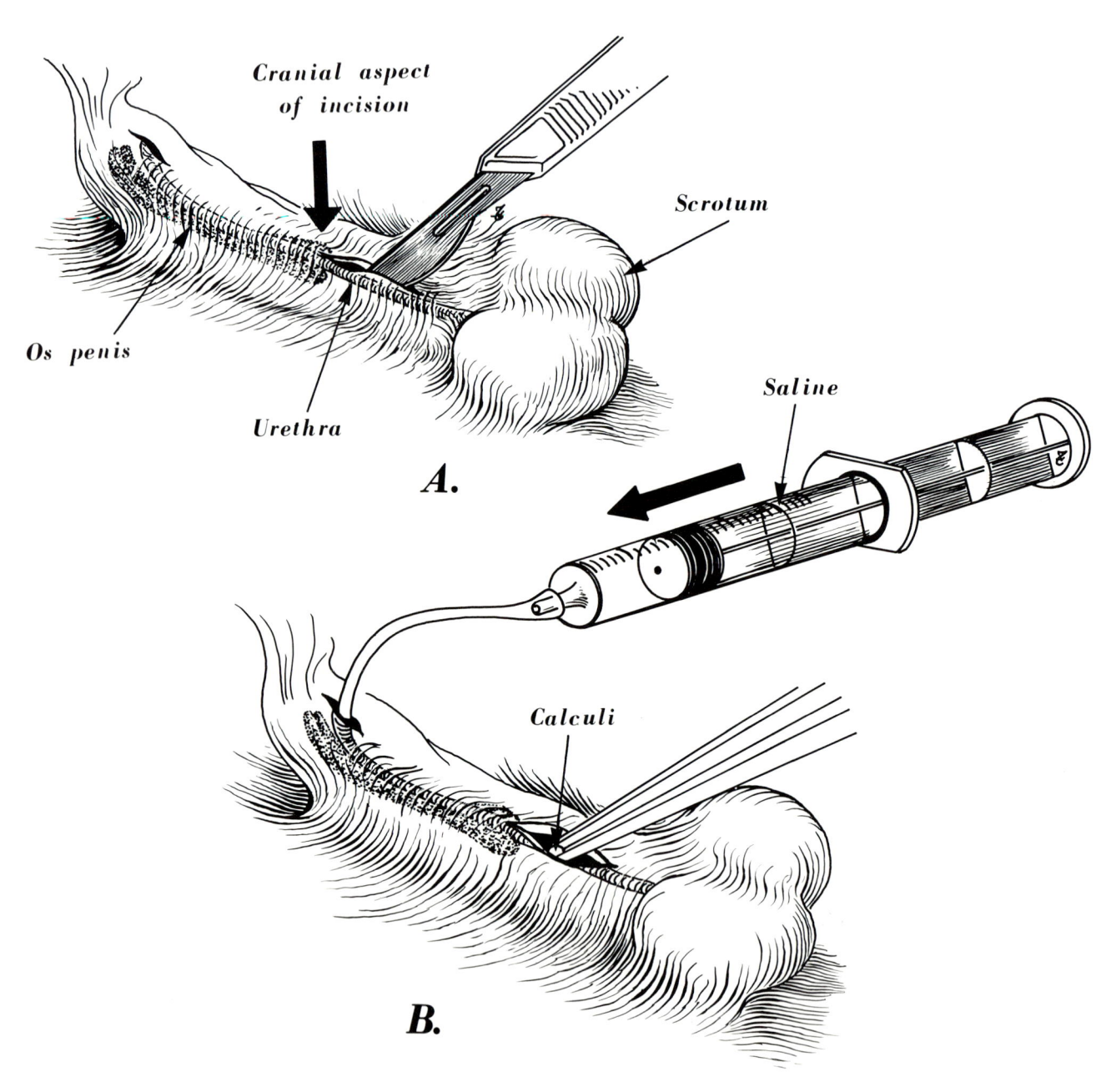

Cranial aspect of incision

Os penis

Urethra

Scrotum

Saline

Calculi

A.

B.

Figure 7–21

7–21 URETHROTOMY

CLARENCE A. RAWLINGS

Indications

Urethrotomy in the dog is indicated for removal of urethral calculi lodged caudal to the os penis. Prior to urethrotomy, counter pulsation of the calculi into the urinary bladder should be attempted.

Anesthesia

A short-acting general anesthetic (e.g., thiobarbiturate, intravenous Innovar-Vet, or halothane induction and maintenance) is required for most patients. Severely depressed patients with postrenal uremia may require only local anesthesia.

Patient Positioning

The patient should be placed in dorsal recumbency.

Operative Preparation

Prior to the urethrotomy and during anesthesia, the penis should be prepared for sterile urethral catheterization. Prior to catheterization, sterile lubricant is injected into the urethra. An urethral catheter is advanced, and counterpulsation is applied to force the calculi retrograde. If the calculi are forced into the urinary bladder, the urethral catheter is left in place. The calculi are removed by cystotomy (Procedure 7–20), and the urethrotomy is not performed.

Details of Procedure

Figure 7–21A. A midline incision is made over the urethra and between the os penis and the scrotum. The urethra is incised on the ventral midline. Palpation of the calculi or an urethral catheter aids in identification of the urethra.

Figure 7–21B. The urethral calculi are flushed through the urethrotomy. Following calculi removal, the catheter should be passed into the urinary bladder. The urethrotomy should be left open to heal by granulation.

Postoperative Considerations

The urethrotomy is left open to drain. Hemorrhage is common but seldom produces clinically significant hypovolemia. Further diagnostic studies are done to determine if other calculi and/or a urinary tract infection is present. When cystic calculi are present, the dog should be prepared for anesthesia, and a cystotomy should be performed when the animal is well hydrated. Between the time of urethrotomy and cystotomy for removal of small calculi, a urethral catheter should be positioned. Therapy should be initiated to reduce the likelihood of recurrence of calculi.

NOTES:

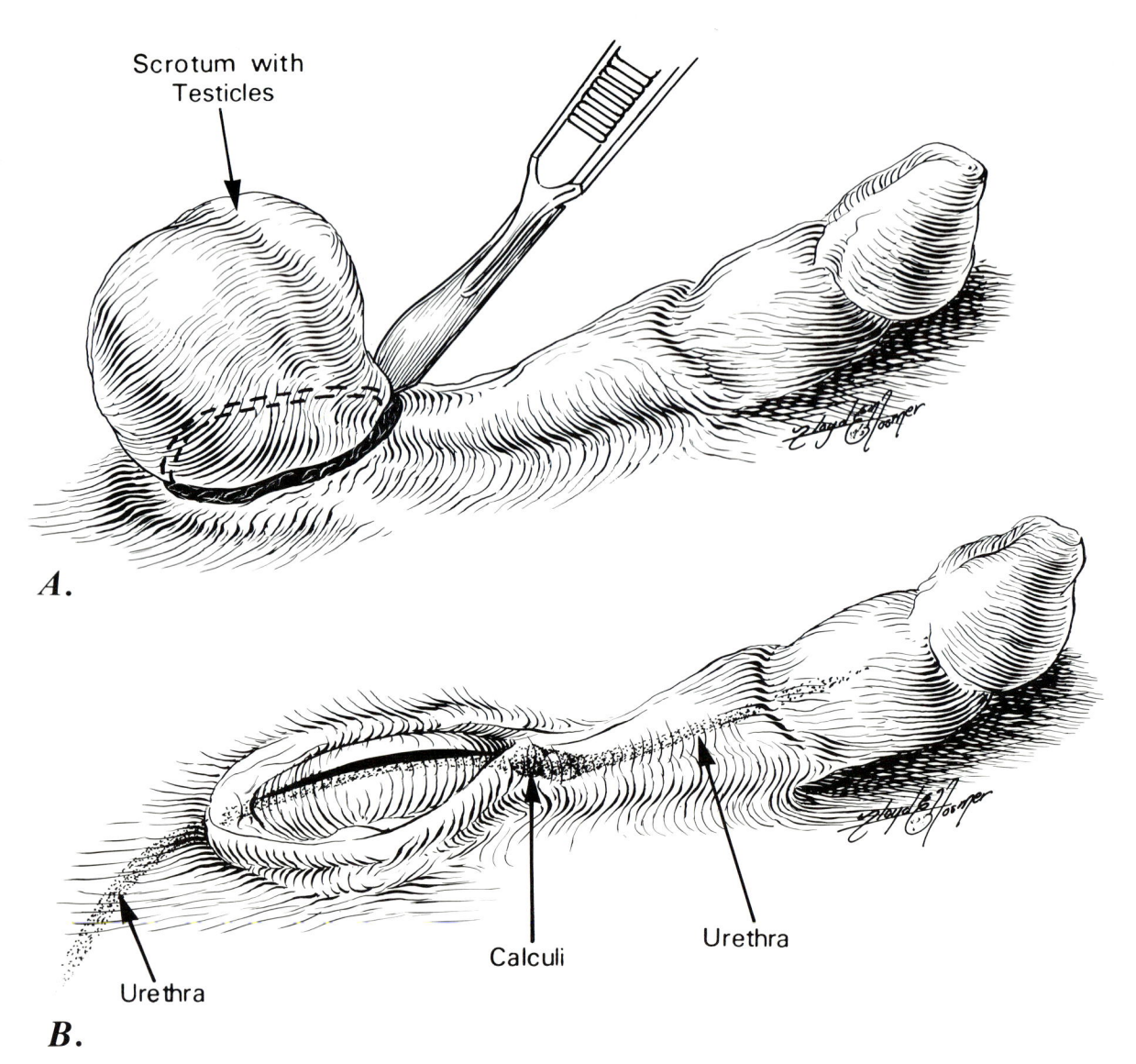

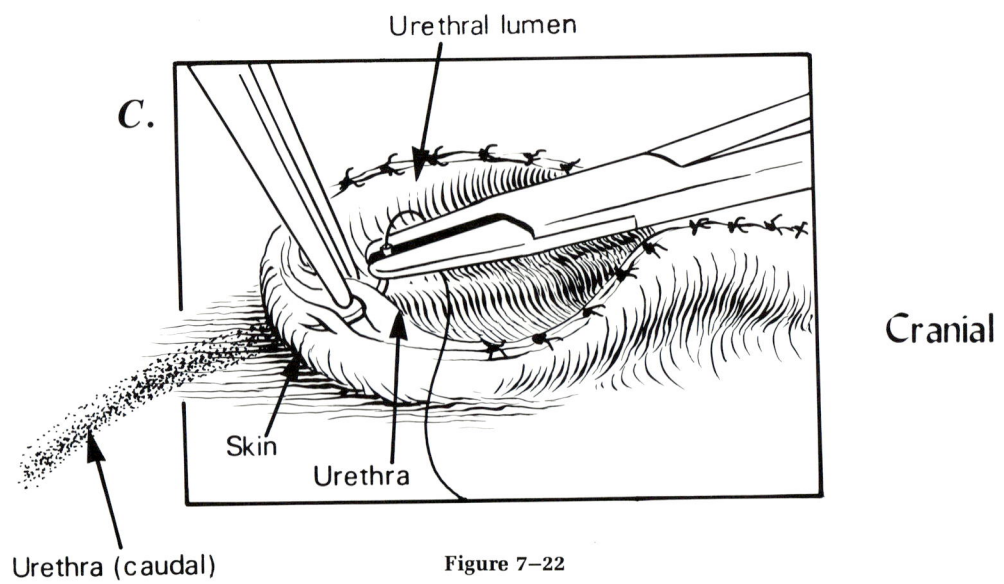

118   SOFT TISSUE SURGERY

A. Scrotum with Testicles

B. Urethra — Calculi — Urethra

C. Urethral lumen — Skin — Urethra — Cranial

Urethra (caudal)

Figure 7–22

7–22 SCROTAL URETHROSTOMY

Clarence A. Rawlings

Indications

Scrotal ablation and a permanent urethrostomy are indicated in dogs with severe urethral trauma or stricture due to urethral calculi or in dogs with recurrent urethral calculi.

Anesthesia

General anesthesia is required. Preoperative management should reduce or eliminate postrenal uremia.

Patient Positioning

The patient is placed in dorsal recumbency.

Operative Preparation

Suture Material. Nonabsorbable (4-0) and absorbable (2-0 to 3-0) suture materials with swaged needles are used.

Details of Procedure

Figure 7–22A. The approach to a scrotal urethrostomy is through a scrotal ablation incision. The castration is performed either through the ablation incision or by a bilateral scrotal incision technique (Procedure 7–29).

Figure 7–22B. The scrotal ablation is continued on a midline to the urethra. Either a catheter within the urethra or calculi should be palpated to identify the lumen. The urethra is incised on the ventral side as far caudally as the caudal aspect of the scrotal ablation incision.

Figure 7–22C. A row of simple interrupted sutures (2-0 or 3-0 absorbable suture material) is used to appose the subcutaneous layer to the penile muscles. This suture line reduces tension on the urethral mucosa-to-skin sutures. Simple interrupted sutures of 3-0 or 4-0 nonabsorbable suture material are used to appose the skin to the urethral mucosa.

Postoperative Considerations

Hematuria and hemorrhage should be anticipated, but they seldom produce clinically significant hypovolemia. The urinary calculi and any urinary tract infection should be treated to prevent recurrence.

NOTES:

7–23 FELINE PERINEAL URETHROSTOMY

Clarence A. Rawlings

Indications

Urethrostomy of the male cat is indicated after repeated urethral obstruction due to the feline urological syndrome (FUS). Other indications would include a distal urethral obstruction due to trauma, inflammation, or neoplasia.

Anesthesia

Preanesthetic management should include urinary catheterization, hydration, and volume diuresis in the cat with postrenal uremia. General anesthesia with a nonrebreathing system with endotracheal intubation is required. Because of operative positioning and the elevation of the cat's rear quarters, assisted ventilation three to four times per minute is required to prevent hypercarbia, and periodic sighing with a high inspiratory pressure reduces the development of atelectasis.

Patient Positioning

The patient is positioned in ventral recumbency, with the rear quarters slightly elevated. Following initial surgical preparation, a pursestring suture is placed around the anus, and the surgical site is prepared again for aseptic surgery.

Operative Preparation

Specialized Instruments. The lengthwise urethral incision should be performed with straight iris scissors. Delicate cardiovascular or ophthamological tissue forceps and needle holders are needed.

Suture Material. The urethral mucosa is sutured to the skin with either 4-0 silk, Polydek, or polyglycolic acid (Dexon).

NOTES:

SOFT TISSUE SURGERY 121

Details of Procedure

Figure 7–23A. The intact cat should be castrated by either an open or closed technique (Procedure 7–30). An eliptical incision is made around the scrotum and prepuce. The dorsal aspect should be halfway between the anus and the dorsal aspect of the scrotum. The ventral aspect should be where the prepuce is reflected from the perineal skin. The lateral aspect should be approximately 1 cm lateral to the scrotum.

NOTES: *(Continued)*

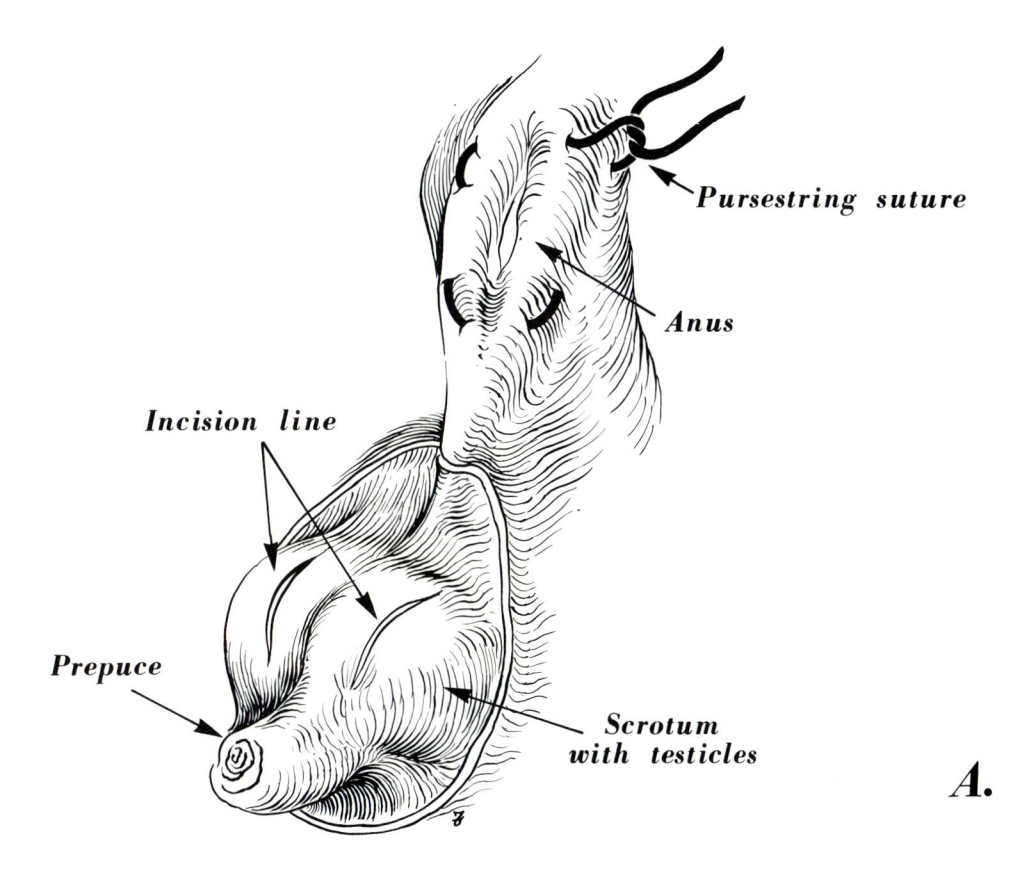

Figure 7–23
Illustration continued on following page.

Figure 7–23 Continued
Illustration continued on opposite page.

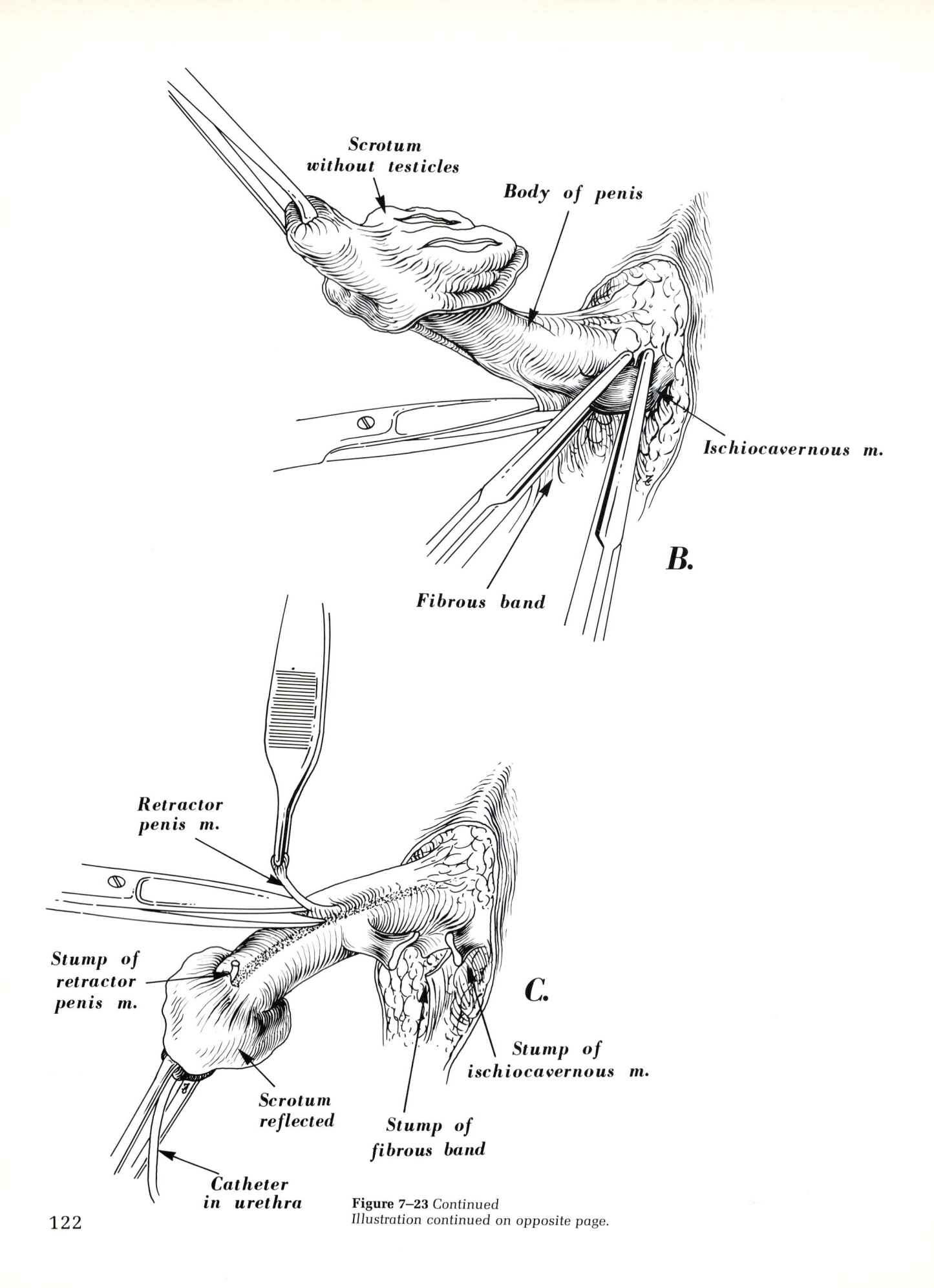

SOFT TISSUE SURGERY

Figure 7–23B. The incision is developed in a plane directed toward the level of the penis to which the ischiocavernous muscles are attached. The ischiocavernous muscles are identified, and crushing forceps are applied to them. The muscles are incised. A plane of dissection is developed near the penis, with special emphasis to incise the ventral fibrous attachment to the pubis. This should loosen the penile attachments sufficiently to permit the caudal traction of the penis.

Figure 7–23C. A urethral catheter is positioned. The retractor penis muscles and associated fascia are dissected as far cranially as the cranial aspect of the ischiocavernous muscles.

Figure 7–23D. The dorsal portion of the penis is partially incised to the level of the urethral catheter. This incision should be at the level of the desired penile amputation. The urethra is incised on the midline with iris scissors to beyond the level where the urethral lumen widens. This is at the level of the bulbourethral glands that are located just cranial to the ischiocavernous muscles. A temporary tourniquet of 1-0 suture material placed around the penis 1.0 cm caudal to the cranial commissure of the urethrotomy reduces hemorrhage during the initial closure of the urethral mucosa and skin. The two initial sutures of 4-0 suture material are placed at a 30-degree angle from the end of the urethral incision. These sutures should be placed from inside to outside the urethra and then be sutured to the skin. Both sutures are preplaced prior to tying. Care must be taken to directly appose the urethral mucosa to the perineal skin. A suture placed at the 12 o'clock position may be utilized to further open the urethral orifice.

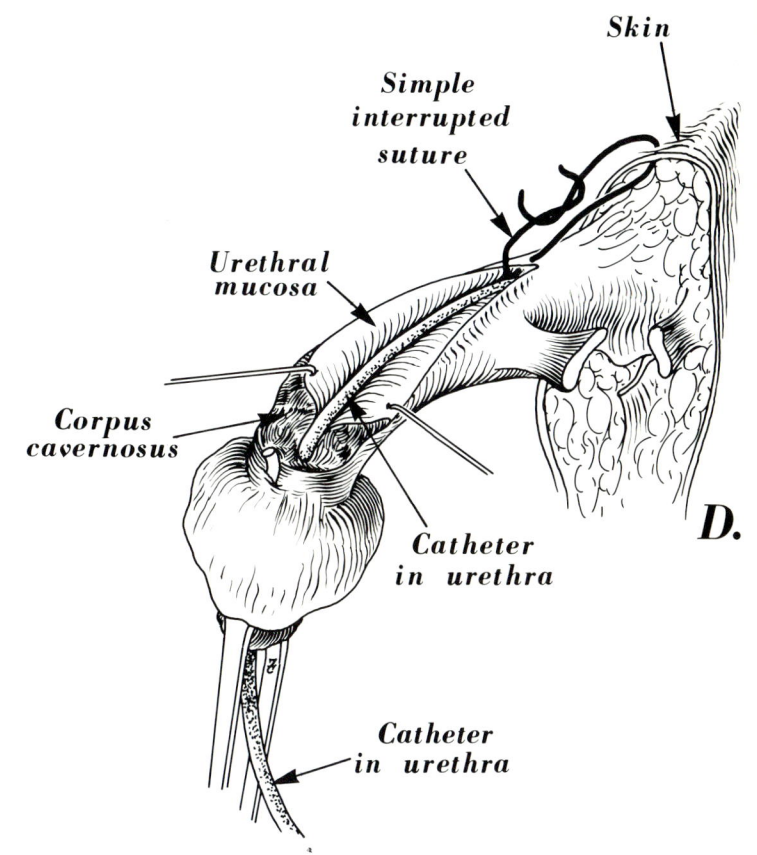

Figure 7–23 Continued
Illustration continued on following page.

NOTES: *(Continued)*

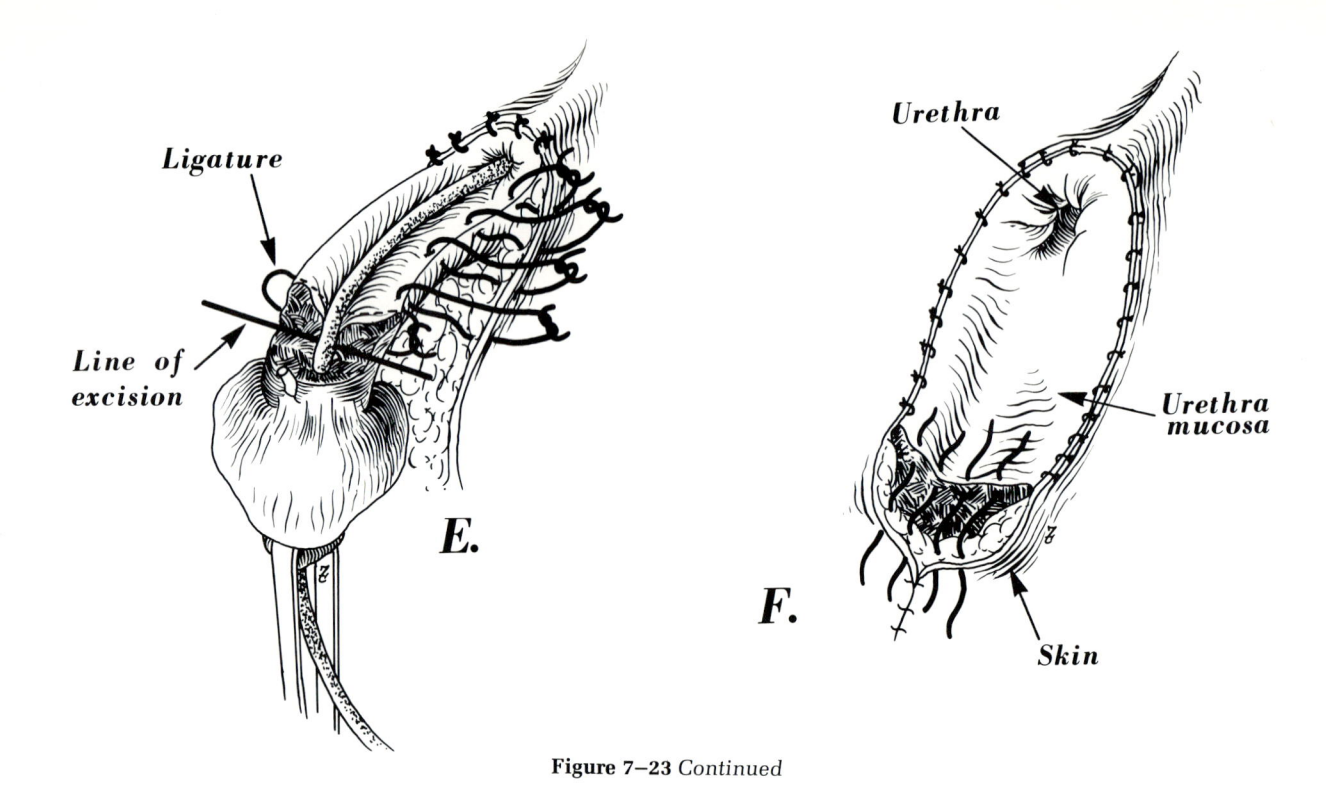

Figure 7–23E. Simple interrupted sutures are used to appose the urethral mucosa to the skin. An absorbable ligature is passed beneath the urethral mucosa to encircle the deep portion of the penile urethra. The penis is amputated distal to this ligature.

Figure 7–23F. The urethral skin suture line is continued, and the ventral aspect of the incision is closed. No catheter is left in the urethra. Following surgery, petrolatum is applied to the suture line to keep the sutures soft and to provide a moisture barrier.

NOTES: (Continued)

Postoperative Considerations

No catheter is necessary following surgery. Since a high number of cats with feline urinary syndrome have a urinary tract infection, the urine should have been cultured prior to surgery. Antibiotics should be initiated and later adjusted based upon bacterial sensitivities.

7–24 RUPTURED URETHRA

Clarence A. Rawlings

Indications

Reapposition of the urethral wall and mucosa is indicated for traumatic lacerations, prostatectomies, urethral neoplasias, and some urethral calculi.

Anesthesia

Animals with traumatically induced fistulae frequently require preoperative management to reduce the effects of uremia, sepsis, anorexia, and dehydration. Once the animal is properly prepared for surgery, a variety of general anesthetic regimens are satisfactory.

Patient Positioning

Most urethral lesions are best approached with the patient in dorsal recumbency.

Operative Preparation

Special Draping. The operative site should be isolated by moist laparotomy pads to reduce peritoneal contamination.

Specialized Instruments. Self-retaining retractors (Balfour) are necessary for maintaining abdominal exposure. A smaller self-retaining retractor (baby Finochietto) is useful for pubic-splitting procedures. Urethral catheters are necessary.

Suture Materials. The urethra is closed with sutures of a 4-0 synthetic absorbable or nonabsorbable material. Closure of the pubic osteotomy is with orthopedic stainless steel wire (18 to 20 gauge).

Incision and Exposure

A caudal midline laparotomy is performed to expose the pelvic and abdominal urethra. To more fully expose the pelvic urethra, a reflection of the pubis or splitting of the pubic symphysis is helpful.

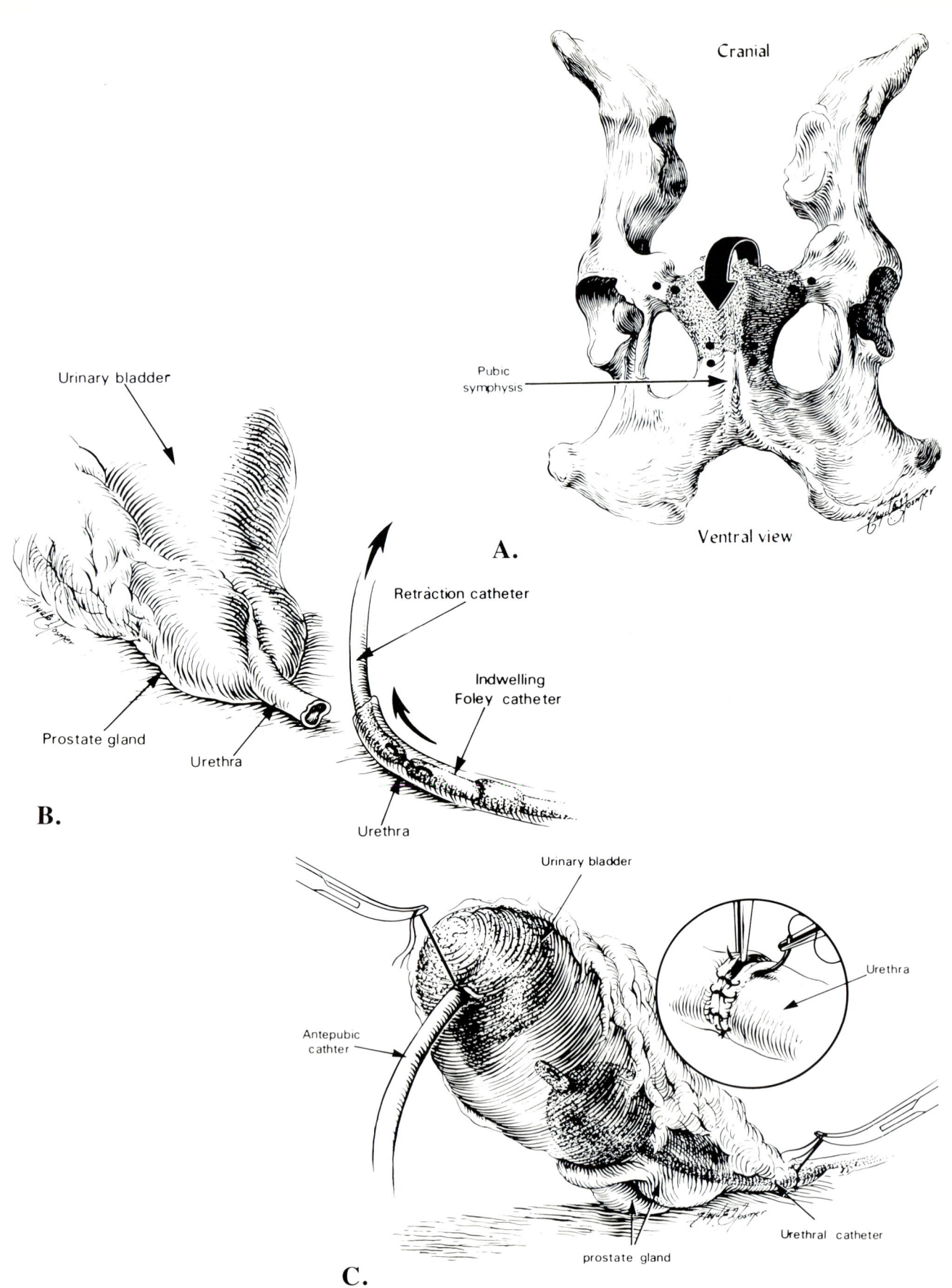

Figure 7–24
Illustration continued on page 128.

126

SOFT TISSUE SURGERY

Details of Procedure

Figure 7–24A. To improve exposure of the pelvic urethra, a pubic splitting or reflection of a portion of the pubis, as demonstrated, may be required. Holes for wire sutures should be drilled prior to osteotomy.

Figure 7–24B. Following identification and debridement of the urethral tear, the urethra should be reapposed over an indwelling urethral catheter. To facilitate catheter retention and to provide traction on the urinary bladder, a Foley catheter should be positioned. The Foley catheter can be withdrawn into the surgical site by attaching it to and retracting it with a stiff urethral catheter that is passed from the inside (bladder) to the outside (urethral tear). The catheter is then passed into the urinary bladder. A cystotomy may be required to position the catheter.

Figure 7–24C. The balloon should be inflated and the Foley catheter retracted to improve apposition of the urethral segments. Simple interrupted sutures of a 4-0 synthetic absorbable suture material are placed through the full thickness of the urethral wall. An antepubic catheter may also be used to decompress the urinary bladder and to redirect urine flow from the repaired urethra.

NOTES:

128　　　　　　　　　　　　　　　　　　　　　　　　　　　　　　　SOFT TISSUE SURGERY

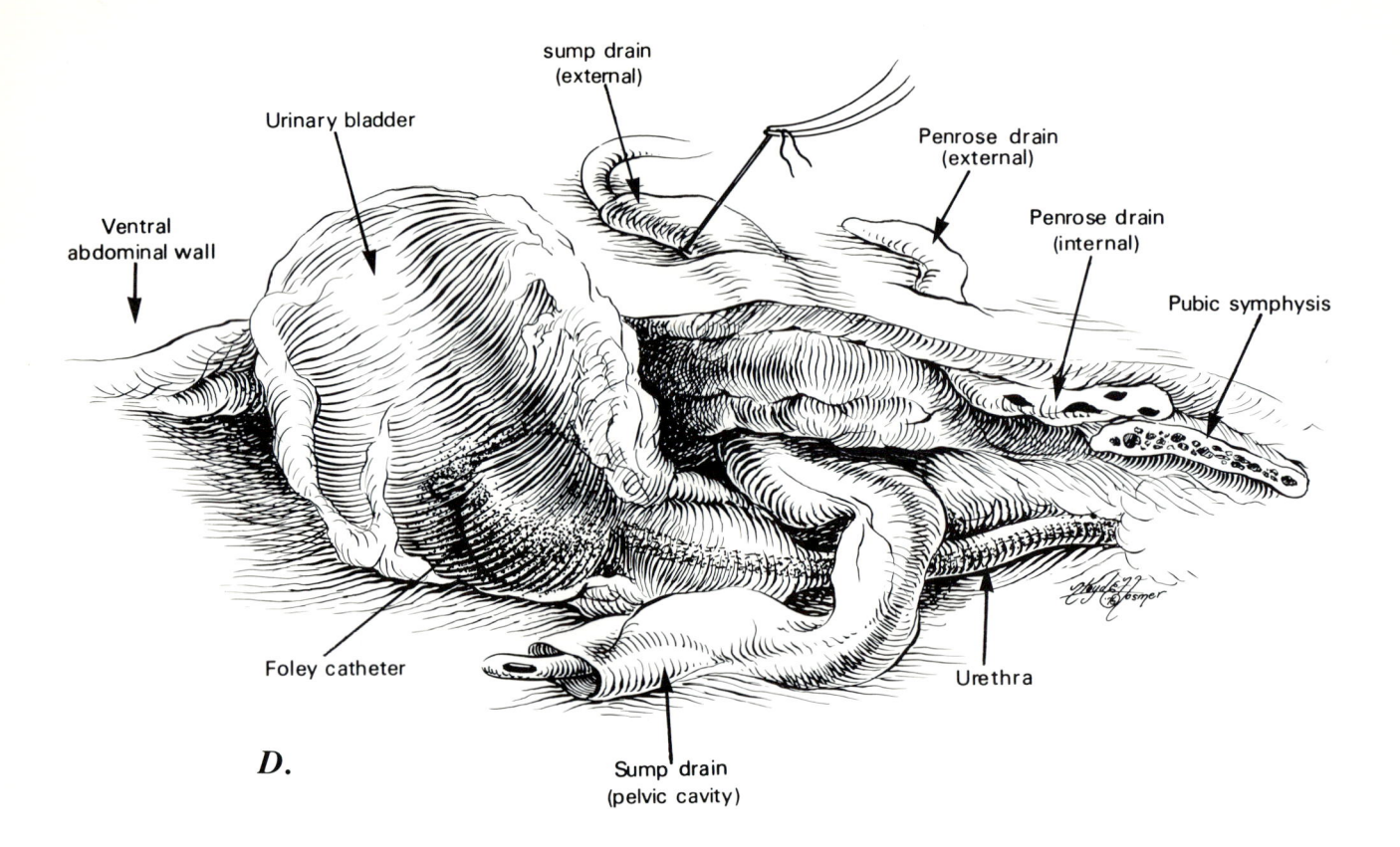

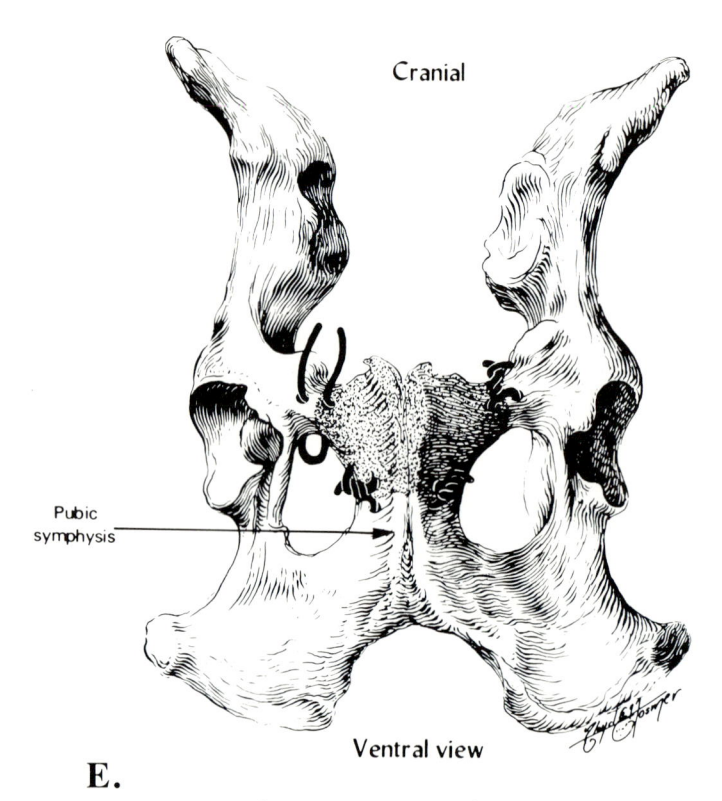

D.

Labels: Ventral abdominal wall; Urinary bladder; sump drain (external); Penrose drain (external); Penrose drain (internal); Pubic symphysis; Foley catheter; Sump drain (pelvic cavity); Urethra

E.

Labels: Cranial; Pubic symphysis; Ventral view

Figure 7–24 Continued

Figure 7–24D. Prior to closure, the operative site should be thoroughly lavaged with warm saline. During closure, drainage catheters, such as sump drains and/or Penrose drains, are positioned in the subcutaneous tissues of the abdomen.

Figure 7–24E. During closure, the reflected pubic segment can be wired together using the predrilled holes and 18-to-20-gauge orthopedic wires.

Postoperative Considerations

The urethral catheter is left in place for 7 to 10 days. Care should be taken to reduce ascending infection. As an alternative, a prepubic catheter can also be left in place for the same period of time. Because these animals are frequently severely depressed and anorectic, forced feeding and other patient management techniques are required. A leukogram, blood urea nitrogen, and urinalysis should be performed at regular intervals.

NOTES: *(Continued)*

7–25 URETHRAL PROLAPSE

CLARENCE A. RAWLINGS

Indications

Amputation of the penile mucosa is indicated for correction of urethral prolapse.

Anesthesia

General anesthesia is required.

Patient Positioning

The animal is placed in dorsal recumbency.

Operative Preparation

Specialized Instruments. A tourniquet of heavy suture material or umbilical tape is placed around the penis.

Suture Material. Swaged 4-0 silk is used for the urethral mucosa to penile epithelium suture.

Details of Procedure

Figure 7–25. The penile mucosa is partially incised through the full thickness into the lumen. Simple interrupted 4-0 silk sutures are used to appose the urethral mucosa to the penile epithelium. The amputation is continued by alternately incising and suturing. The tourniquet and catheter are removed.

Postoperative Considerations

The urethral catheter may be left in place for a few hours, but this is generally unnecessary. Recurrence of this condition is not unusual. Special emphasis should be placed on assessing a possible urethritis as the cause of the prolapse.

NOTES: *(Continued)*

SOFT TISSUE SURGERY 131

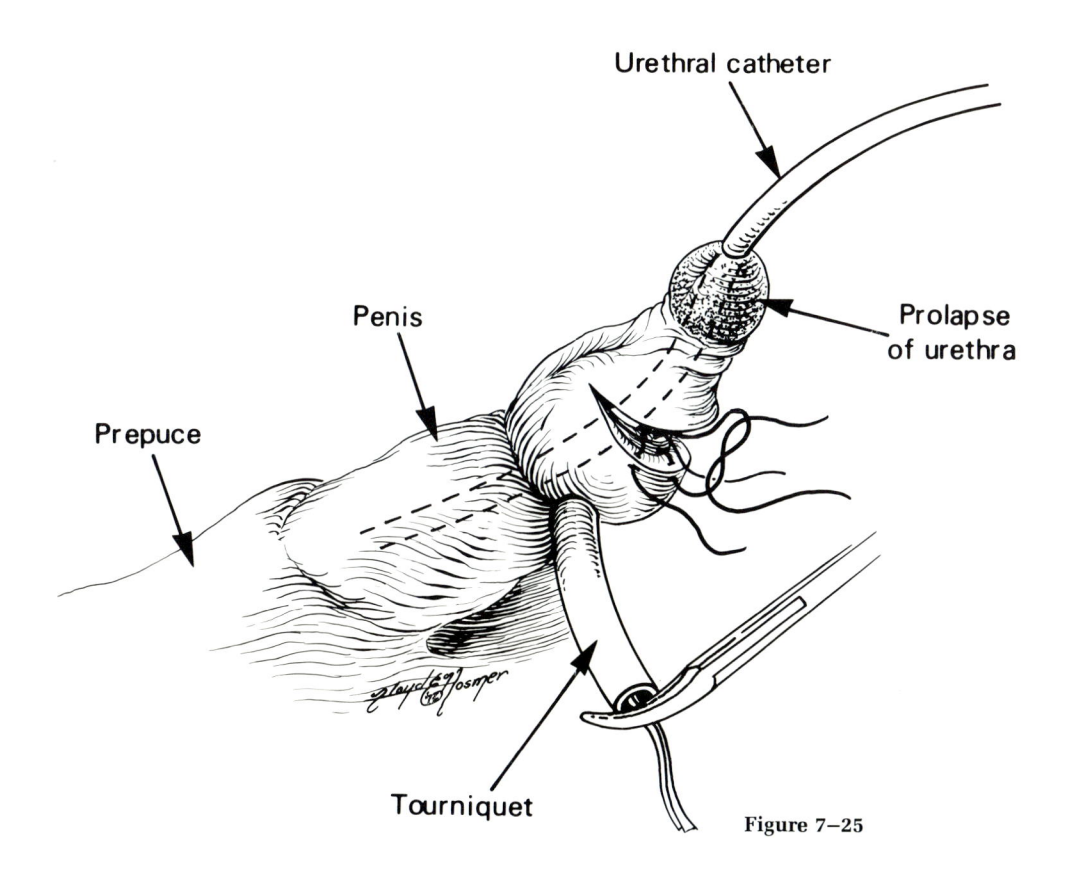

Figure 7–25

7-26
OVARIOHYSTERECTOMY

Eberhard Rosin

Indications

Ovariohysterectomy is indicated for sterilization and for treatment of pyometra, infection, neoplasia of the genital tract, or hyperplasia and neoplasia of the mammary glands. It is also indicated for management of diabetic patients and those dystocia patients with a devitalized uterus.

Anesthesia

The elective ovariohysterectomy patient can be operated on under a general anesthesia of the surgeon's choice. Ovariohysterectomy of the patient with either pyometra or toxic uterus during dystocia can be more difficult. In both cases, the patient may have prerenal uremia, and the pyometra patient may have an immune mediated glomerulopathy. Preanesthetic evaluation of fluid balance and renal function are critical. In both cases, the patient should be partially rehydrated and operated on within two to four hours of presentation. These patients should be managed as renal patients. Anesthesia may consist of either (1) inhalant induction and maintenance, (2) epidural anesthesia, if the patient is rehydrated, or (3) narcotic and nitrous oxide induction and maintenance.

Patient Positioning

The patient is positioned in dorsal recumbency.

Operative Preparation

No special instruments are required except an ovariohysterectomy hook and Carmalt forceps. The ovarian pedicle, the broad ligament, and the body of the uterus are ligated with chromic catgut.

Incision and Exposure

Exposure for ovariohysterectomy is through a midventral abdominal incision started at the edge of the umbilicus and continued caudally for approximately 4 to 10 cm, depending on the size of the animal.

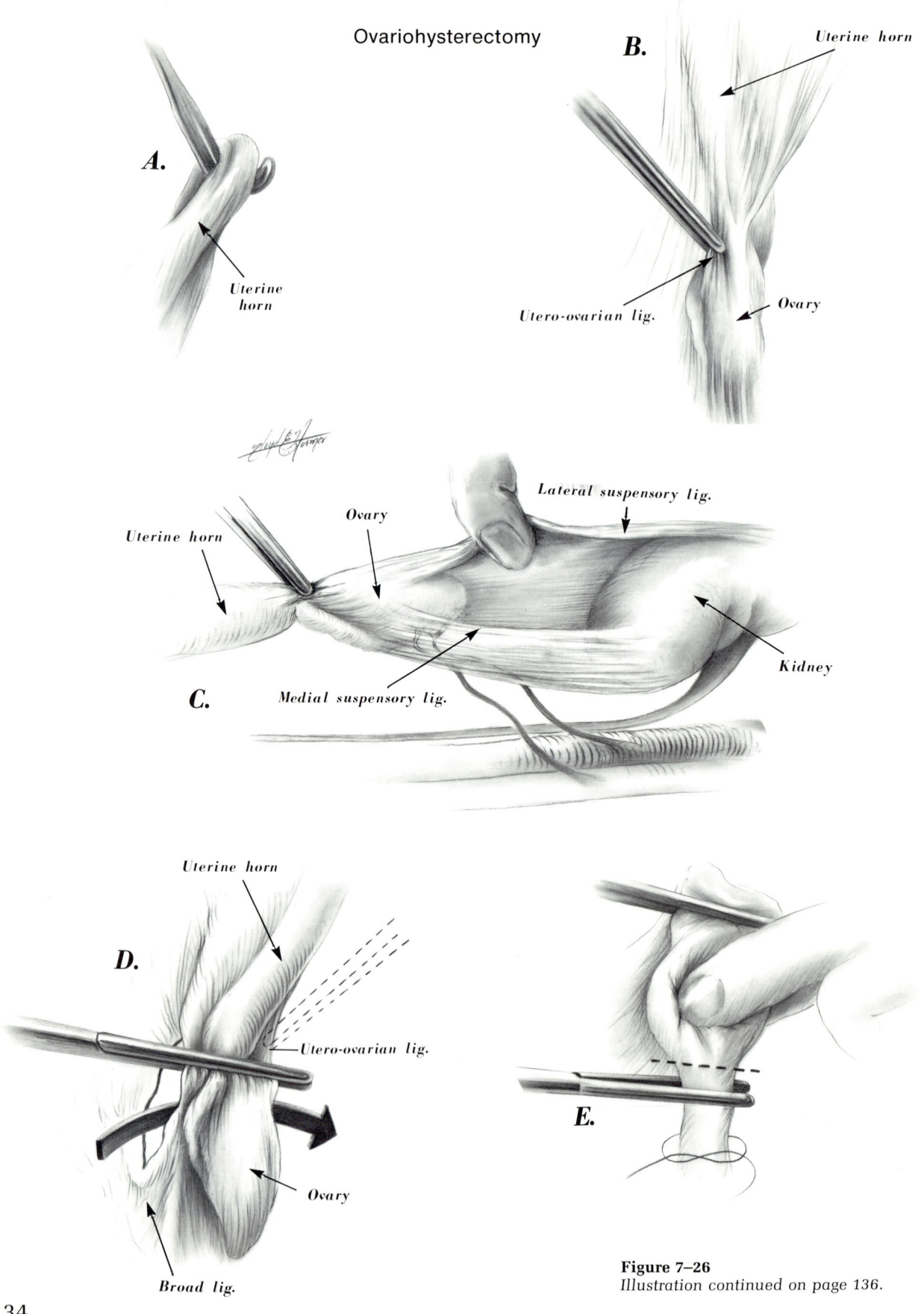

Ovariohysterectomy

A.
Uterine horn

B.
Uterine horn
Utero-ovarian lig.
Ovary

C.
Uterine horn
Ovary
Lateral suspensory lig.
Kidney
Medial suspensory lig.

D.
Uterine horn
Utero-ovarian lig.
Ovary
Broad lig.

E.

Figure 7–26
Illustration continued on page 136.

SOFT TISSUE SURGERY

Details of Procedure

Figure 7–26A. The uterine horn is extracted from the abdomen using an ovariohysterectomy hook. The right side of the abdomen is initially explored in an effort to avoid the spleen, which is on the left side. The hook is inserted toward and along the abdominal wall. Upon reaching the dorsum, the hook is rotated 180 degrees and then gently withdrawn in a caudal, medial direction. Upon presentation, the uterine horn is grasped with a gauze sponge.

Figure 7–26B. Carmalt forceps are clamped on the utero-ovarian ligament.

Figure 7–26C. The index finger is placed in the hammock formed by the lateral suspensory ligament and the mesovarium and is slid cranially toward the kidney. The suspensory ligament is torn by applying traction toward the body wall. Care must be taken to avoid tearing more than the suspensory ligament.

Figure 7–26D. The Carmalt forceps are removed and used to fenestrate an avascular region of the broad ligament just caudal to the ovary. The Carmalt forceps are reapplied to the utero-ovarian ligament through the fenestration.

Figure 7–26E. A second Carmalt forceps are placed through the fenestration and clamped across the ovarian pedicle proximal to the ovary. Palpation of the ovary before placing the clamp will assure complete removal.

The pedicle is transected on top of the second forceps with scissors, using the index finger as a guide to help protect adjacent structures.

The pedicle is ligated with absorbable suture material placed as a modified clove hitch. When done correctly, this knot is self-retaining and thus can replace the classic "three-forceps" method of pedicle ligation.

The forceps are removed from the pedicle, and the other uterine horn and ovary are handled in a similar fashion, except that the ovariohysterectomy hook is not required.

NOTES:

Ovariohysterectomy

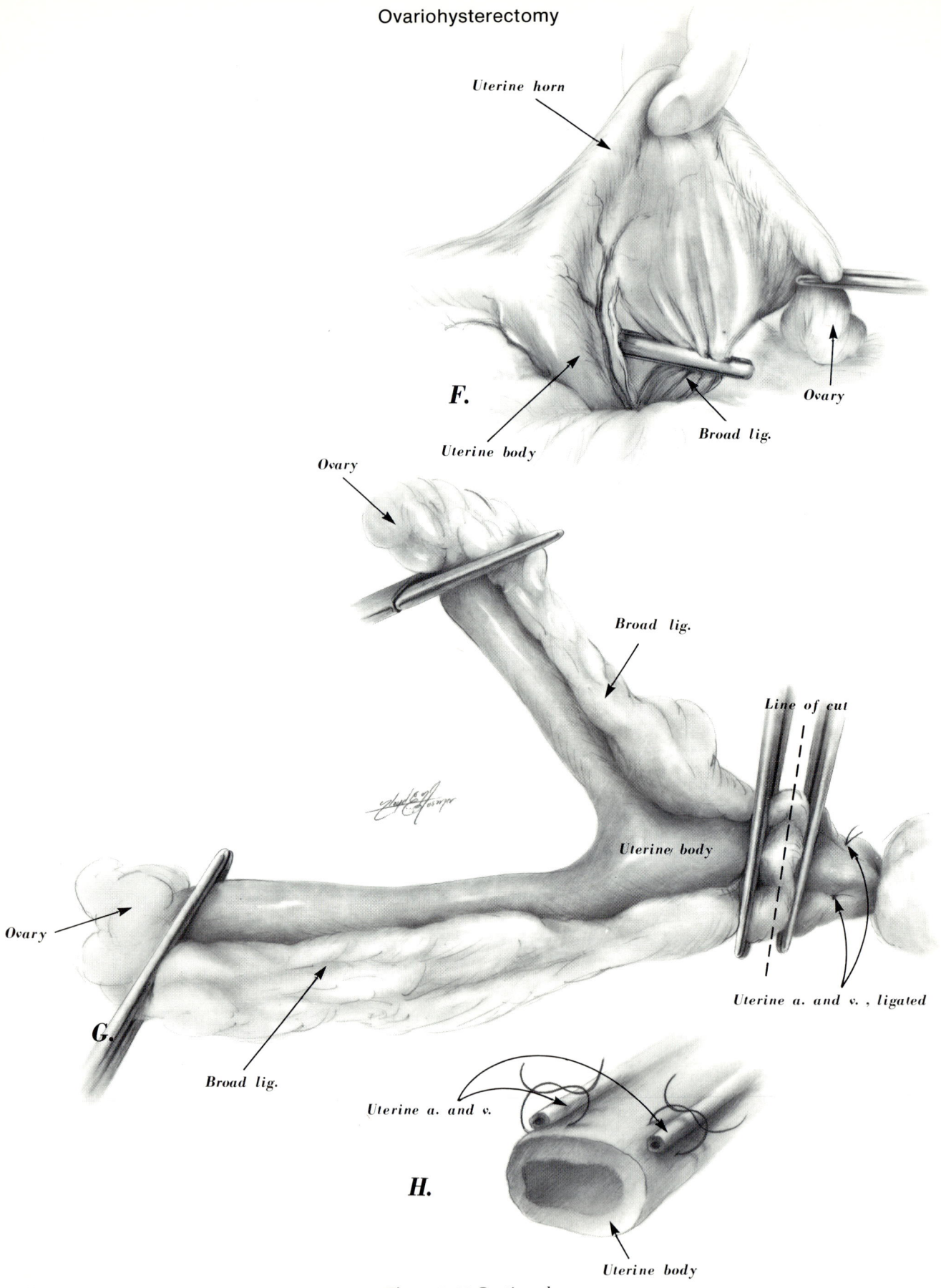

F.
- Uterine horn
- Ovary
- Broad lig.
- Uterine body

G.
- Ovary
- Broad lig.
- Uterine body
- Line of cut
- Uterine a. and v., ligated
- Ovary
- Broad lig.

H.
- Uterine a. and v.
- Uterine body

136   **Figure 7–26** Continued

SOFT TISSUE SURGERY

Figure 7–26F. The broad ligament may be ligated by fenestrating adjacent to the body of the uterus (but not including the uterine artery and vein) and placing Carmalt forceps through the fenestration and across the broad ligament. The broad ligament is transected on top of the forceps with scissors and ligated below the forceps, using absorbable suture material placed as a modified clove hitch.

Figure 7–26G. The body of the uterus is doubly clamped between the bifurcation and the cervix.

Figure 7–26H. The uterine vessels are transfixed separately by passing a suture needle with absorbable suture material into the edge of the uterine wall. The uterus is cut between the forceps and a modified clove-hitch ligature is placed around the stump in the area of the transfixion ligatures. The remaining clamp is removed, and the abdomen is closed in a routine manner.

Postoperative Considerations

The incision is monitored for swelling or discharge; exercise is restricted for 10 to 14 days; and skin sutures are removed in 6 to 8 days.

NOTES: *(Continued)*

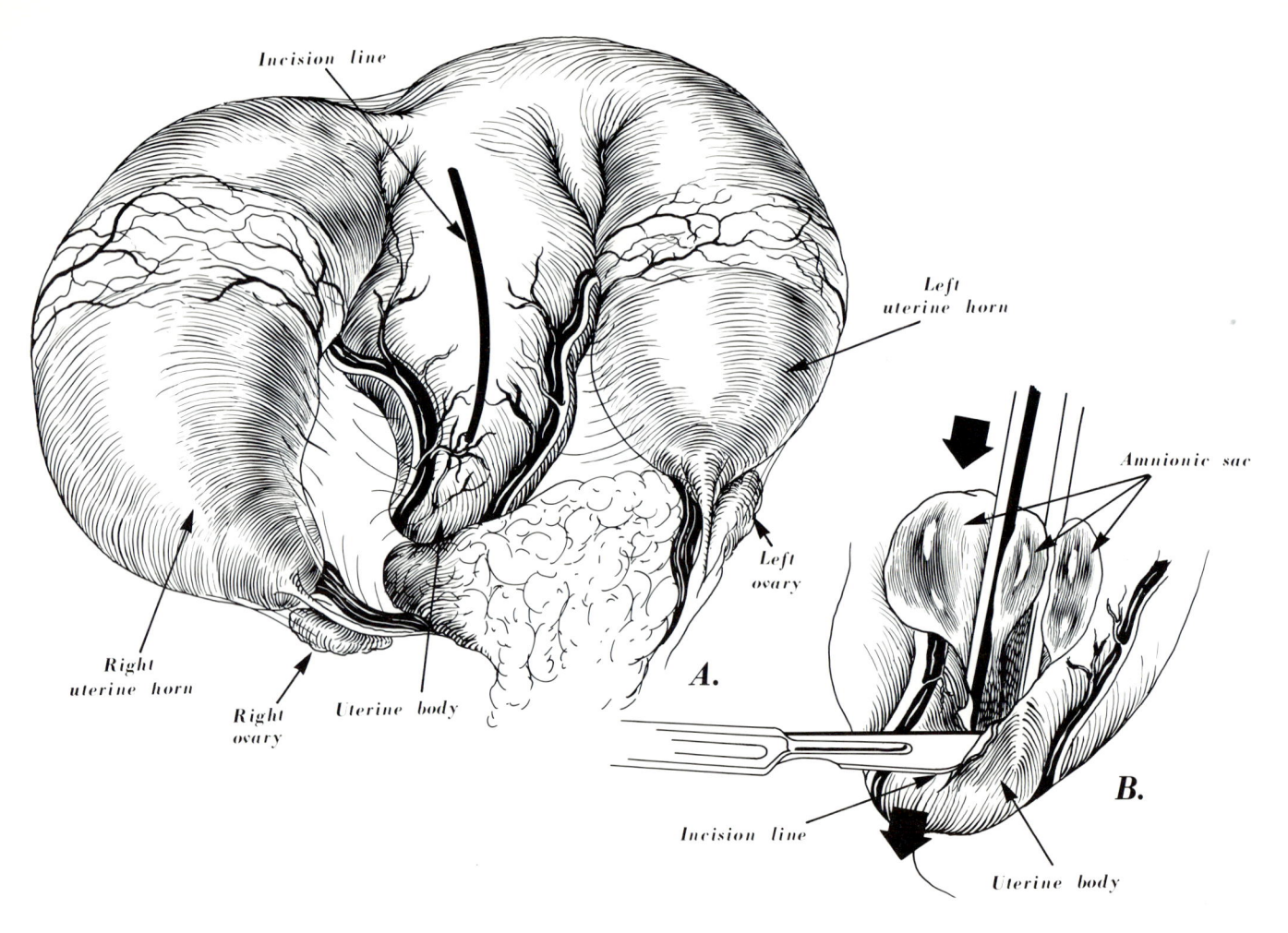

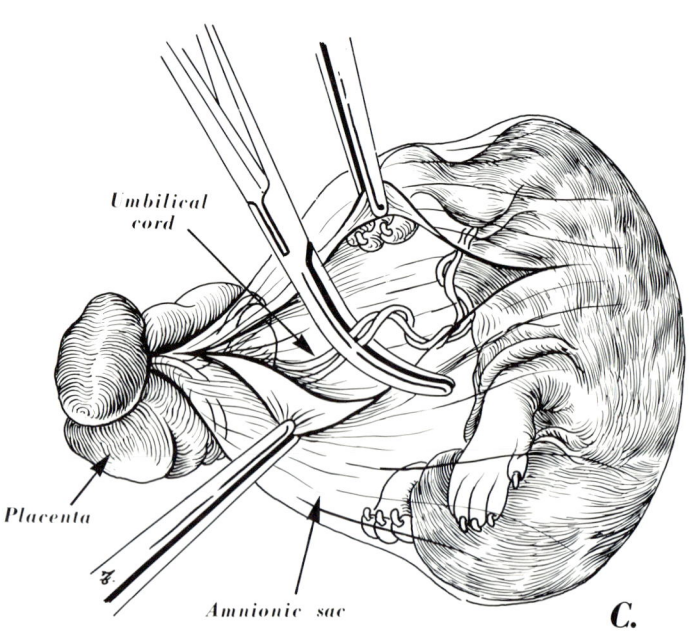

Figure 7–27
Illustration continued on page 140.

7–27 CESAREAN SECTION

JONATHAN N. CHAMBERS

Indications

Cesarean section is indicated when normal birth is impossible or when nonsurgical measures have failed to resolve a dystocia.

Anesthesia

During preanesthetic evaluation, special attention should be given to the fluid status of the patient. A prolonged dystocia can produce fluid loss, metabolic acidosis, and toxic depression. These animals need to be rehydrated. Dystocias of longer than 24 hours in a toxic bitch should probably be treated by partial correction of the fluid imbalance, shock dosages of corticosteroids, and antibiotics, and then surgically treated by an ovariohysterectomy. Patients with dystocias lasting between 12 and 24 hours may also be candidates for an ovariohysterectomy. Many clients also prefer an ovariohysterectomy to a hysterotomy.

When the client desires to save the newborns, anesthetic considerations are compounded. Nearly all anesthetic drugs cross the placental membrane to produce fetal depression and, possibly, death. One of three anesthetic regimens is suggested:

1. Inhalant induction and maintenance with halothane and nitrous oxide.
2. A tranquilizer-narcotic combination supplemented with a local anesthetic. A narcotic-reversing agent can be administered to the newborns if they appear depressed. Following removal of the newborns, anesthesia can be supplemented with inhalant anesthesia.
3. Epidural anesthesia supplemented with a sedative for restraint.

Patient Positioning

The patient is placed in dorsal recumbency.

Operative Preparation

When the newborns are delivered, adequate help should be available to assist in their resuscitation.

Incision and Exposure

The surgical approach is through a liberal, caudal midline abdominal incision. Care must be taken to avoid injury to the enlarged mammary glands and the gravid uterus.

Details of Procedure

Figure 7–27A. The uterus is exteriorized and isolated with surgical towels. The standard incision site is on the dorsal midline of the uterine body. The incision should be long enough to allow easy removal of the newborns.

Figure 7–27B. Thumb forceps or a groove director are used to protect the underlying fetal membranes. The fetus and placenta are gently advanced to the hysterotomy by applying pressure through the uterine wall.

Figure 7–27C. Upon presentation, the fetus is removed from the uterus, and the fetal membranes are removed. The umbilical vessels are clamped or ligated, and the newborn is handed to an assistant for resuscitation.

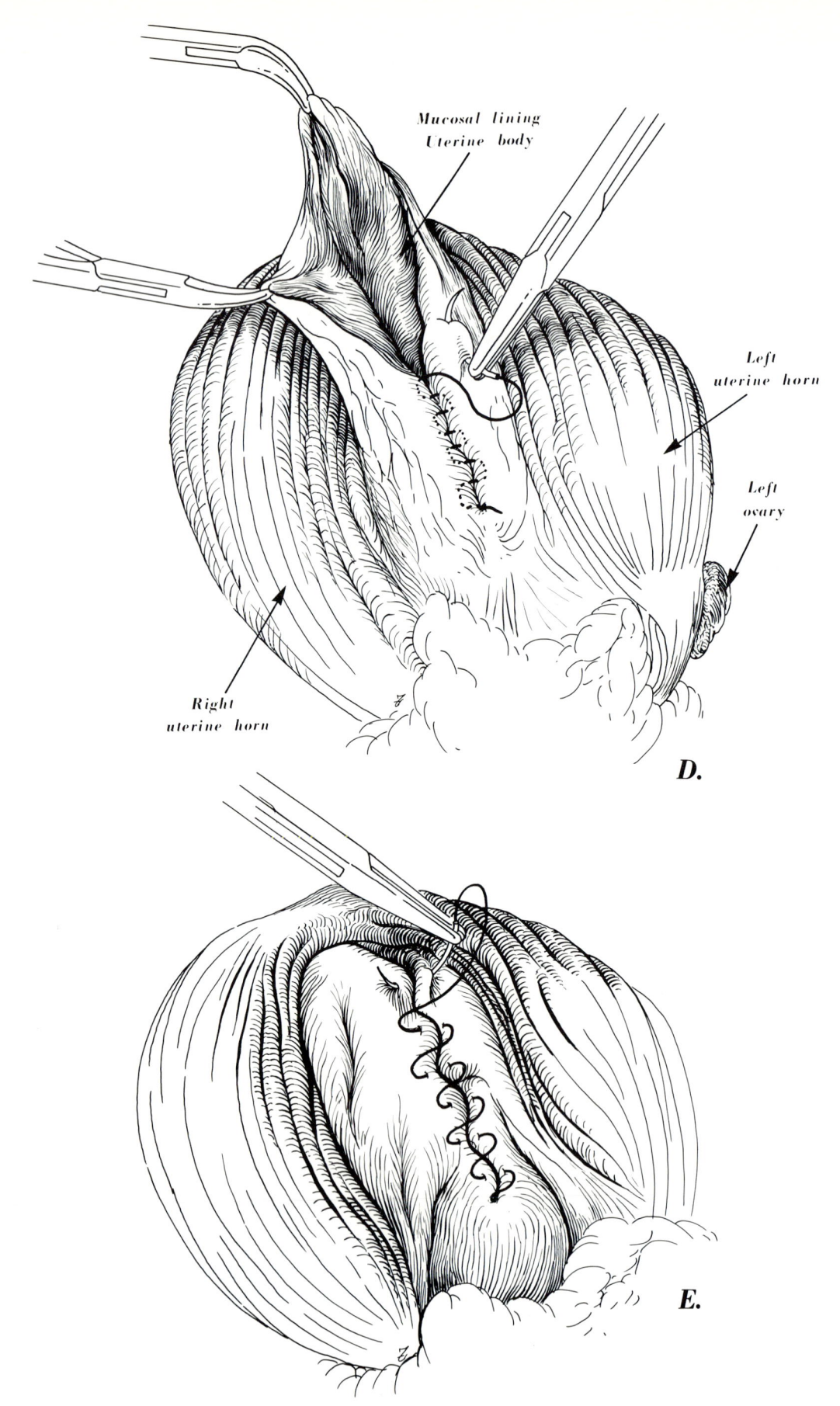

Figure 7–27 Continued

SOFT TISSUE SURGERY

Figure 7–27D. The hysterotomy is closed in two layers with absorbable suture material. The first layer is a Cushing pattern to appose the wound edges.

Figure 7–27E. The second layer is a Halsted pattern. The surgical towels are removed; the uterus is replaced; and the abdomen is closed in a routine manner.

Postoperative Considerations

The mother and newborns are returned to the home environment as soon as they are stable. Delayed healing of the skin incision is not unusual owing to the constant irritation of nursing.

NOTES: *(Continued)*

Figure 7–28
Illustration continued on page 144.

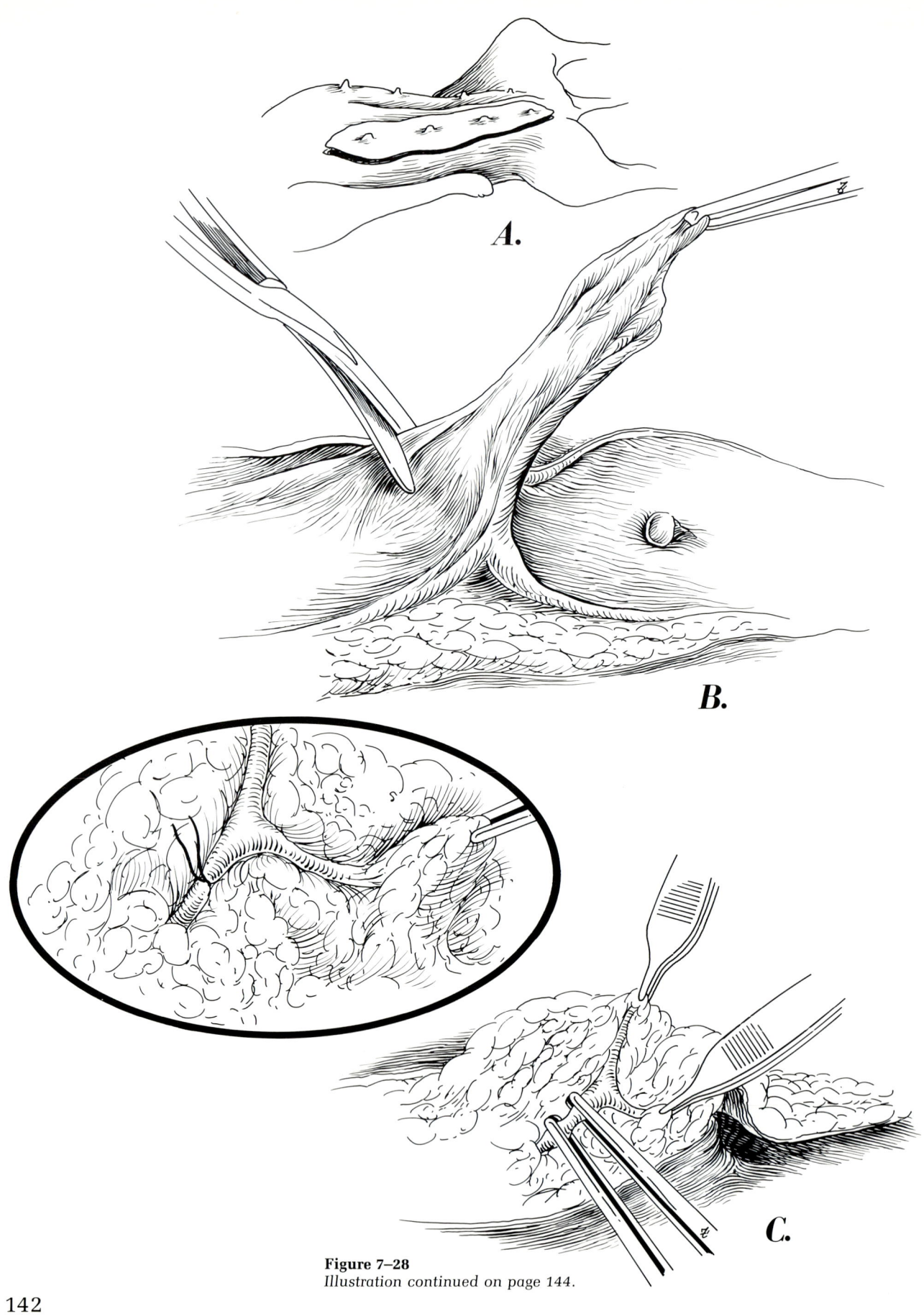

7–28 MASTECTOMY

ANDREW J. FREY

Indications

Mastectomy is performed for removal of mammary gland neoplasms, severely lacerated glands, or abscessed mammary tissues.

Anesthesia

Choice of anesthetic regimen is based upon the patient's overall condition.

Patient Positioning

The patient is placed in dorsal recumbency.

Operative Preparation

Specialized Instruments. Several small hemostatic forceps are necessary for control of hemorrhage. Electrocautery may also be used.

Suture Material. Ligation of blood vessels is performed with 4-0 Dexon or chromic catgut.

Details of Procedure

Figure 7–28A. The dog is positioned in dorsal recumbency, with its legs gently abducted. Sharp skin incisions are begun cranial to the first mammary gland and are extended caudally in an elliptical shape on each side of the mammary glands. The incisions are ended caudal to the last mammary gland.

Figure 7–28B. The mammary glands may be grasped with Allis tissue forceps and retracted caudally as the glands are bluntly dissected from the abdominal fascia. The cranial and caudal thoracic glands receive their blood supply from sternal branches of the internal thoracic artery and the intercostal and lateral thoracic arteries. The cranial abdominal gland is supplied by the cranial superficial epigastric artery and anastomotic branches from the caudal superficial epigastric artery. The veins follow a similar pattern. When these vessels are encountered, they are ligated with 4-0 suture material. Careful hemostasis is an important factor in the prevention of postoperative fluid accumulation. After the cranial mammae have been dissected free, the exposed muscle and fascia are covered with moist gauze sponges, and the dissection is continued caudally.

Figure 7–28C. The caudal abdominal and inguinal mammae are supplied by the caudal superficial epigastric artery and vein, which are branches of the external pudendal artery and vein. The external pudendal vessels are carefully isolated and doubly ligated with 4-0 suture material as they exit from the inguinal canal. The superficial inguinal lymph node(s) are situated in the fat underlying the fourth and fifth glands and are not easily identified. Excision of the mammary glands and underlying fat usually results in excision of these lymph nodes.

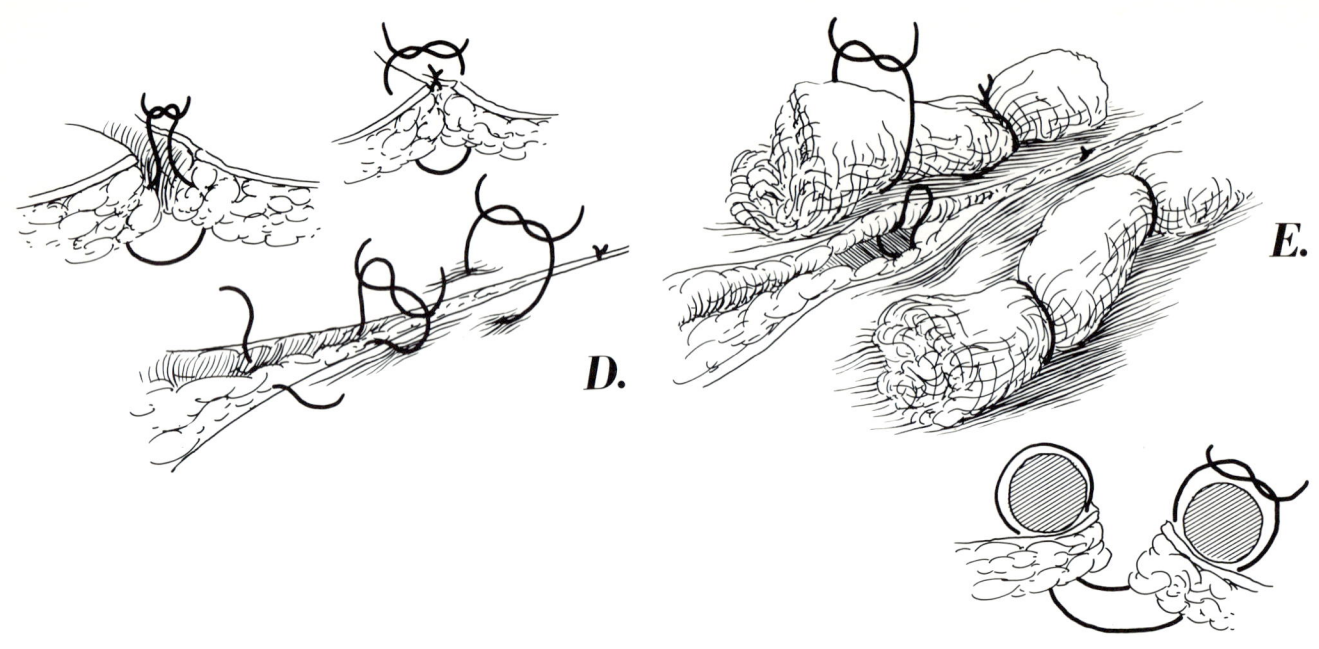

Figure 7–28 Continued

Figure 7–28D. After excision of the mammary glands, the skin defect is closed in two layers. The first layer is a simple interrupted subcutaneous suture pattern of 2-0 chromic catgut. This layer should be applied so that the skin sutures are under no tension. The second layer is a simple interrupted skin suture pattern of a nonabsorbable suture material.

Figure 7–28E. If excessive tension is present in the thoracic region, tension sutures may be employed. Large vertical mattress sutures tied over rolled gauze sponges can be effective. The sutures are placed at least 1 cm from the skin edges. A nonabsorbable suture material is used. If excessive dead space cannot be obliterated in the inguinal region with subcutaneous sutures, a Penrose drain may be used.

Postoperative Considerations

A body wrap may be applied to relieve excess tension on the incision.

NOTES:

SOFT TISSUE SURGERY 145

7–29 CANINE CASTRATION
Charles William Betts

Indications

Castration is done for sterilization, to correct or eliminate obnoxious behavior, prevent roaming, and decrease opportunities for fights in the young dog. The dog should be given sufficient time for development of secondary sexual characteristics prior to castration. Older dogs may require castration in conjunction with or as therapy for other related problems, i.e., benign prostatic hypertrophy.

Anesthesia

General anesthesia is required.

Patient Positioning

The dog is placed in dorsal recumbency, with the rear limbs gently abducted.

Preoperative Preparation

The inner thighs, the caudal two thirds of the shaft of the penis, and the scrotum should be gently clipped with particular care taken to avoid any clipper burns or abrasions of the scrotum.

Operative Preparation

Special Draping. Three corner draping is sufficient, with the base of the triangle immediately cranial to the scrotum and the apex of the triangle over the shaft of the penis caudal to the prepuce.

Suture Material. Three to 4-0 chromic catgut or Dexon is recommended for subcutaneous closure. The skin should be closed with 3-0 to 4-0 nylon, Prolene, or fine Vetefil. If a satisfactory subcuticular closure is done, skin closure is not necessary.

Details of Procedure

Figure 7–29A. One of the testicles is displaced cranially by finger manipulation through the caudal drape. It is positioned ventral to the penis immediately cranial to the scrotum and held with sufficient pressure to cause the testicle to bulge under the skin. A midline incision is made over the testicle with sharp dissection through the subcutaneous tissue. Do not incise through the common tunic.

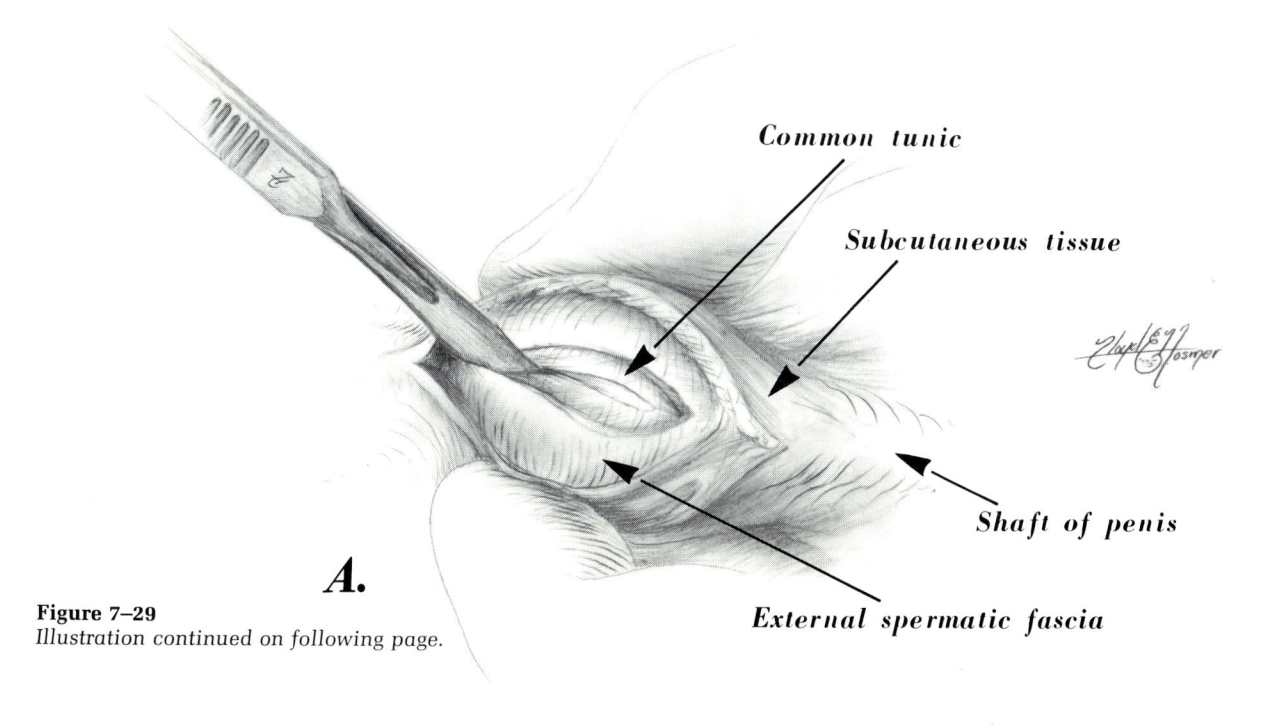

Figure 7–29
Illustration continued on following page.

Testicle

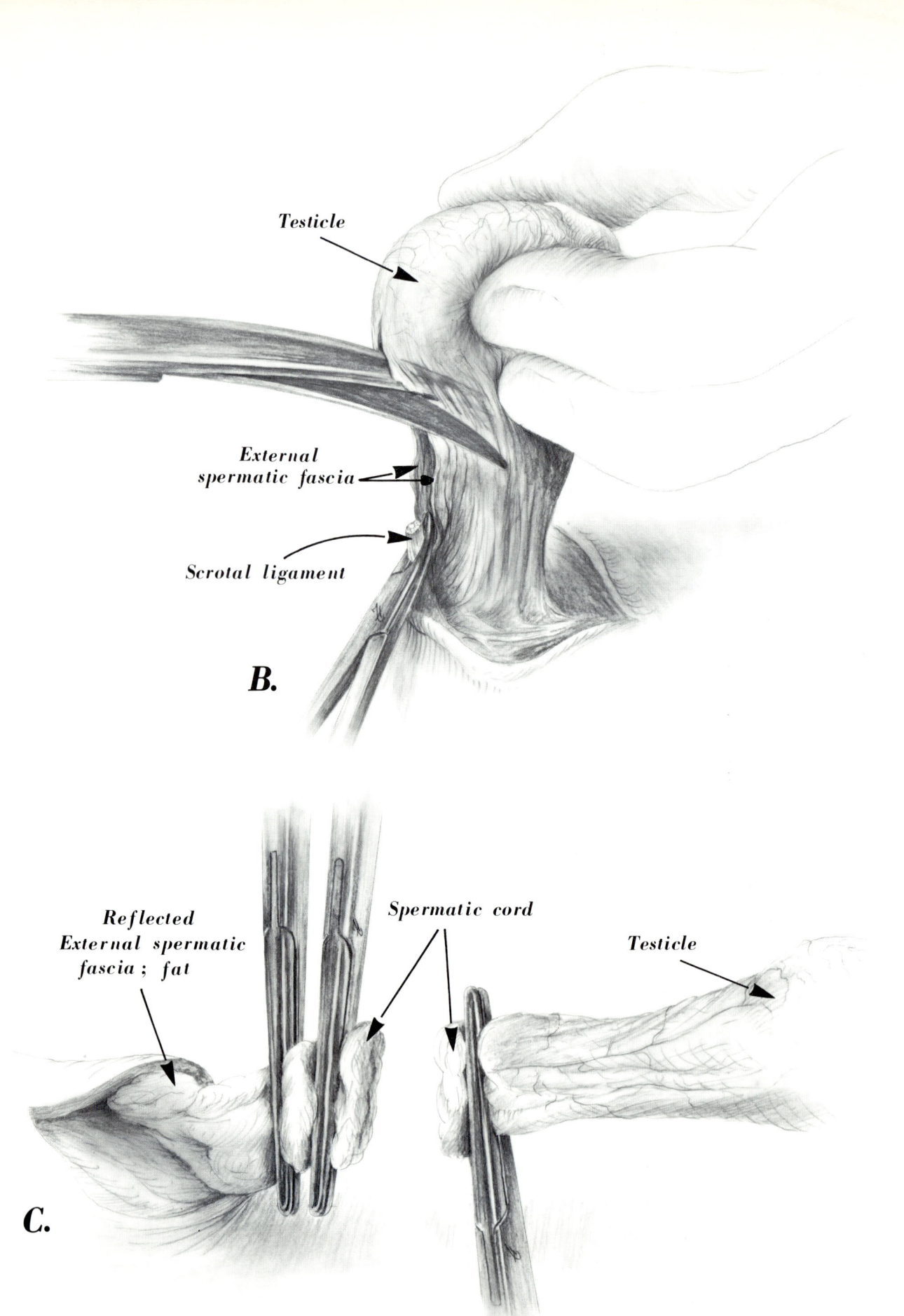

External spermatic fascia

Scrotal ligament

B.

Reflected External spermatic fascia; fat

Spermatic cord

Testicle

C.

Figure 7–29 Continued.

Figure 7–29B. The incision is made large enough to cause the testicle to "pop" through the subcutaneous tissue. The gubernaculum or scrotal ligament is clamped and incised. This opens a pocket at the caudal aspect of the testicle through which the external spermatic fascia can be incised on each side of the testicle and dissected free to the external inguinal ring. A gauze sponge can also be used to strip the fascia and fat from the spermatic cord.

Figure 7–29C. The scrotal ligament is checked for bleeding and is released. Three Carmalt forceps are placed on the spermatic cord still enclosed within the common tunic. The spermatic cord and testicle are removed by incising between the outer two clamps. A Miller's knot is placed around the two remaining clamps and slipped over the pedicle. The clamp farthest from the external inguinal ring is checked to be sure it has a secure grasp on the tissue. As the Miller's knot is tightened, the bottom clamp is simultaneously released and removed, allowing the knot to slip into the crushed groove previously occupied by the clamp. Grasp the pedicle with the thumb forceps, remove the last clamp, relax the tension on the pedicle, and check carefully for hemorrhage. Place the pedicle in the inguinal area. The procedures above are repeated on the remaining testicle. The wound is closed with a subcuticular stitch and a simple interrupted stitch in the skin.

Postoperative Considerations

The dog should have moderate restriction of exercise. The incision should be checked daily for swelling or discharge. If the vessel in the scrotal ligament bleeds or subcutaneous hemorrhage is excessive, the scrotum may fill with blood that forms a palpable blood clot. This problem is usually self-limiting. The most common problem after surgery is scrotal dermatitis initiated by rough clipping or harsh scrubbing and perpetuated by the dog's licking.

NOTES:

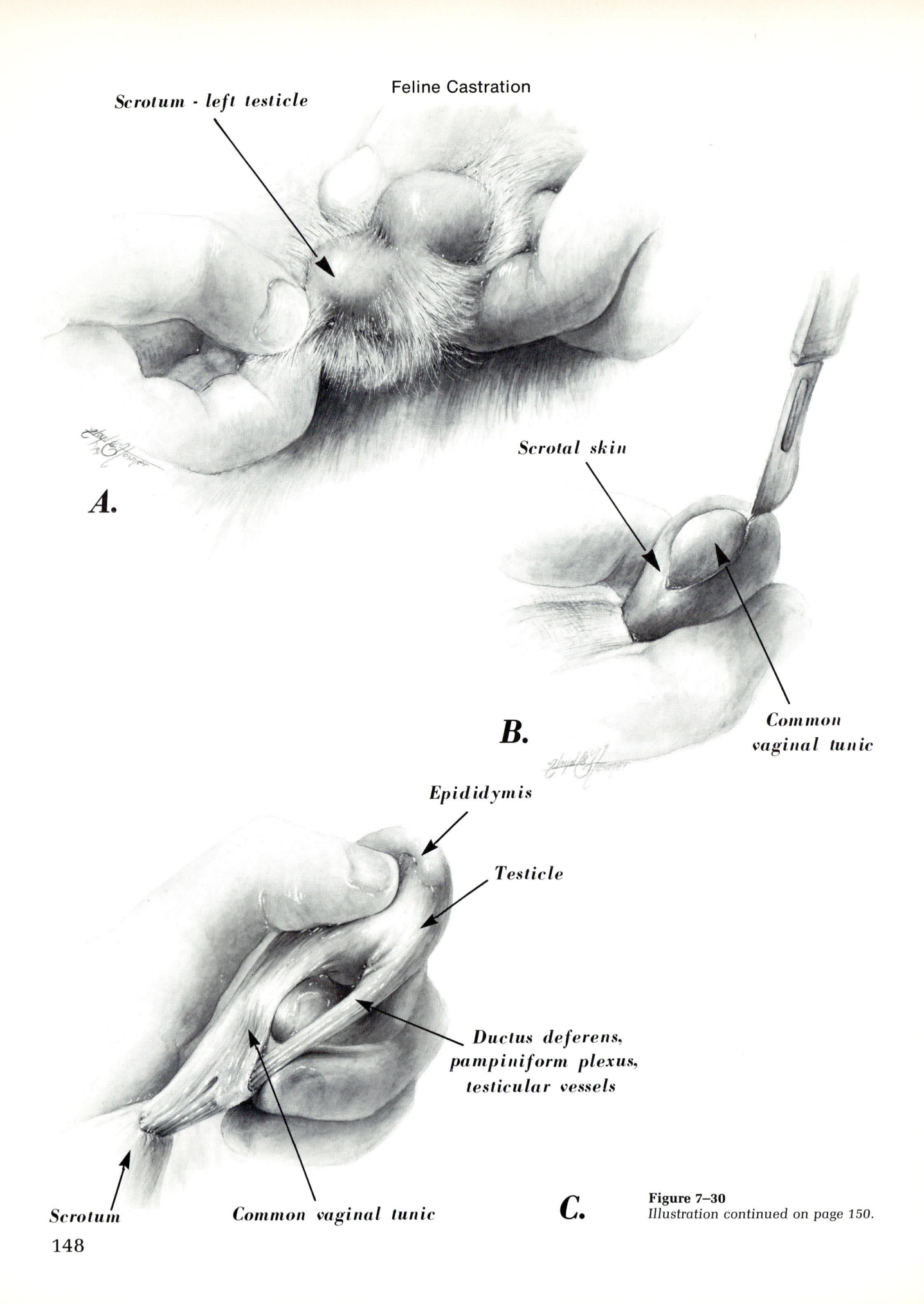

Feline Castration

A. Scrotum - left testicle

B. Scrotal skin / Common vaginal tunic

C. Epididymis / Testicle / Ductus deferens, pampiniform plexus, testicular vessels / Scrotum / Common vaginal tunic

Figure 7–30
Illustration continued on page 150.

7–30 FELINE CASTRATION

Clarence A. Rawlings

Indications

Castration is indicated as an elective procedure to prevent impregnation and reduce the characteristic odor of a tomcat and for behavior modification.

Anesthesia

General anesthesia or heavy sedation is indicated.

Patient Positioning

The patient is placed in lateral recumbency.

Operative Preparation

Specialized Instruments. Hemostatic clips (e.g., Versa clips) are more efficient than suture ligatures.

Details of Procedure

Figure 7–30A. The hair is "plucked" from the scrotal skin.

Figure 7–30B. The scrotal skin is liberally incised in a vertical direction over the more dependent testicle. A closed castration is performed without penetrating the common vaginal tunic. To perform an open castration, the tunics are incised.

Figure 7–30C. The testicle is forcefully withdrawn from the scrotal incision. The incision in the common vaginal tunic is continued proximally, and the area of ductus deferens, pampiniform plexus, and testicular vessels is identified.

NOTES:

Feline Castration

Epididymis
Testicle
Incision
Scrotum
Ligature
Ductus deferens, pampiniform plexus, testicular vessels
Common vaginal tunic

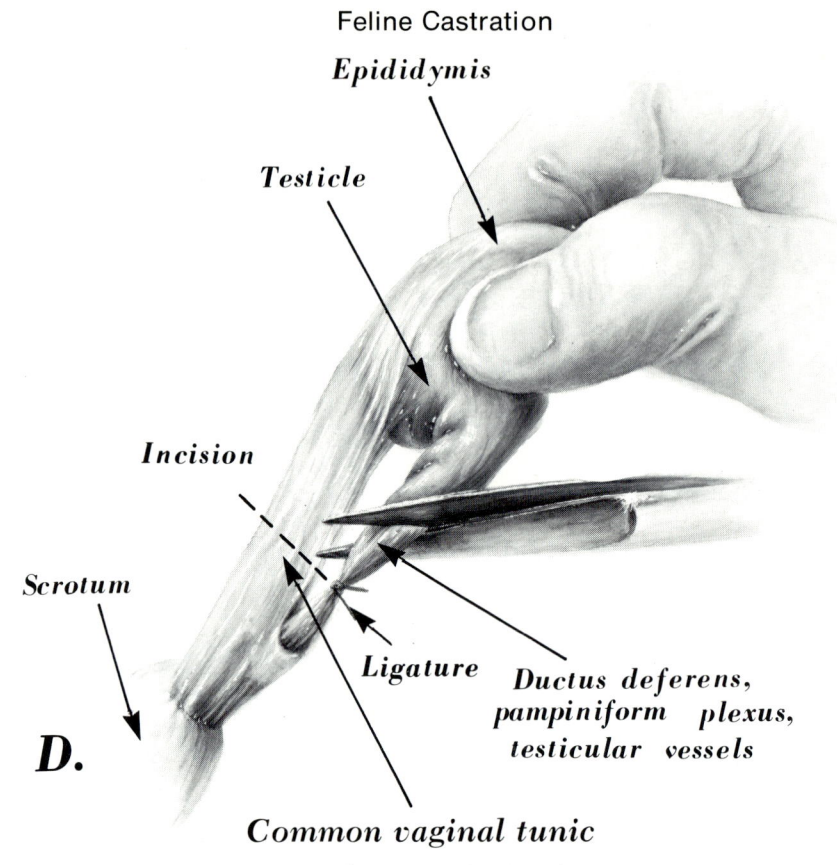

D.

Figure 7–30 Continued

Figure 7–30D. A ligature of absorbable suture material or a hemostatic metal clip is placed around the area of the ductus deferens, pampiniform plexus, and testicular vessels. This tissue is excised and replaced into the common vaginal tunic, and the excessive tunic tissue is excised. The scrotal incision is allowed to heal by second intention.

NOTES: (Continued)

Postoperative Considerations

The scrotal area should be examined daily for evidence of swelling, discharges, pain, and heat.

7–31 LATERAL EAR RESECTION

Wayne E. Wingfield

Indications

Resection of the lateral wall of the external ear canal will provide effective drainage. Chronic otitis externa is frequently noted in dogs with long, floppy ears. Moisture and debris may accumulate in the ear canals of these patients, making adequate cleansing and medication difficult. As chronic otitis progresses, the otic tissues become hyperplastic, further decreasing the size of the vertical and horizontal ear canals. With resection of the lateral wall of the vertical canal, the ear is allowed to drain, air is more available for drying the ear, medication is more easily administered, and the horizontal canal becomes accessible for cleansing.

Anesthesia

Routine inhalation anesthetics are administered following assessment of anesthetic risk.

Preoperative Preparation

The hair is removed from both sides of the pinna as well as ventral to the opening of the external ear canal. Thoroughly cleanse the ear canal before proceeding with the surgical scrub. This is best accomplished with a warm water and pHisohex flush. Follow the flushing procedure with a cleansing and drying of the ear canal using cotton swabs.

Patient Positioning

The patient is positioned in lateral recumbency in preparation for surgery.

Operative Preparation

Special Draping. Quadrant draping with the pinna exposed is used for a lateral ear resection. Extend the ventral drape to an area below the horizontal ear canal. (Figure 7–31A shows the location of the incision.)

Specialized Instruments. Cartilage of the ear canal becomes quite thickened or even ossified with chronic otitis. Be prepared to cut through this material. Heavy dissecting scissors or cartilage scissors are useful for this part of the procedure.

NOTES:

SOFT TISSUE SURGERY

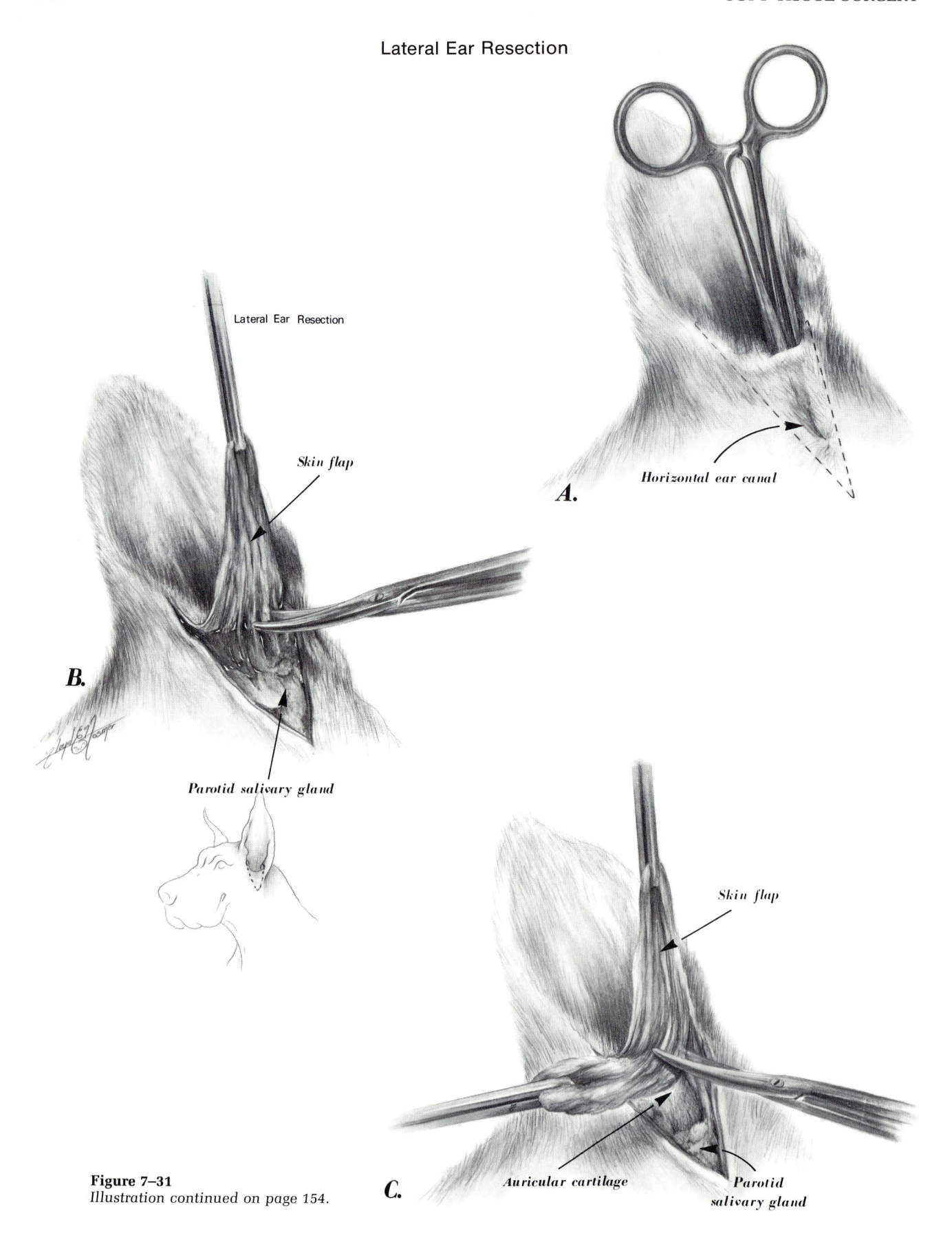

Lateral Ear Resection

A. Horizontal ear canal

B. Lateral Ear Resection — Skin flap; Parotid salivary gland

C. Skin flap; Auricular cartilage; Parotid salivary gland

Figure 7–31
Illustration continued on page 154.

SOFT TISSUE SURGERY

Incision and Exposure

Figure 7–31A. A skin incision is extended ventrally from the cranial and caudal aspects of the lateral ear canal wall. This incision is carried ventral to the horizontal ear canal. The exact level of this canal may be determined by first inserting curved forceps into the vertical ear canal and palpating the forceps' points as they reach the level of the horizontal canal. The incision of the skin may be either triangular or rectangular. The intertragic and tragohelicine incisures are landmarks for the caudal and cranial incisions. Extend these incisions to a level approximately one and a half to two times the length of the vertical canal.

Details of Procedure

Figure 7–31B. Continue the skin incision through the subcutaneous tissues. Care must be taken to avoid the underlying parotid salivary gland. Dissect the salivary tissue free from the subcutaneous tissue. The skin flap, subcutaneous tissues, and auricular muscles are reflected dorsally.

Figure 7–31C. After removal of these tissues, the cartilage of the lateral wall is easily visualized.

NOTES: *(Continued)*

154 SOFT TISSUE SURGERY

Lateral Ear Resection

D.
A
1/2 of AB
20° angle
Skin flap removed for illustrative purpose
B
A'
Parotid salivary gland
Auricular cartilage

E.
Horizontal ear canal
Auricular cartilage

F.
Auricular cartilage

G.
Skin flap
Auricular cartilage
Parotid salivary gland

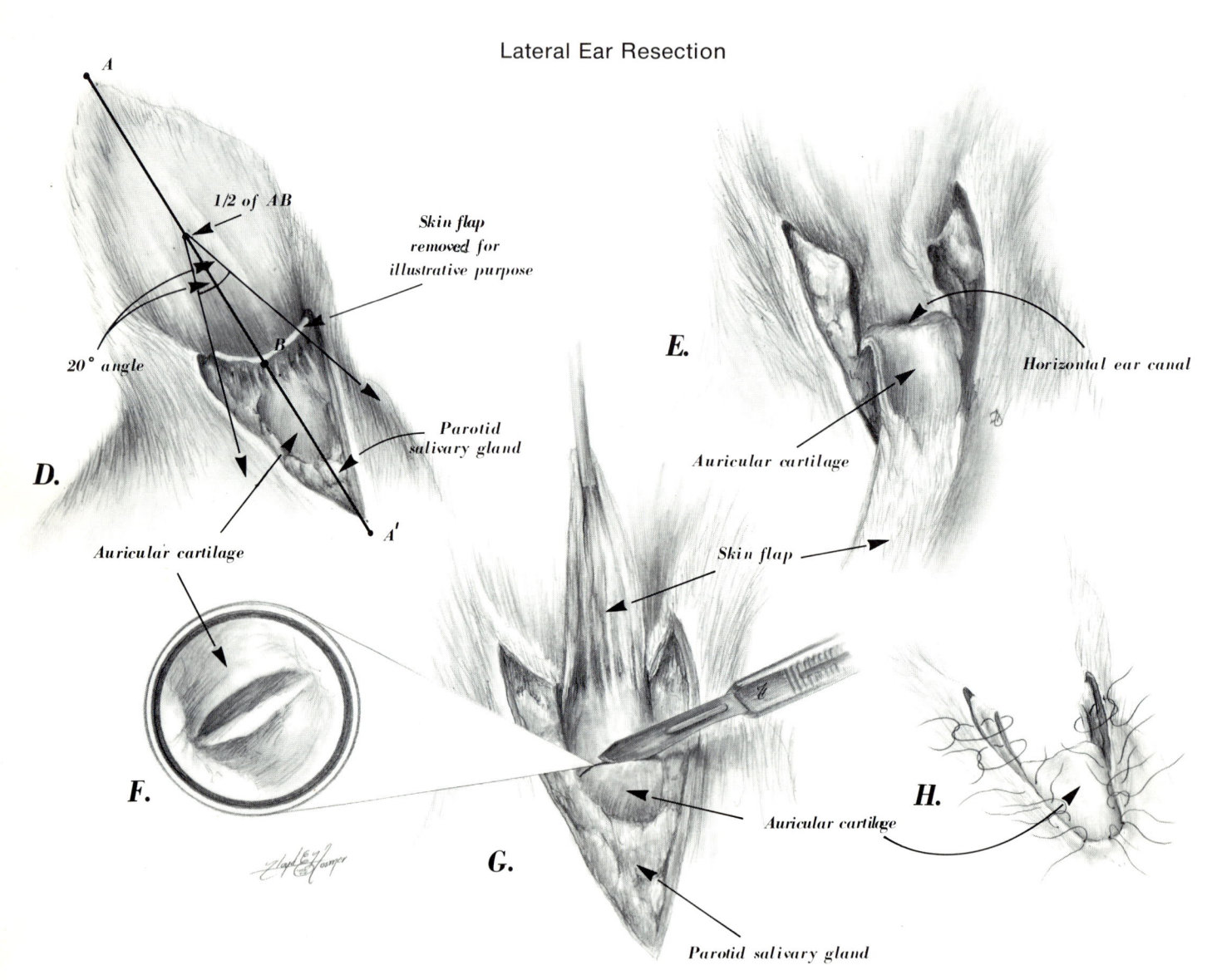

H.

Figure 7–31 Continued

Figure 7–31D. Two incisions are made in the lateral cartilage wall of the vertical ear canal. The incision is directed caudally at a 20-degree angle from a point approximately half the distance from A to B. Extend this cartilage incision along this imaginary line to the level of the horizontal ear canal. Cartilage scissors or heavy dissecting scissors are used to make this incision. Use the same angle and approach to make the rostral incision. This incision is begun at the tragohelicine incisure and extended ventrally to the meatus of the horizontal canal. Extending the cartilage incisions caudally and rostrally helps to avoid making a narrow cartilage flap at the level of the horizontal canal.

Figure 7–31E. Reflect the cartilage flap ventrally to expose the horizontal ear canal. This flap will be utilized to form a drainage board ventral to the horizontal canal.

Figures 7–31F and 7–31G. To enable the cartilage flap to lay flat against the head, a "V" is removed from the cartilage at the ventral aspect of the horizontal meatus. The "V" need not extend completely through the cartilage.

The attached skin and one third to one half of the cartilage are excised. This leaves a ventrally attached cartilage flap.

Figure 7–31H. Closure of the incision utilizes a simple interrupted pattern and 4-0 nonabsorbable suture material. Begin the closure by suturing the skin to the cartilage flap on the ventral portion of the incision. It is desirable to provide a slight amount of ventral traction on the cartilage by the skin. With the "V" of the cartilage removed ventral to the horizontal canal, this cartilage flap should lay flatly against the head. Each interrupted suture is passed through the skin edge and through the edge of the cartilage. Continue suture placement until the entire surgical incision has been closed.

Postoperative Considerations

The incision must be protected from mutilation by the animal. The pinnae are placed over the top of the head and taped in place. A stockinette covering is used to maintain this position and to protect the incision from dirt, debris, and soiling. Additional restraint devices, such as tape hobbles and collars, are often required to prevent the animal from scratching at the incision.

Few complications usually result. In providing ear drainage, it is imperative that the surgery promote an adequate meatus to the horizontal canal following lateral resection of the vertical canal wall.

NOTES: *(Continued)*

NEUROLOGICAL SURGERY CHAPTER 8

8–1 STABILIZATION OF ATLANTOAXIAL SUBLUXATION

JONATHAN N. CHAMBERS

Indications

This technique utilizing nonmetallic suture material is indicated for use in toy breeds with atlantoaxial subluxation due to agenesis or separation of the dens (Fig. 8–1A). This subluxation will allow a laxity of the two vertebrae to exert pressure on the spinal cord (Fig. 8–1B). The same exposure can be used for exploration and decompression of other lesions involving the C-1 to C-2 area.

Anesthesia

The location of the lesion and the animal's surgical position require special anesthetic considerations. Some surgeons may request a preoperative myelogram. Because of the possibility of a myelogram-induced seizure, preanesthetic anticonvulsant agents (phenobarbitol, diazepam) should be considered. Before, during, and after anesthesia, the lack of cervical stability dictates careful, gentle manipulation of the neck. Induction should not require forceful restraint, and intubation should be performed without hyperextension of the neck — i.e., perform with the animal in lateral recumbency.

During anesthesia, the head and neck should be positioned so that venous flow within the external jugular veins is not retarded. The patient should be hyperventilated in an effort to reduce the arterial partial pressure of carbon dioxide and, consequently, reduce cerebral blood flow and brain size. When an insult is inflicted on the medullary control center (an area close to the surgical site), bradycardia can result. Heart rate needs to be monitored closely.

Patient Positioning

The patient is positioned in sternal recumbency in preparation for surgery, with a sandbag supporting the chin. The head or ears are secured to the table with tape to prevent rotation and to maintain symmetry during the operation.

Operative Preparation

Specialized Instruments. A self-retaining retractor, such as a Weitlaner, Beckman, or Gelpi, is needed to maintain good exposure.

Incision and Exposure

The skin is incised on the dorsal midline from the occiput to the midcervical region. The complex of paraspinal muscles is incised through the median raphe and gently elevated from the dorsal arch of the atlas and dorsal spinous process of the axis. A self-retaining retractor is inserted to afford continual exposure of the vertebrae.

NEUROLOGICAL SURGERY 157

A.

Labels: Atlanto-Occipital articulation; Dorsal Atlanto-Occipital membrane; Incision site; Dorsal Atlanto-Axial ligament; Dorsal Atlanto-Axial membrane; ATLAS; AXIS; Atlanto-Axial joint capsule

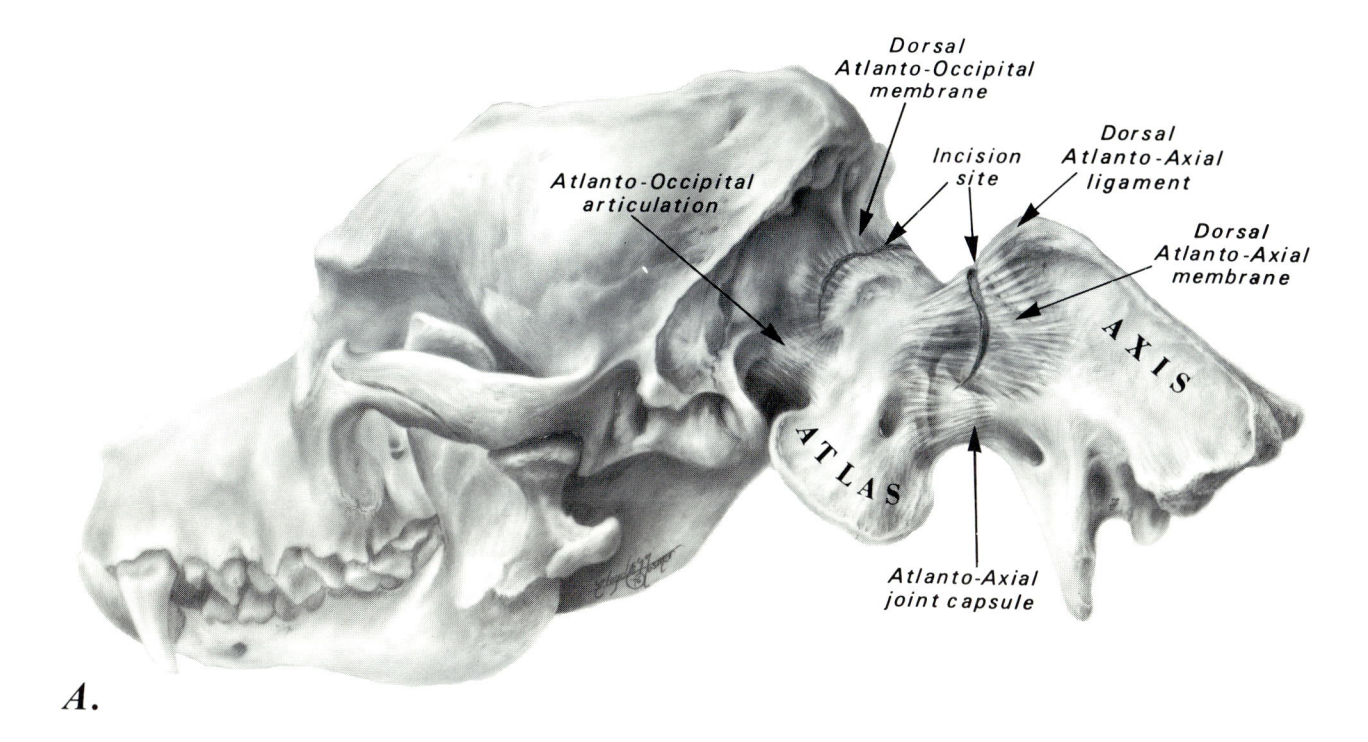

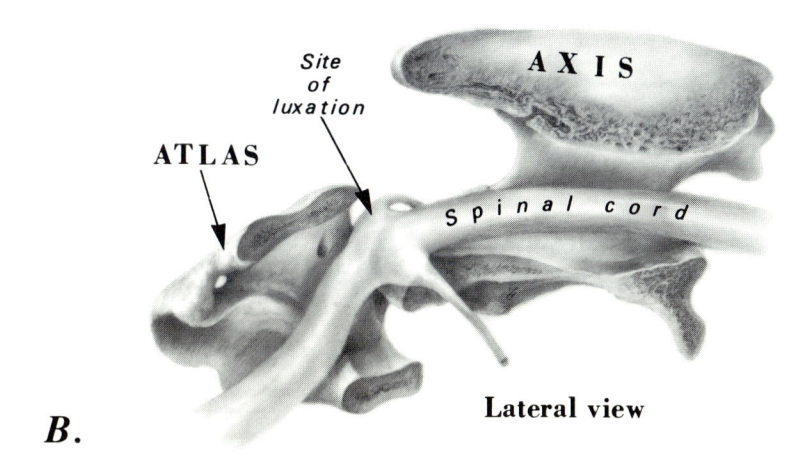

B. Lateral view

Labels: ATLAS; Site of luxation; AXIS; Spinal cord

Figure 8–1
Illustration continued on following page.

Details of Procedure

<u>Figure 8–1A</u>. Entrance to the epidural space is gained through incisions in the dorsal atlanto-occipital and atlantoaxial membranes. This is best accomplished with an inverted No. 11 Bard-Parker knife blade. Care must be taken not to penetrate the underlying dura (Fig. 8–1*B*).

NOTES:

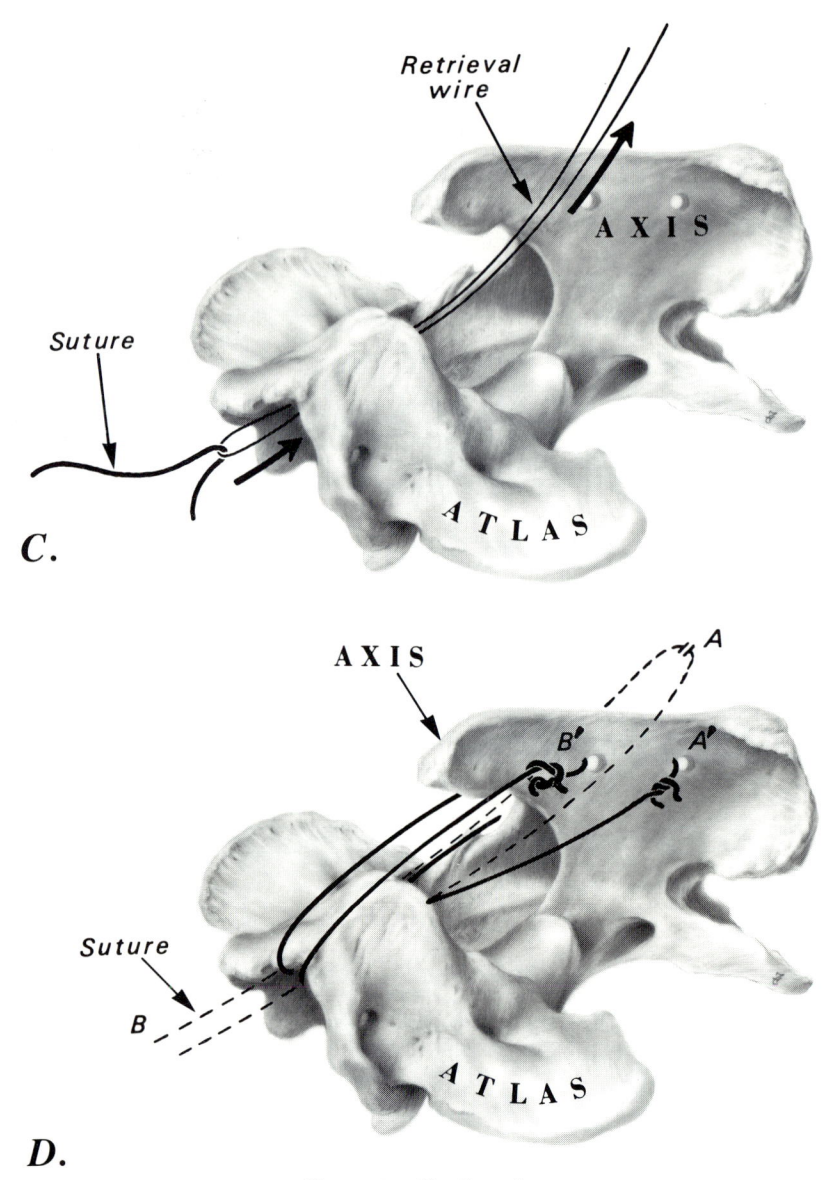

Figure 8–1 Continued
Illustration continued on opposite page.

A loop of fine stainless steel wire is passed under the arch of the atlas from caudal to cranial. As the loop appears at the foramen magnum, a strand of nonmetallic, nonabsorbable suture material (Numbers 0 to 2-0 nylon or impregnated silk — "silky" Polydek —or Dacron — Tevdek, Deknatel) is threaded through the loop and drawn back under the roof of the atlas (Fig. 8–1C). The strand is cut at its midpoint, creating two parallel strands.

Figure 8–1D. Two holes are drilled in the dorsal spine of the axis with a 0.045 Kirschner wire. The suture is tied caudally at point A,

NOTES: (Continued)

AXIS

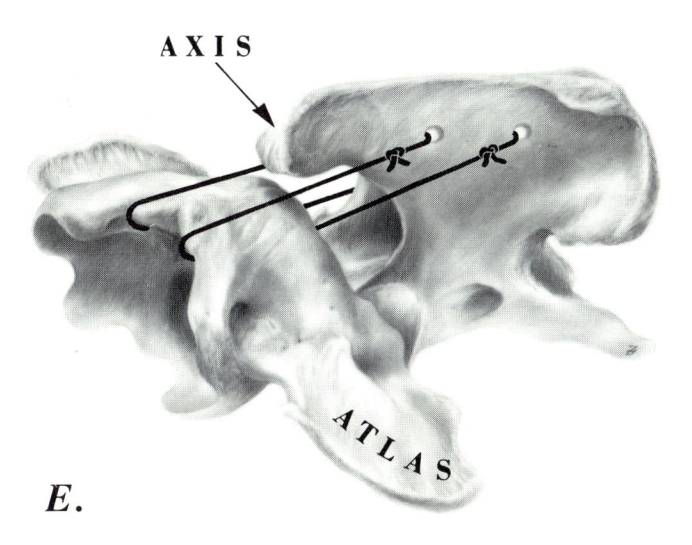

ATLAS

E.

Figure 8–1 Continued

A¹. The cranially emerging suture is then used to correct the subluxation and tied (B¹).

It is important to gently depress the cranial aspect of the axis ventrally while determining the desired amount of tension necessary to reduce the subluxation. The correct alignment is shown in Figure 8–1E.

An alternative method is to drill a hole on both sides of the roof of the atlas approximately midway from cranial to caudal. The suture is then passed transversely under the roof of the atlas and tied to the axis as illustrated.

The wound is closed by simple apposition of the paraspinal muscles with simple interrupted sutures. The subcutaneous tissue and skin are closed in a routine fashion.

Postoperative Considerations

Support of the neck with a brace or bandage is optional, depending on the stability afforded by the surgery. Some animals may require medication for pain following surgery.

NOTES: *(Continued)*

8–2 BULLA OSTEOTOMY

Wayne E. Wingfield

Indications

Bulla osteotomy involves the opening of the osseous bulla in animals with otitis media. Generally, the otitis media has become chronic, and less radical attempts at therapy have failed or have produced unsatisfactory results. With chronic otitis media, the bulla may be filled with inflammatory exudate or granulation tissue or may have begun to ossify. Occasionally, a neoplasm is encountered in this area, necessitating surgical exposure of the tympanic bulla.

Anesthesia

General anesthesia with tracheal intubation and maintenance on inhalation anesthetics is required after assessing operative risk.

Patient Positioning

The patient is placed in dorsal recumbency, with the head and neck extended. Tape is applied over the tip of the mandible to stabilize the head. The forelimbs are extended caudally and tied in place.

Preoperative Preparation

Hair is clipped from the ventral head, cranial cervical region, and along the side of the face to the external auditory meatus on the affected side. Lavage with soapy, warm water is used to clean the external ear canal, and cotton swabs are used for additional cleansing and drying.

Operative Preparation

Special Draping. Quadrant draping is used to expose the intermandibular area down to the external auditory meatus.

Specialized Instruments. Routine operative instruments will be utilized. In addition, a 3 to 4 mm drill, equipment to provide drilling capabilities (hand drill, power drill, or Jacobs chuck), and a piece of ¼-inch Penrose drain or latex rubber tubing will be utilized. A used, ¼-inch Steinmann pin with a small hole drilled in one end will help facilitate passage of the tubing during the operative procedure. Self-retaining retractors are useful.

Incision and Exposure

An incision is made medial and parallel to the digastricus muscle on the affected side.

NEUROLOGICAL SURGERY

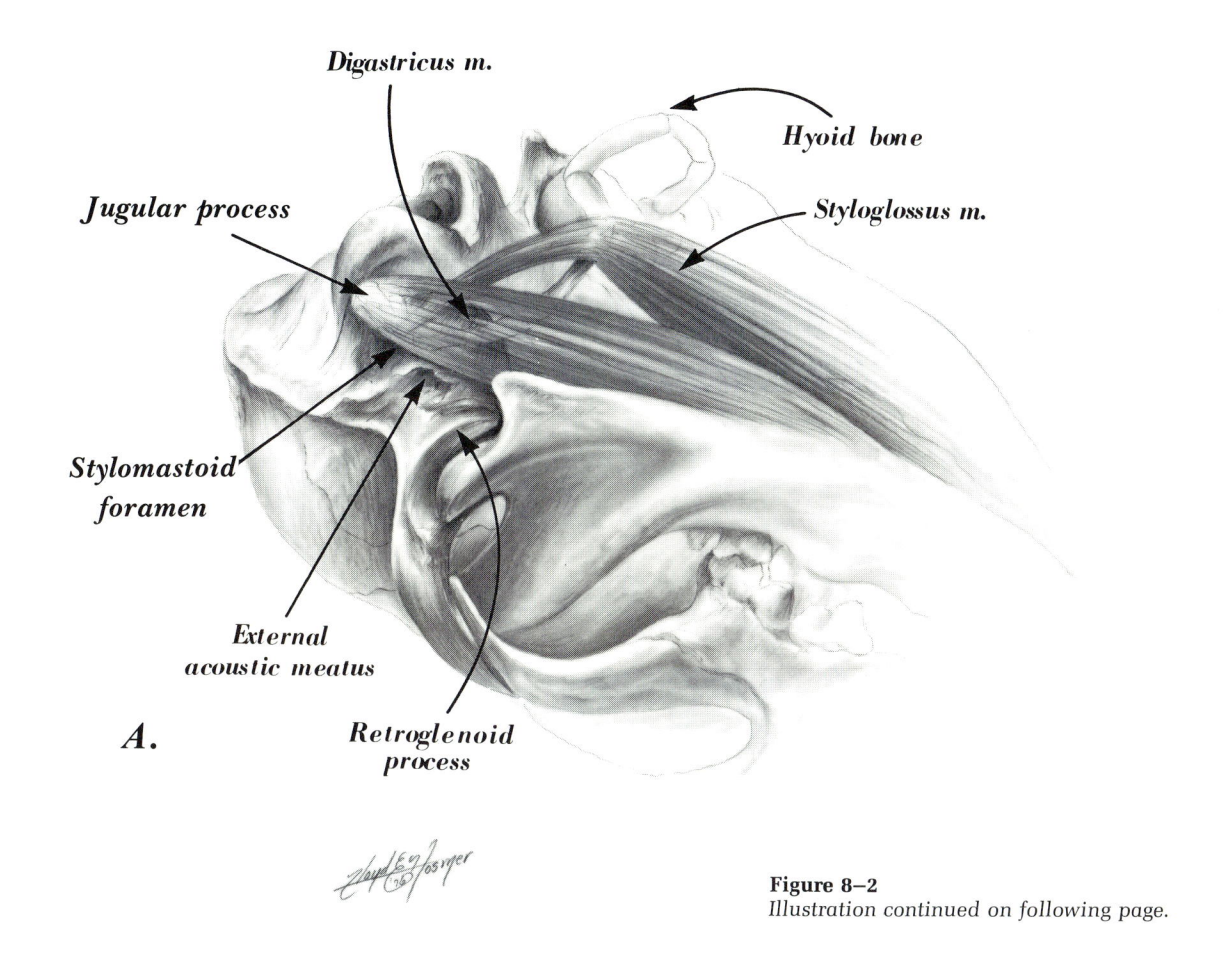

Figure 8–2
Illustration continued on following page.

Details of Procedure

Figure 8–2A. Continue the incision through the subcutaneous tissue until the digastricus muscle is exposed. The mylohyoid muscle is overlying the digastricus muscle and must be incised. Bluntly dissect between the digastricus muscle and the more medial styloglossus and hyoglossus muscles. Avoid damaging the large hyoglossal nerve, salivary ducts from the mandibular and sublingual glands, and carotid arteries.

The osseous bulla is located by palpating the muscular process of the basioccipital and stylohyoid bones located just lateral to the bulla.

NOTES:

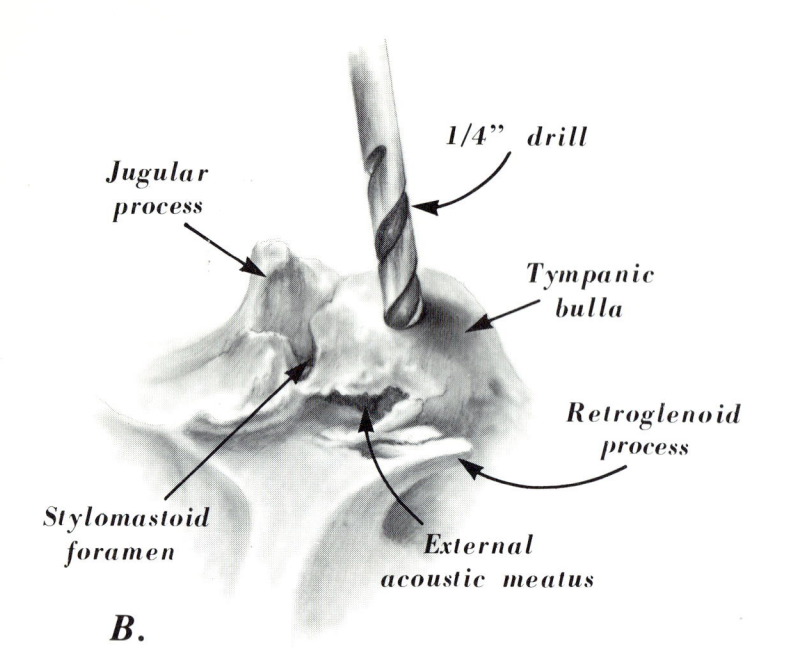

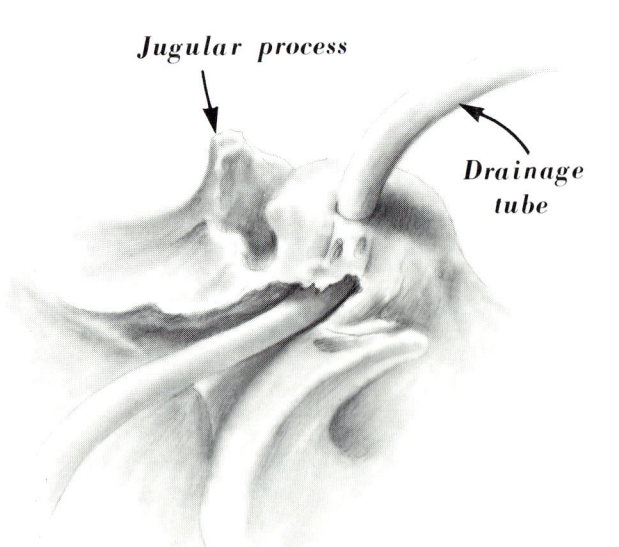

Figure 8–2 Continued

Figure 8–2B. After palpating and identifying the bulla, the self-retaining retractors are inserted to separate the digastricus and styloglossus muscles. The drill bit is used to open the ventral bulla. Additional exposure may be required, and a bone rongeur should be used to enlarge the ventral opening.

Additional treatment depends upon the cause of the problem. Foreign bodies are removed, and granulation or neoplastic tissue is excised. With purulent material, adequate drainage is provided by inserting a tube through the bulla, out the tympanic membrane, and through the external ear canal.

Figure 8–2C. A ¼-inch Steinmann pin with a hole drilled in one end is inserted through the external ear canal and the tympanum. A piece of suture material is passed through the hole in the pin and through the drainage tubing to be used. The pin is pulled back through the external ear canal pulling the tubing along.

Figure 8–2D. Bacterial cultures and histopathology samples are taken from the open bulla. Fenestration of the tube allows for the flushing of appropriate solutions to hasten recovery.

Closure of the incision involves suturing the mylohyoid muscle, subcutaneous tissue, and skin. The tubing is affixed to the ventral and otic skin with horizontal mattress sutures.

Leave the drainage tube in place for approximately five days. Use of the bulla osteotomy should be reserved for chronic, unresponsive patients. It provides relief of symptoms in most cases, but occasionally, a patient is not helped by this surgery.

NOTES: *(Continued)*

Postoperative Considerations

Lavage may be performed through the inserted tubing. This tubing is usually removed after five to seven days. Appropriate antibiotics are administered systemically in the presence of infection.

8–3 CERVICAL DISK FENESTRATION

Wayne E. Wingfield

Indications

Ventral fenestration of the cervical intervertebral disks is indicated with the protrusions of these disks, in cervical spondylopathy patients, in spinal fusion procedures, occasionally in cervical trauma patients, and during ventral cervical decompressive procedures.

Anesthesia

Intubation of all patients undergoing cervical disk fenestration is manditory. Choice of anesthetics is according to the surgeon's personal preference, but caution should be exercised in the use of neuromuscular blocking agents. With these agents, the spinal cord will be unresponsive to iatrogenic trauma.

Patient Postioning

The patient is positioned in dorsal recumbency, with padding placed beneath the neck to slightly arch the neck toward the surgeon. Tape is placed over the mandible to secure the head and to help maintain the neck positioning. The forelegs are pulled caudally and tied in place.

Operative Preparation

Specialized Instruments. A claw-type dental tartar scraper is used to fenestrate the cervical disks. This tartar scraper is first ground to make its width more narrow and then is blunted slightly. Because this is done, the instrument may be utilized in the small to larger breeds of dogs.

Use of a self-retaining retractor will facilitate good surgical exposure. Examples of adequate retractors include the Frazier, Weitlaner, hinged-Weitlaner, and Beckman retractors.

Incision and Exposure

A midventral cervical skin incision is made from the larynx to the manubrium of the sternum. Better asepsis will be afforded if the surgeon sews in water-repellent drapes to avoid potential skin contamination during the operative procedure.

Details of Procedure

Figure 8–3A. The skin incision is carried through the subcutis to expose the paired sternohyoideus muscles. These muscles form a ventral covering over the trachea. At the caudal portion of the incision, the paired sternomastoideus muscles overlie the sternohyoideus muscles.

Figure 8–3B. The paired bellies of the sternohyoideus muscles are separated along the midline, exposing the underlying trachea, esophagus, and carotid sheaths. A self-retaining retractor is inserted to retract the esophagus and left carotid sheath to the left and the trachea and right carotid sheath to the right.

At this point in the procedure, the surgeon must identify landmarks to locate appropriate intervertebral spaces. The common landmarks are the wings of the atlas (C-1), the large transverse processes of C-6, and the direction of the muscle fibers of the longus colli muscles.

There is no intervertebral disk located at the C-1 to C-2 intervertebral space. To palpate

Cervical Disc Fenestration

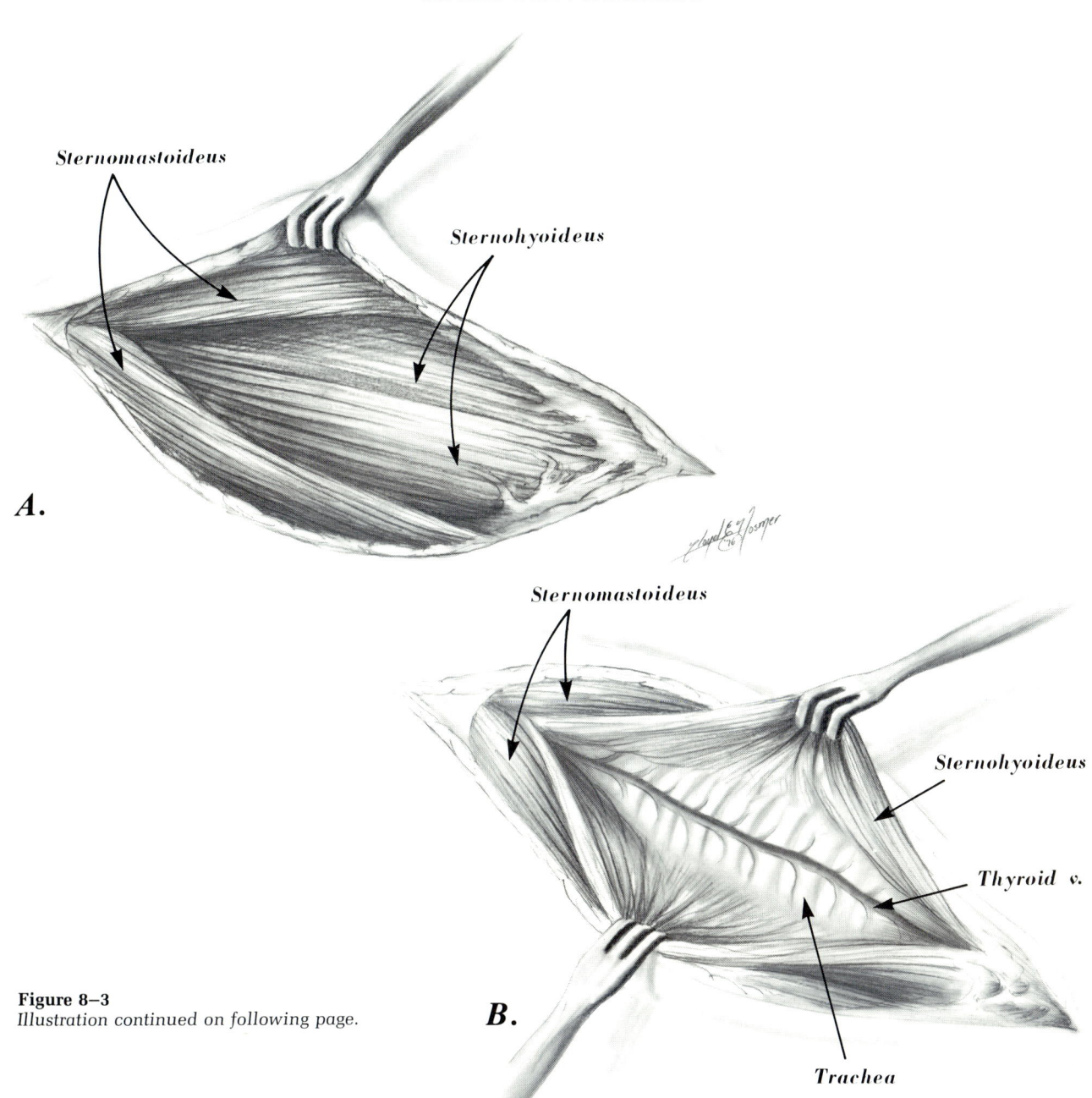

A.
Sternomastoideus
Sternohyoideus

B.
Sternomastoideus
Sternohyoideus
Thyroid v.
Trachea

Figure 8–3
Illustration continued on following page.

the wings of C-1, one must gently insert a finger under the skin until the C-1 wings are palpated and then carefully count backwards to the C-2 to C-3 space. A large ventral tubercle is palpated on C-1.

A better landmark is the easily palpated C-6 transverse processes. These large processes extend ventrally, and immediately cranial to these processes is the C-5 to C-6 intervertebral space.

NOTES:

Cervical Disc Fenestration

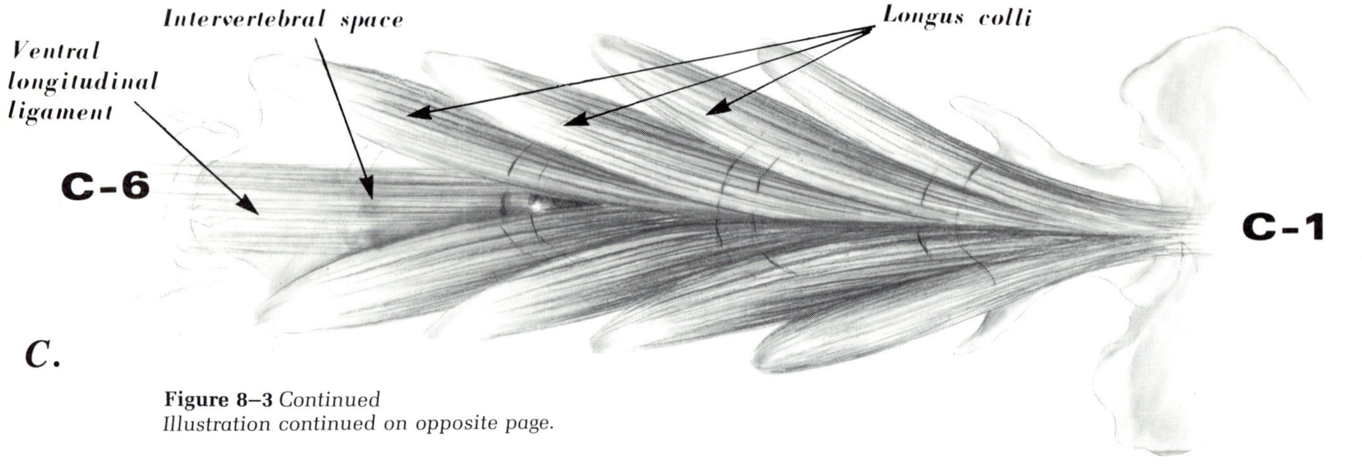

Figure 8–3 Continued
Illustration continued on opposite page.

Figure 8–3C. The muscle fibers of the longus colli form a cranially oriented "V" shape. Each ventral tubercle located on the caudal, ventral aspect of the adjacent cervical vertebrae serves as a point of insertion for the longus colli muscles.

Using the two lateral processes and the centrally located ventral tubercle, the position of the intervertebral disk may be located. The longus colli muscles cover the ventral entrance to the intervertebral space and must be retracted. Using a mosquito hemostat, the longus colli muscles are separated just caudal to the ventral tubercle. By forcing the hemostat downward, the muscles may be retracted with minimal hemorrhage. Following retraction, the ventral longitudinal ligament is exposed as a white, shiny structure.

NOTES: (Continued)

Cervical Disc Fenestration

Ventral tubercle

Annulus fibrosus

D.

Transverse process

Figure 8–3 Continued
Illustration continued on following page.

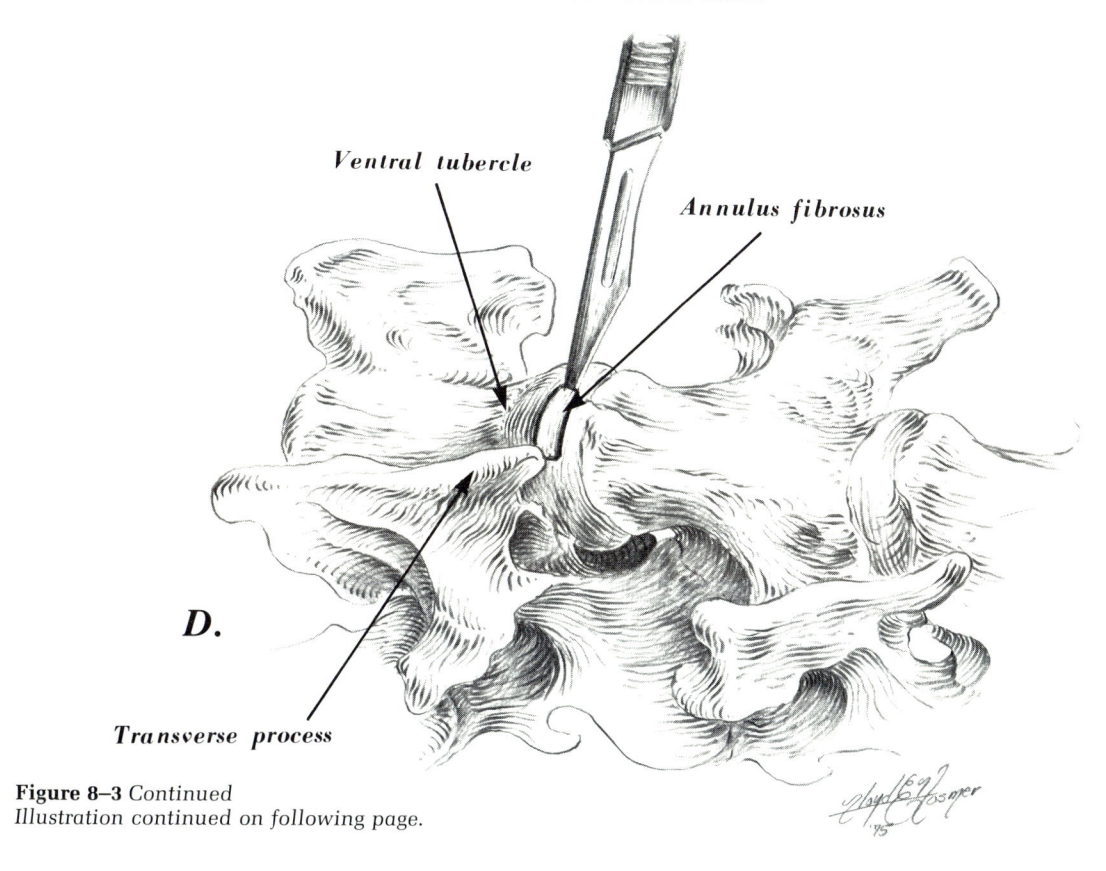

<u>Figure 8–3D.</u> A No. 11 Bard-Parker blade is used to excise a small window in the ventral longitudinal ligament and the ventral annulus fibrosus.

NOTES: *(Continued)*

Cervical Disc Fenestration

Nucleus pulposus

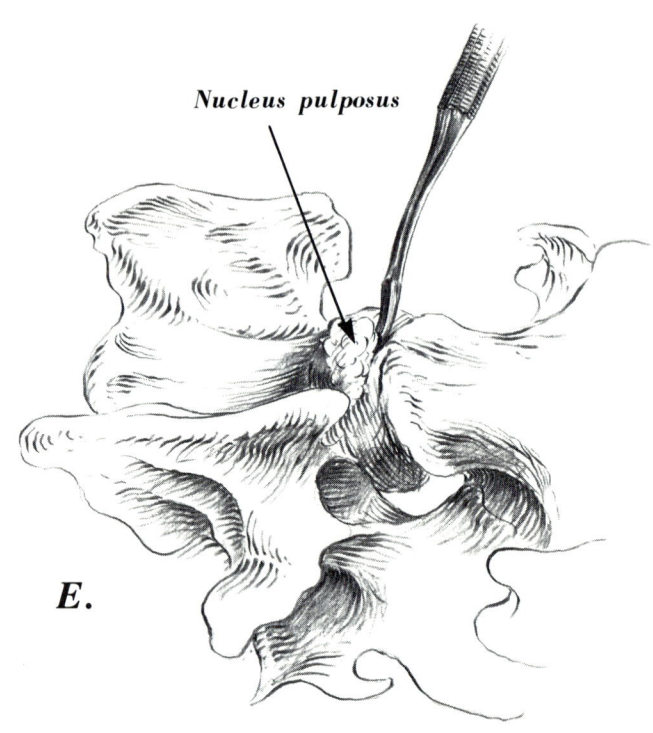

E.

Figure 8–3 Continued

Figure 8–3E. Using a modified curved tartar scraper, the nucleus pulposus is removed. Care is taken to avoid pressure directed toward the spinal cord. Intervertebral spaces C-2 to C-3, C-3 to C-4, C-4 to C-5, and C-5 to C-6 are normally fenestrated.

Should hemorrhage be encountered in retracting the longus colli muscles, the source is generally the laceration of the muscle fibers. Packing of the area with a gauze sponge while continuing with other fenestrations will usually result in adequate hemostasis upon returning to the area.

The incision is closed with simple interrupted sutures in the fascia of the sternohyoideus muscles using 3-0 or 4-0 chromic catgut. The separated sternomastoideus muscles are closed similarly, and the subcutis is closed with a subcuticular pattern and 4-0 catgut. The skin is closed with a nonabsorbable suture material and a simple interrupted pattern.

Postoperative Considerations

With postoperative pain, analgesics should be employed. If disk material was not forced into the spinal canal and an excessive amount of disk material was not present prior to surgery, relief of symptoms is expected in 14 to 21 days.

NOTES: *(Continued)*

8-4 CERVICAL VENTRAL DECOMPRESSION

CHARLES WILLIAM BETTS

Indications

This procedure is necessary to relieve spinal nerve root pain for cord pressure in the cervical region caused by extruded disk material. In some dogs, a surprising amount of disk material can be in the cervical spinal canal with minor effect. In other dogs, it may cause quadriplegia. The disk material in the canal is not removed by routine fenestration, and cervical ventral decompression will often be successful when a fenestration has failed.

Patient Positioning

The dog is placed in dorsal recumbency, with the rear legs extended caudally.

Anesthesia

General anesthesia, as discussed in Procedure 8-1, is required.

Operative Preparation

Special Draping. Four corner draping is used to expose the ventral cervical midline.

Specialized Instruments. Gelpi retractors, pediatric Beckman retractors, an air drill and accessories, and suction are required.

Incision and Exposure

The excision and exposure are the same as those for cervical disk fenestration to the point of identifying the disk. Once the correct disk is localized, the longus colli muscles are separated by sharp dissection through the ventral midline over the length of the two adjacent vertebrae. Subperiosteal reflection is used to reflect the muscles laterally, and the retractors are placed caudal and cranial to the disk. The insertions of the longus colli muscles are then transected.

Figure 8–4

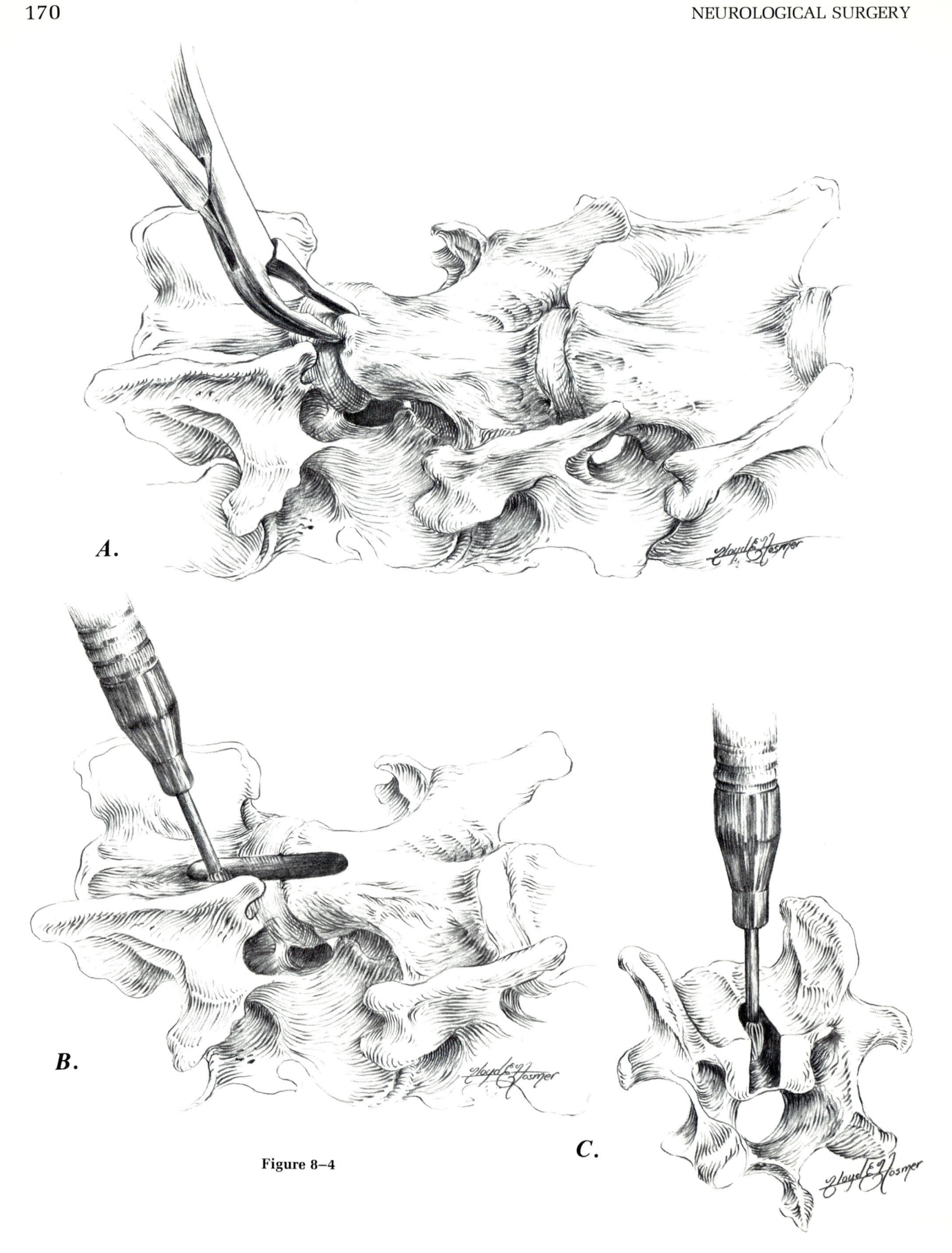

Details of Procedure

Figure 8–4A. The disk can be fenestrated as illustrated, or the ventral slot can be made without fenestration. The caudal tubercle is rongeured off prior to use of the air drill.

Figure 8–4B. A longitudinal slot is burred through the vertebral body. The vertebral vein often encountered about halfway through the bone is easily plugged with bone wax.

Figure 8–4C. Once the inner cortical shelf is reached, small rongeurs and a bone curette or tartar scraper may be used to remove the bone. The decompression should be widest over the disk space, as the vertebral sinuses diverge here. The sinuses should be avoided to prevent hemorrhage. Gelfoam or a muscle plug can be used to stop sinus hemorrhage with occasional success. The dorsal annulus fibrosus and dorsal longitudinal ligament can be incised (carefully) with a No. 11 Bard-Parker blade to provide access into the spinal canal. Disk material is removed with small mosquito hemostats or suitable thumb forceps.

A few interrupted sutures (3-0 Dexon) are placed in the longus colli muscles. The rest of the closure is the same as that for cervical disk fenestration.

Postoperative Considerations

Strict confinement is necessary. Some dogs will require a soft, padded neck bandage to restrict neck rotation. Many animals will do amazingly well 24 to 48 hours after surgery. They should be weaned off steroids 24 to 48 hours after surgery. Wound management is routine.

NOTES:

8–5 THORACOLUMBAR HEMILAMINECTOMY AND INTERVERTEBRAL DISK FENESTRATION

CHARLES WILLIAM BETTS

Indications

Hemilaminectomy has proven to be an effective technique for spinal cord decompression and for removal of extruded disk material in dogs with intervertebral disk disease. Surgical candidates must be properly selected. Fenestration of the involved disk should prevent further extrusion of disk material. Fenestration of adjacent disks considered statistically prone to rupture may be beneficial as a means of prophylaxis. Select cases with unrelenting or frequent episodes of pain may respond to prophylactic fenestration without decompression.

Anesthesia

General anesthesia is required.

Preoperative Preparation

The dog should be clipped over the dorsal midline to the junction of the proximal and middle third of the body. The area clipped should extend from the proximal third of the thorax to the tuber coxae.

Patient Positioning

The dog is placed in ventral recumbency. The vision of the assistant is improved by tilting the dog 20 to 30 degrees toward the assistant.

Operative Preparation

Special Draping. Double four corner draping is encouraged. Steridrapes may be placed over the skin. I prefer to sew in waterproof drapes to the subcutaneous tissue.

Specialized Instruments. Instruments suggested include a Weitlaner or Beckman pediatric self-retaining retractor, a Gelpi self-retaining retractor, a medium and a small bone rongeur of good quality (3 to 5 mm bite), a Hall air drill (or similar product) — this item is expensive and optional, or a Michelle trephine. Nerve root retractors and tartar scrapers are necessary to remove disk material from the canal and for disk fenestration. A good periosteal elevator (Adson) is valuable.

Incision and Exposure

A dorsal midline incision over the dorsal spinous processes is made from T-9 to T-10 to

L-4 to L-5 if a prophylactic fenestration is to be done. If only a decompression is to be done, the incision should extend two vertebrae cranial and caudal to the involved interspace.

HEMILAMINECTOMY

After the skin and subcutaneous layer are incised, the thoracolumbar fascia is incised just lateral (1 to 2 mm) to the tip of the dorsal spinous process. Subperiosteal reflection of the multifidus muscle from the dorsal spines from caudal to cranial is done next. Tendinous insertions of the multifidus lumborum should be incised adjacent to the dorsal spine below the supraspinous ligament as each successive dorsal spine is exposed. The origin of the multifidus muscle at the cranial aspect of each respective mammillary process is then incised starting at the caudal facet and proceeding cranially after reflecting the musculature with the periosteal elevator. If necessary, the insertion of the longissimus muscle can be transected 3 to 5 mm from the accessory process to facilitate lateral retraction of the epaxial musculature. Care should be taken to avoid severing the small artery beneath the tendinous insertion. I prefer to fracture the accessory process at its base with a bone rongeur and then depress it ventrally. Proper exposure of the bone provides a neat, clean field hampered by minimal hemorrhage. The self-retaining retractors can be placed at this time. The involved interspace is identified by identifying the dorsal costotransverse ligament attaching the thirteenth rib to the vertebral body of T-13. A hypodermic needle can also be "walked" up the rib until its position correlates with the dorsal spine of T-13 if this area is not exposed.

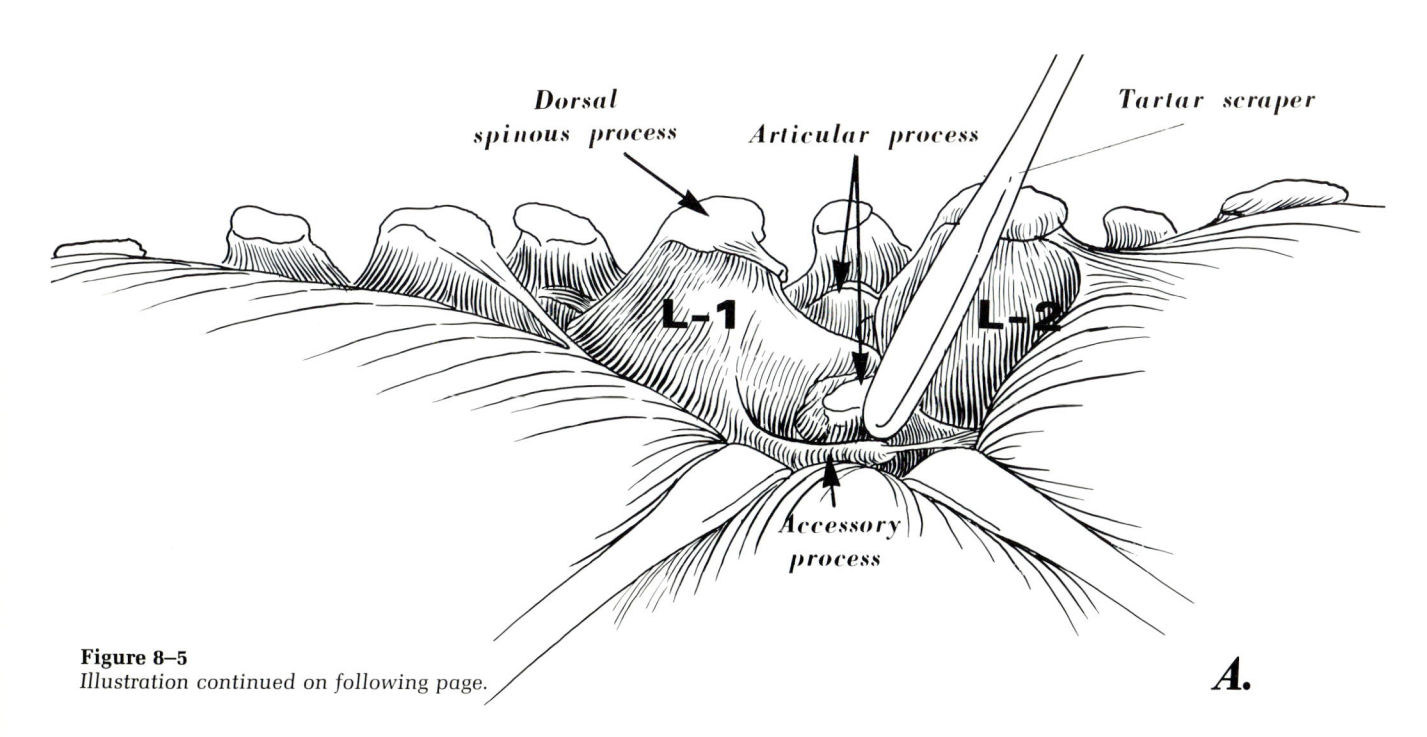

Details of Procedure

Figures 8–5A and 8–5B. The articular facet over the involved disk is now removed using a bone rongeur or bone cutter. Next a window is cut in the bone using an air drill. If

NOTES:

Figure 8–5
Illustration continued on following page.

A.

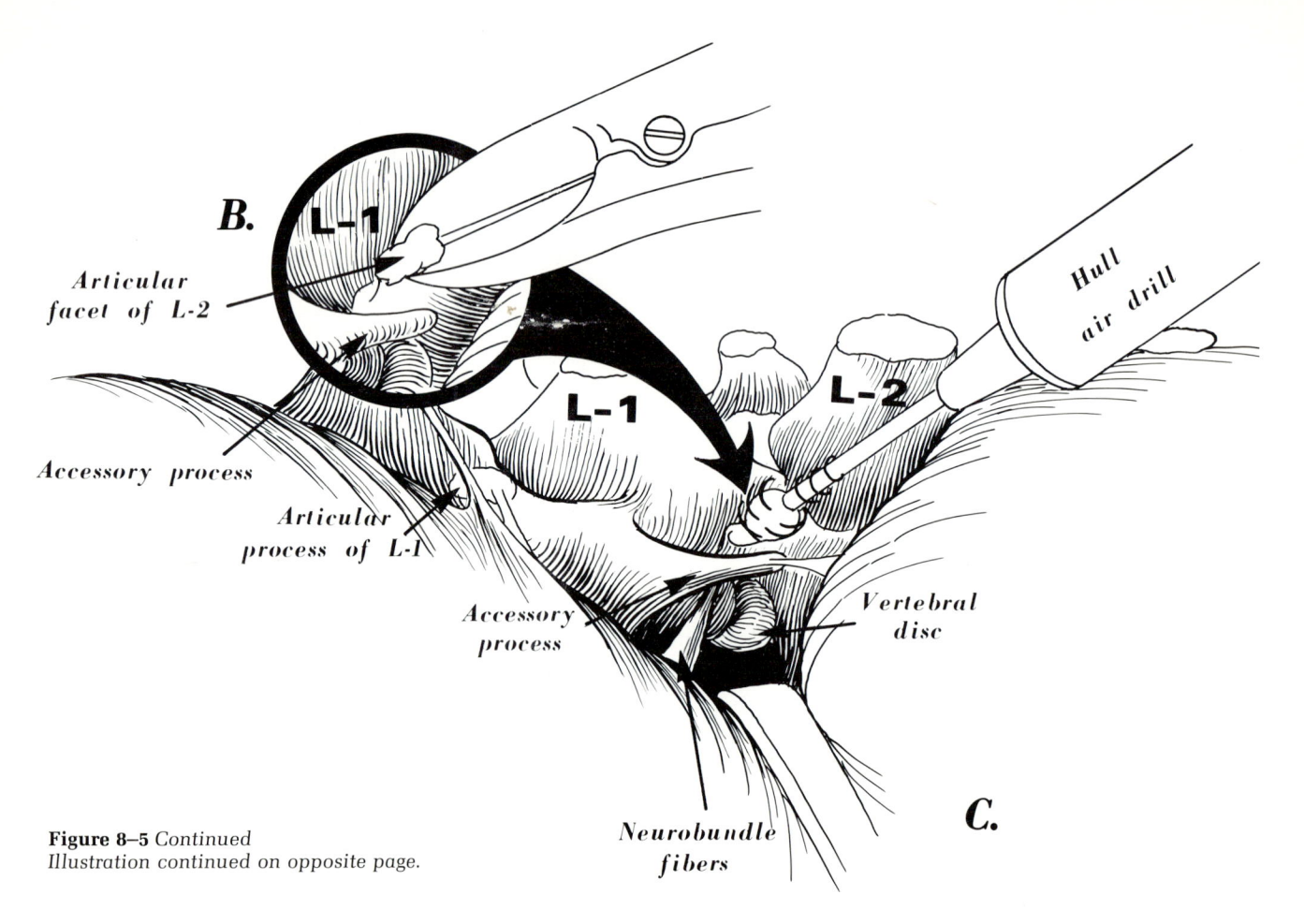

Figure 8-5 *Continued*
Illustration continued on opposite page.

a trephine is used, the articular facet may be used to provide a base for the trephine. Color changes are rated carefully as the air drill cuts away the bone. As the depth of the window increases, the color of the bone changes from white outer cortical bone to red medullary bone and finally to an inner shelf of white cortical bone. At this point caution must be exercised, as the spinal cord may be displaced toward the endosteal side of the inner cortex. It is possible to brush the bone away with the air drill to the level of the endosteum, which usually has a slight purplish tinge. The final layer of inner cortical bone and/or endosteum is carefully removed with small bone rongeurs to expose the spinal cord. The decompression should extend from the caudal limit of the cranial facet of the cranial vertebra to the cranial limit of the caudal facet of the caudal vertebra. It is now possible to examine the spinal cord and remove disk material from the spinal canal.

Figure 8-5C. Fenestration of the involved disk can be done by reflecting the longissimus muscle from the proximal, cranial aspect of the transverse process to identify the intervertebral disk immediately cranial to the junction of the transverse process and the vertebral body. Care should be exercised to avoid the neurovascular bundle emerging from the intervertebral foramen slightly cranial and dorsal to the disk below the accessory process. The procedure is the same in the thoracic region, except that the rib is used for a landmark instead of the transverse process.

Figure 8-5D. Fenestration may be accomplished through a muscle separation technique. In the lumbar region, the mammillary process is palpated. The lumbar fascia is incised over the mammillary process, which exposes the muscle plane between the multifidus muscle dorsally and the longissimus muscle ventrally. The articular process

Figure 8–5 Continued

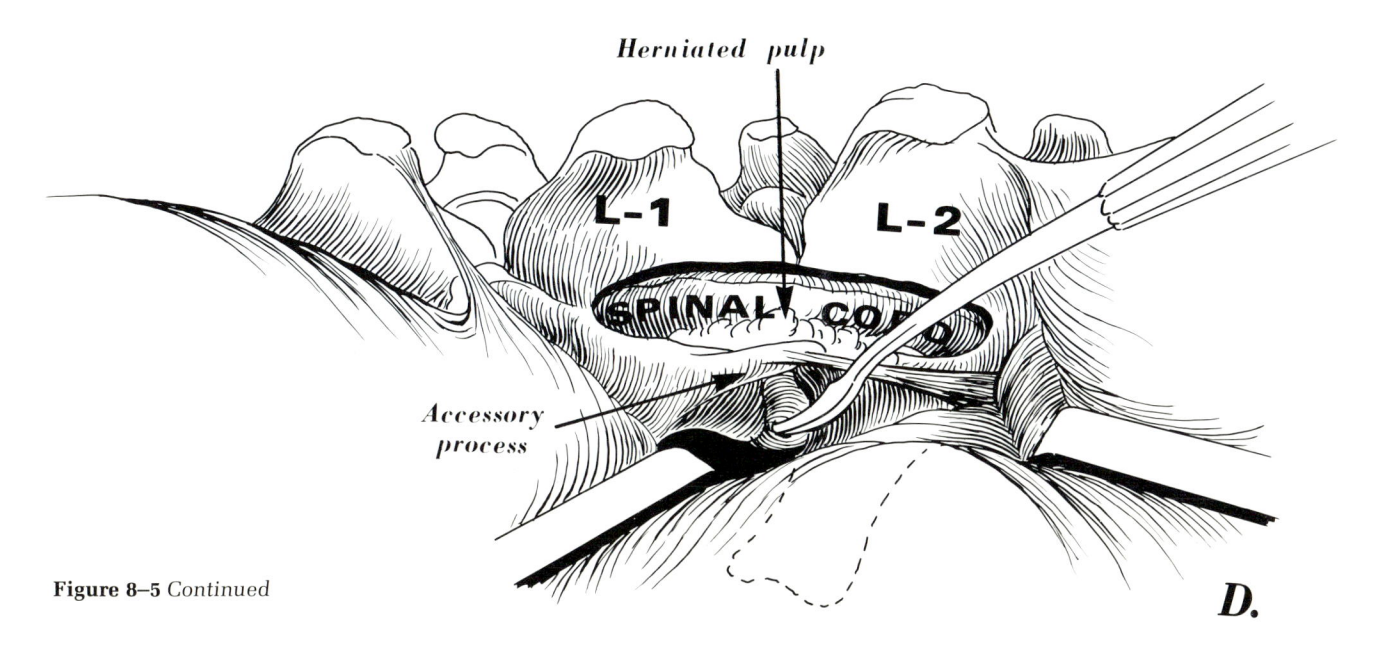

is palpated, and the musculature is subperiosteally reflected ventrally from the lateral aspect of the articular process to the accessory process. The tendinous insertion of the longissimus muscle on the accessory process can be seen. The periosteal elevator is moved laterally over the insertion on the accessory process and gently pushed through the underlying muscle to the transverse process. Slight lateral reflection of the longissimus muscle exposes the transverse process and a retractor (Senn or Matthieu) is placed ventral to the accessory process using medial dorsal reflection of the insertion of the longissimus muscle. This exposes the junction of the transverse process, with the vertebral body and the dorsolateral aspect of the intervertebral disk immediately cranial to this junction. The fenestration is easily accomplished using a hypodermic needle, a No. 11 Bard-Parker blade, and a tartar scraper.

I modify this approach slightly in the thoracic region by separating ventral to the longissimus muscle over the rib. The rib is exposed to its attachment on the vertebral body, with the overlying musculature being reflected dorsally. The disk is cranial and slightly ventral to the dorsal costotransverse ligament and is not as easily located as in the lumbar area. Having a skeleton available for examination is helpful.

Postoperative Considerations

The important aspects of the convalescent period for back cases are the complications that can arise. Urinary function and micturition must be monitored closely. The dog should be kept in a small area and should receive supervised exercise. Paralyzed animals should be on a padded surface or a grate to minimize pressure sores, and they must be kept clean. Routine wound management is in order, and a pressure bandage may be of benefit to reduce the possibility of seroma formation and to keep the incision clean.

NOTES: *(Continued)*

176　　　　　　　　　　　　　　　　　　　　　　　　　　　　　　　　　　　　　ORTHOPEDIC SURGERY

Approach to Shoulder

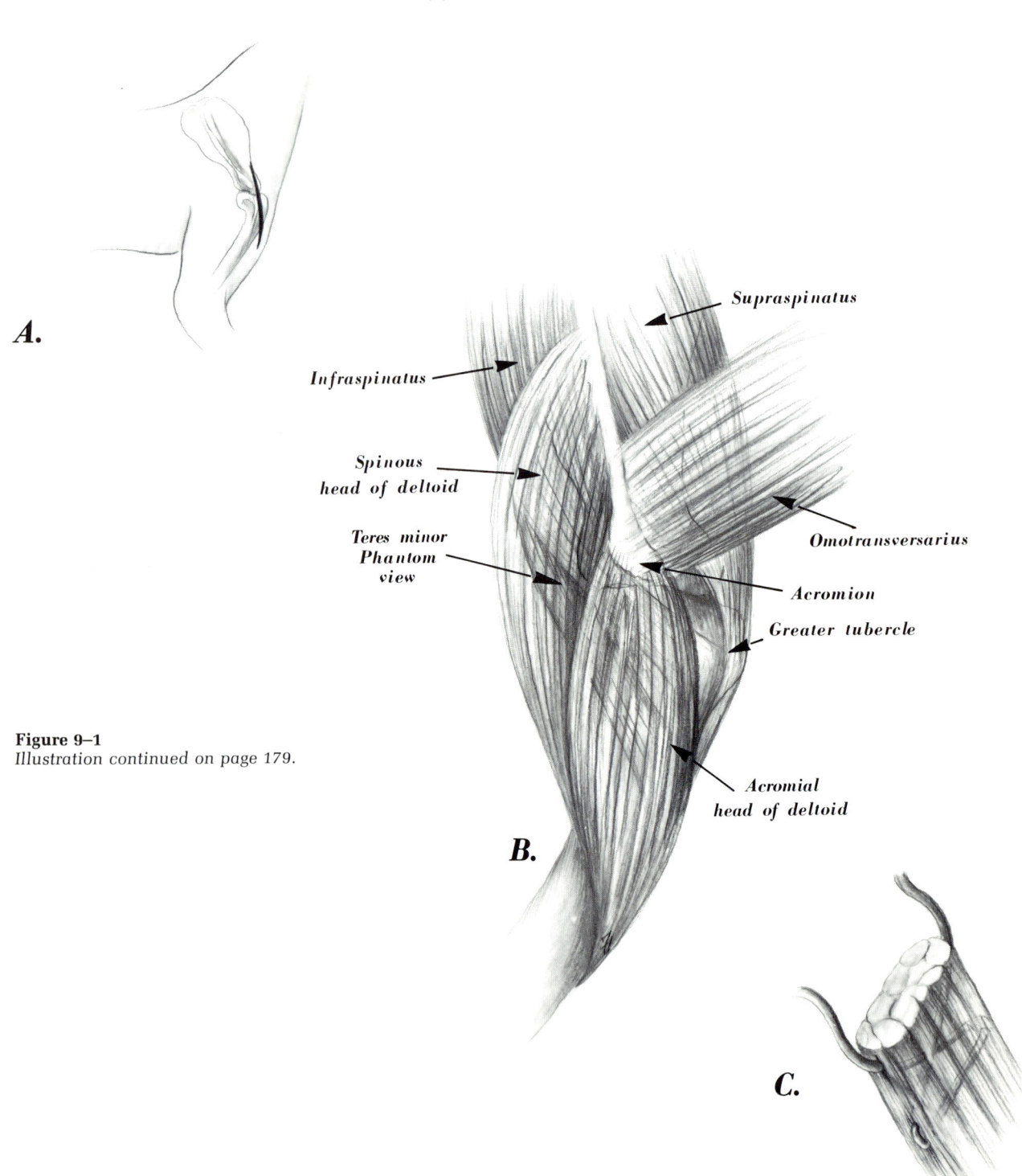

A.

Supraspinatus

Infraspinatus

Spinous head of deltoid

Teres minor Phantom view

Omotransversarius

Acromion

Greater tubercle

Acromial head of deltoid

B.

C.

Figure 9–1
Illustration continued on page 179.

ORTHOPEDIC SURGERY CHAPTER 9

9–1 APPROACH TO THE SHOULDER

Roger A. Rehmel

Indications

The following lateral approach to the canine scapulohumeral joint is utilized primarily for surgical correction of osteochondritis.

Anesthesia

General anesthesia is required.

Patient Positioning

The patient is placed in lateral recumbency.

Operative Preparation

Special Draping. Draping should allow for manipulation of the entire limb.
Specialized Instruments. For correction of osteochondritis, a pair of Army-Navy retractors and a bone curette are necessary.

Incision and Exposure

Figure 9–1A. A curved incision is begun from just craniodorsal to the acromion, crossing over the scapulohumeral joint, and ending approximately at the deltoid tuberosity.

Figure 9–1B. The lateral aspect of the canine shoulder joint is overlaid by deep and superficial musculature that must be dealt with properly to achieve the desired exposure. The ventral border of the omotransversarius muscle is exposed, and its belly is cut transversely to expose the acromion. The deltoid muscle is made up of an acromial and a spinous portion. The cranial boundary of the acromial head of the deltoid muscle is surgically delineated. Its caudal limit is bluntly separated from the fibers of the spinous head of the deltoid muscle by passing a finger underneath the acromial head and palpating for the natural weakness between the two muscular heads. Once located, this division is bluntly extended ventrodorsally.

Figure 9–1C. A partial Bunnell stitch pattern using nonabsorbable suture material is preplaced in the tendon of origin of the acromial head, and tenotomy is performed with a surgical knife.

NOTES:

Figure 9–1D. The acromial head is reflected ventrally, and an Army-Navy retractor is positioned to displace the spinous head caudally. The underlying infraspinous and teres minor muscle insertions are now apparent. Partial Bunnell suture patterns are placed in the tendinous insertion of the infraspinous muscle, and sharp tenotomy is performed. The infraspinous tendon and associated muscles are retracted caudodorsally so that the joint capsule is adequately exposed. The teres minor muscle is carefully delineated for later retraction.

Figure 9–1E. The joint is identified, and a stab incision is made with a surgical knife. This opening is then extended with Mayo scissors to expose the articular surface of the humeral head.

NOTES: *(Continued)*

ORTHOPEDIC SURGERY

Approach to Shoulder

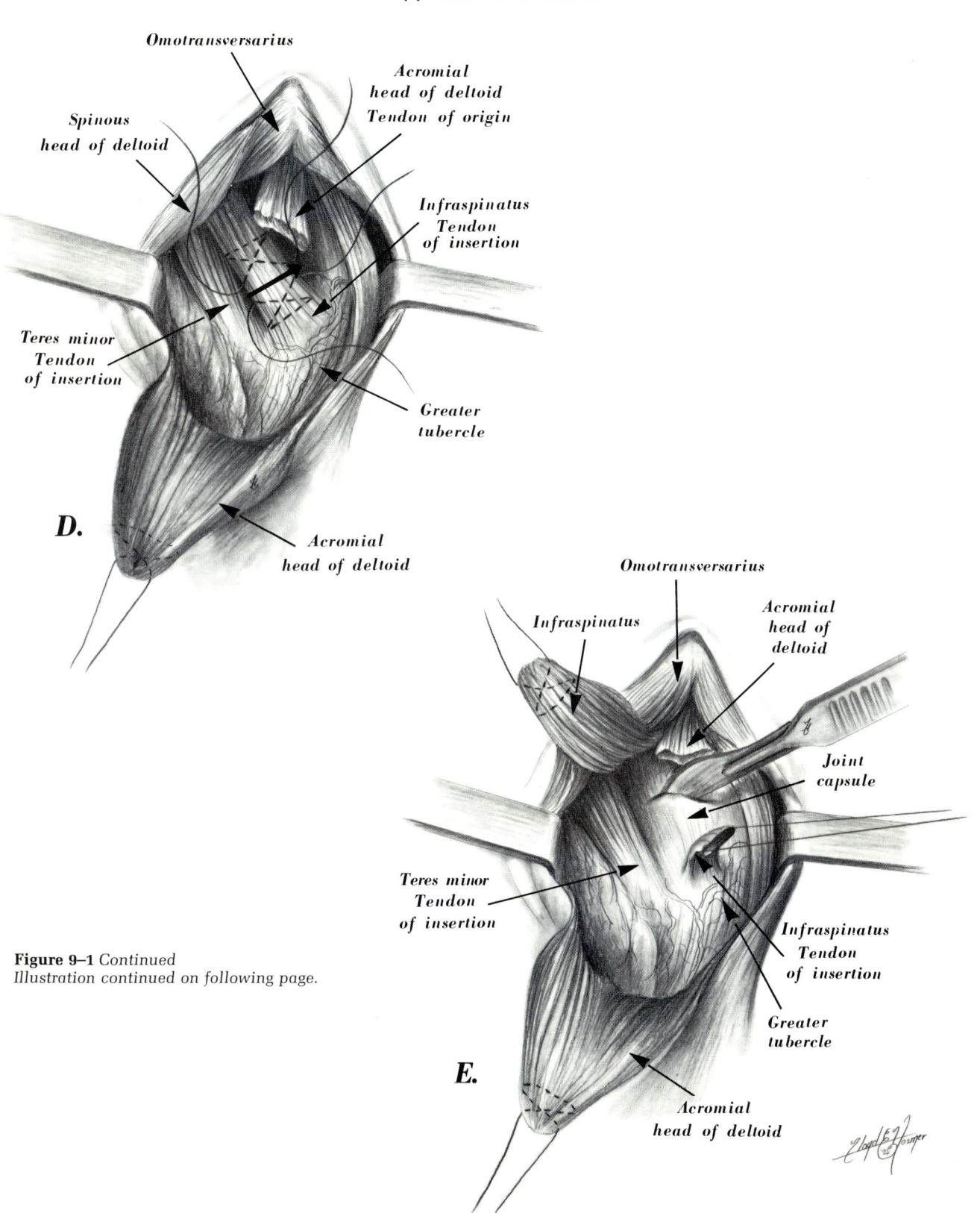

Figure 9–1 Continued
Illustration continued on following page.

Approach to Shoulder

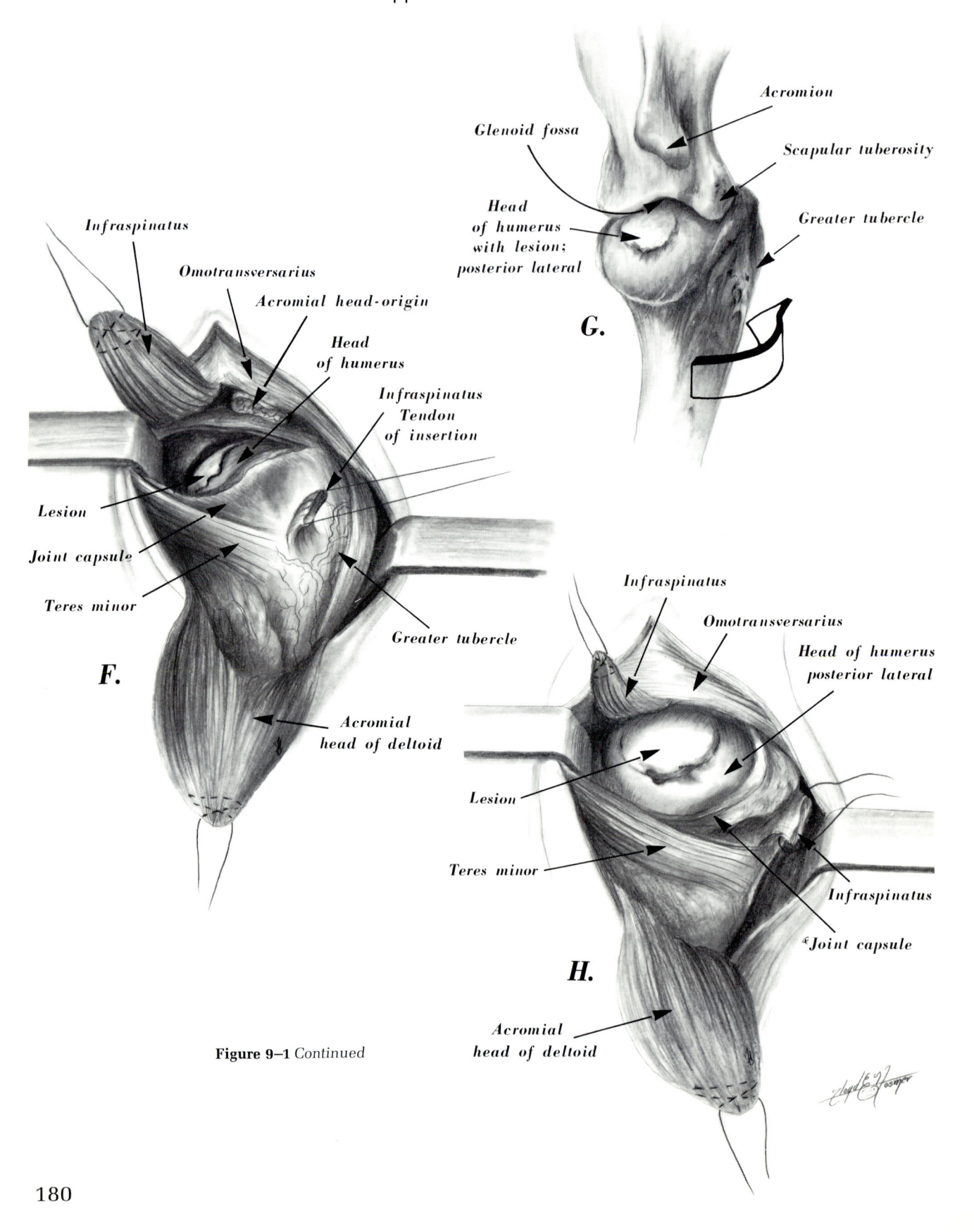

Figure 9–1 Continued

Details of Procedure

Figure 9–1F. Exposure of the humeral head is enhanced by the insertion of an Army-Navy retractor into the caudal joint pouch. This simultaneously retracts the teres minor muscle, the spinous head of the deltoid muscle, and the skin from the surgical field. Many clinical lesions of osteochondritis are partially visible at this stage.

Figures 9–1G and 9–1H. Osteochondritis lesions involving the humeral head are better visualized and exposed for curettage by internally rotating the humerus 90 degrees.

For closure, horizontal mattress sutures of nonabsorbable material are preplaced in the joint capsule and tied. The infraspinous tendon is reunited by externally rotating the humerus and tying the opposing arms of the preplaced partial Bunnell sutures (nonabsorbable material of large size). The acromial head of the deltoid muscle is returned to its origin by placing a mattress stitch utilizing the arms of the preplaced suture. The remainder of the closure is routine, with special diligence in closing all dead space.

Postoperative Considerations

Sutures are removed in seven to ten days. Postoperatively, the patient is cage-confined for the first five to seven days, followed by very limited activity for a month.

NOTES: *(Continued)*

9–2 INTRAMEDULLARY PINNING OF THE HUMERUS

Thomas Earley

Indications

Intramedullary pinning of a fractured humerus is an acceptable means of internal fixation. With a fractured humerus, *always* check radial nerve function prior to surgery.

Anesthesia

General anesthesia is required.

Patient Positioning

The animal is placed in lateral or dorsal recumbency in preparation for a lateral approach to the humerus.

Operative Preparation

Special Draping. An impermeable drape is used to cover the paw and extends to the elbow.

Specialized Instruments. Instruments required are a Gigli saw, an intramedullary pin, and a hand chuck.

Incision and Exposure

Intramedullary pinning of humeral diaphyseal fractures is accomplished through a lateral approach. Distal diaphyseal fractures are approached between the triceps and brachial muscles; mid-diaphyseal and proximal-diaphyseal fractures are approached between the brachial and biceps brachii muscles. With both approaches, identify and protect the radial nerve and cephalic vein.

Details of Procedure

Intramedullary pinning can be accomplished through antegrade or retrograde introduction of the pin. The insertion site for antegrade pinning is on or just distal to the greater tubercle (Fig. 9–2A). Because the intramedullary canal is in direct line with the medial condyle, an appropriate sized pin may be seated into the medial condyle (Fig. 9–2B). However, a pin that is large enough to fill the intramedullary canal at the mid-diaphysis will not fit into the medial condyle (Fig. 9–2C) but will stop just proximal to the supratrochlear foramen.

Closure of the surgical wound involves suturing of the muscle fascia. Subcutaneous tissues and skin are closed routinely.

Postoperative Considerations

Restricted exercise is maintained for four to six weeks. When the fracture site is healed, remove the intramedullary pin.

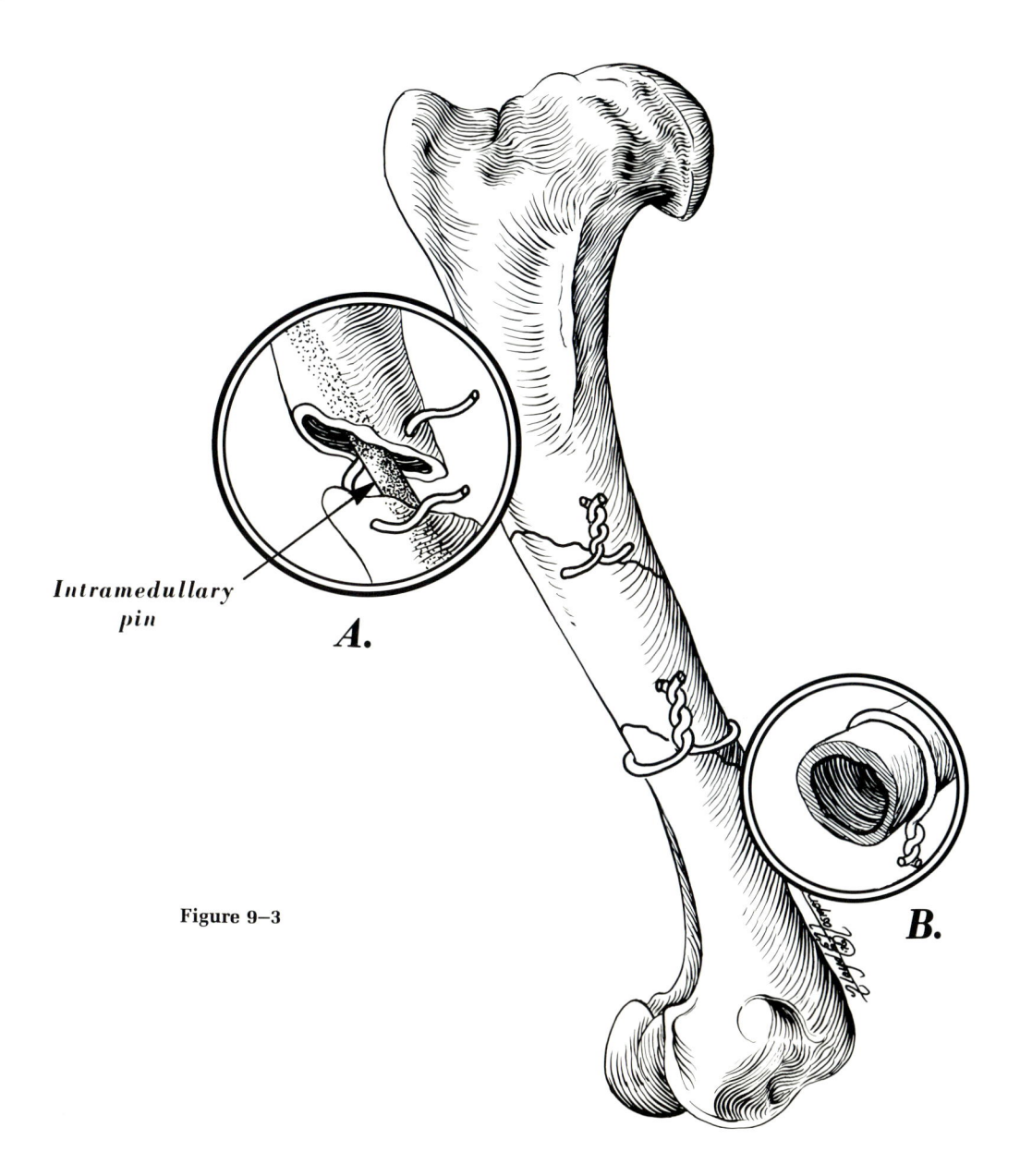

ORTHOPEDIC SURGERY 185

Intramedullary pin

A.

Figure 9–3

B.

NOTES:

9-4
TRANSOLECRANON APPROACH — TENSION BAND WIRING

Thomas Earley

Indications

Tension band wiring is used for fixation of avulsion fractures and for securing certain osteotomy fragments that have been produced in association with special surgical approaches. The purpose of this procedure is to perform an osteotomy of the olecranon and to secure it with a tension band wire.

Patient Positioning

The animal can be placed in either dorsal or lateral recumbency.

Anesthesia

General anesthesia is required.

Operative Preparation

Special Draping. An impermeable leg wrap should cover the paw and the distal third of the antebrachium.

Specialized Instruments. The instruments needed for this procedure are (1) a Gigli saw or an osteotome and mallet to perform the osteotomy; (2) appropriate size Kirschner wires or small Steinmann pins and orthopedic wire (20-gauge) for the tension band wire; (3) a hand chuck and a small pin cutter; and (4) a wire twister or large needle holder.

Incision and Exposure

A slightly curved skin incision that begins at the distal third of the humerus and extends to the proximal third of the antebrachium is made either just lateral or medial to the olecranon. The skin is reflected to expose the triceps tendon. The triceps tendon is defined as it inserts on the olecranon, and the ulnar nerve is identified medially.

Details of Procedure

Curved forceps are passed beneath the triceps tendon and just proximal to the anconeal process of the ulna. One end of the Gigli wire is grasped with the forceps, pulled beneath the triceps tendon, and used to osteotomize the olecranon (Fig. 9–4A). The correct osteotomy site is shown in Figure 9–4B. An osteotome and mallet can also be used to perform the osteotomy.

A 0.045-inch Kirschner wire (in a hand chuck) is used to make a transverse hole in the olecranon, approximately 3 to 4 cm distal to the osteotomy site, for passage of the orthopedic wire. Two Kirschner wires (or small Steinmann pins, depending on the size of bone fragment) are used to secure the osteotomized bone to the ulna, taking care not to drive the pins off the medial (concave) surface of the ulna. The Kirschner wires may be retrograded to insure accurate placement. The Kirschner wires are directed slightly cran-

ORTHOPEDIC SURGERY

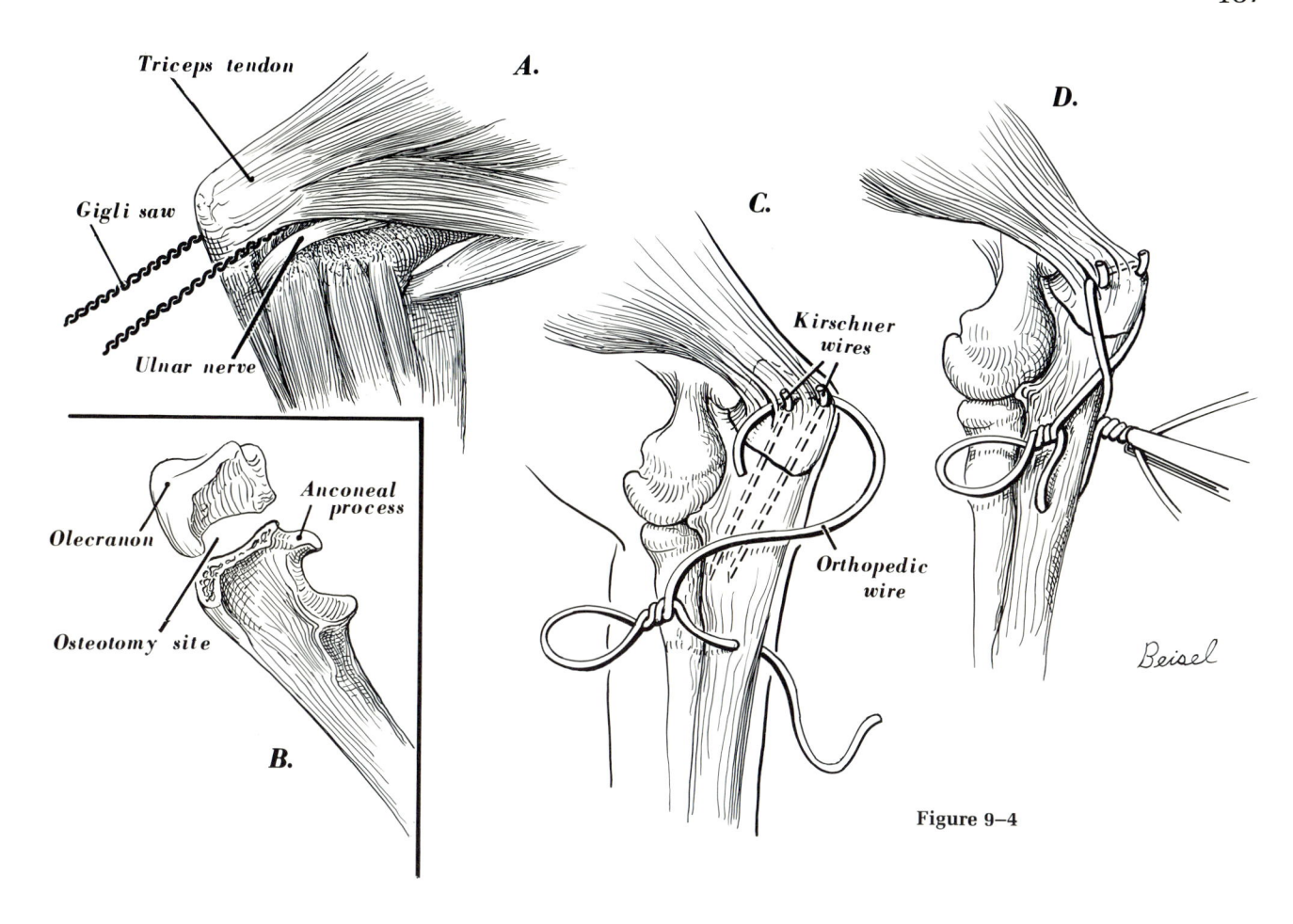

Figure 9-4

ially, and the proximal ends are turned cranially.

A twist is made in the wire, and the wire is directed as seen in Figure 9–4C. Another twist is made in the wire on the opposite side of the ulna, and alternate tightening insures even tension (Fig. 9–4D).

Subcutaneous and skin closures are routine.

Postoperative Considerations

Restricted activity for four to six weeks is recommended. Physical therapy (passive flexion and extension) of the elbow is recommended during the healing phase. There is usually no need to remove the tension band wire.

NOTES:

9–5 FRACTURED HUMERUS — LATERAL CONDYLE: LAG SCREW APPLICATION

THOMAS EARLEY

Indications

The lag screw principle is used when compression between two bone fragments is desired. This compression can be achieved with the use of partially threaded screws alone or with fully threaded screws in specially prepared drill holes.

Anesthesia

General anesthesia is required.

Patient Positioning

The dog may be placed in either lateral or dorsal recumbency.

Operative Preparation

Special Draping. An impermeable leg wrap should cover the paw and distal third of the antebrachium.

Specialized Instruments. The following instruments are required:

- osteotome and mallet
- Gigli saw
- drill bit
- depth gauge
- tap
- cancellous screw
- screw driver
- Kirschner wires
- orthopedic wire (20-gauge)
- hand chuck

Incision and Exposure

The incision and exposure are the same as for tension band wiring (Procedure 9–4). After osteotomizing the olecranon, the anconeus muscle is reflected laterally to expose the distal humerus. (Incise the attachment on the medial condylar ridge.) The lateral condyle of the humerus is osteotomized as in Figure 9–5A.

The first step in securing the lateral condyle is to drive a Kirschner wire across the condyles at a level just proximal to the epicondyles (Fig. 9–5B). This Kirschner wire prevents movement of the lateral condyle during the lag screw application and offers rotational stability postoperatively.

Details of Procedure

The following steps outline the procedure for lag screw fixation: (1) drill a hole through both condyles, entering just cranial and distal to the lateral epicondyle and exiting just cranial to the medial epicondyle (Fig. 9–5B). (2) Using a depth gauge, measure the length of the hole (Fig. 9–5C). (3) Tap (precutting the thread path for the screw) the drill hole (Fig. 9–5D). (4) Select the appropriate screw (cancellous screw) and tighten it in the drill hole (Fig. 9–5E). Make sure that the threads of the screw purchase entirely in the medial condyle to afford compression at the fracture site.

ORTHOPEDIC SURGERY

Closure, with the exception of suturing the medial border of anconeus muscle, is identical to the tension band wiring closure (Procedure 9–4).

Postoperative Considerations

Postoperative care is the same as that for the tension band wiring (Procedure 9–4).

NOTES:

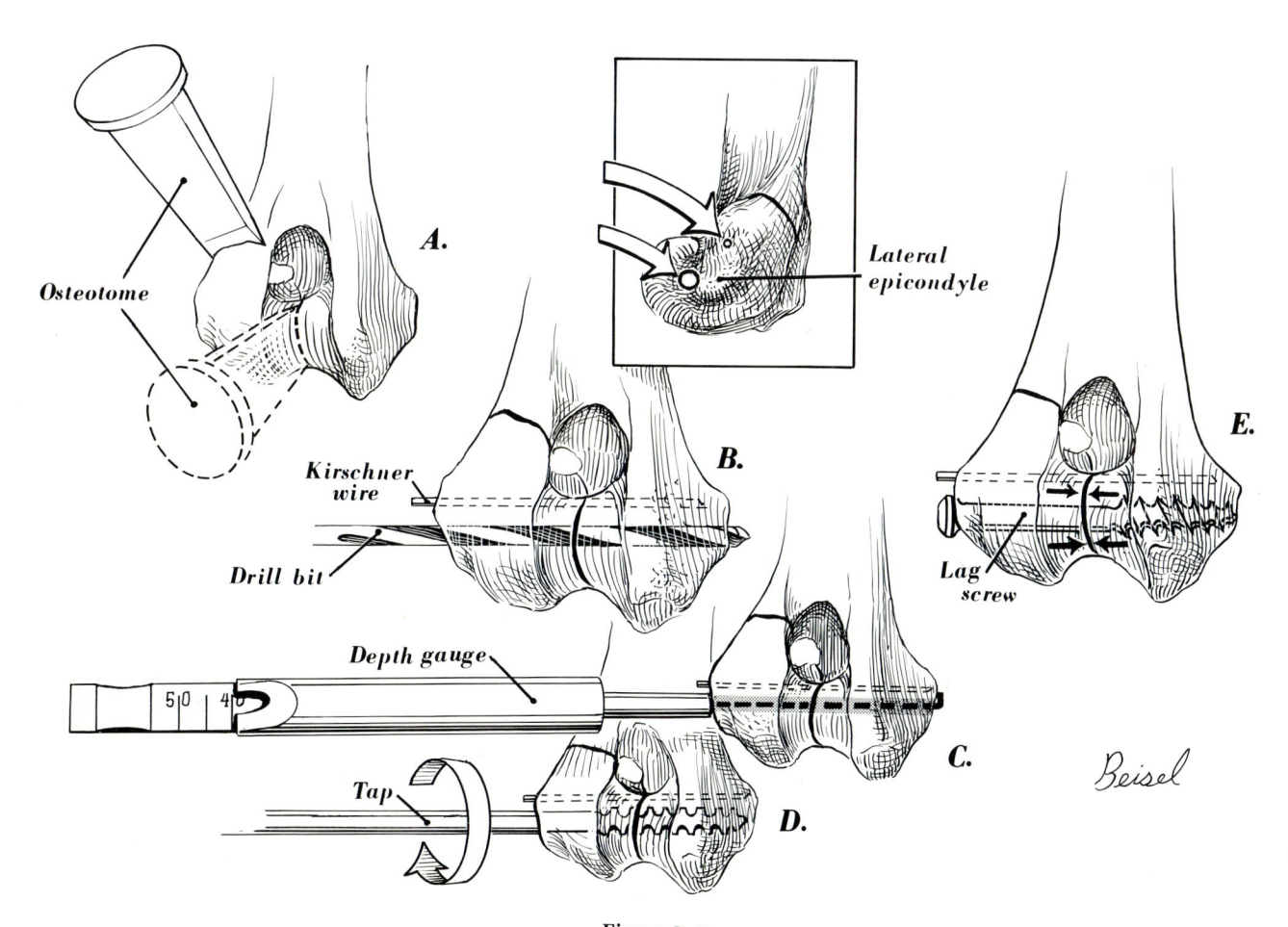

Figure 9–5

9-6 INTRAMEDULLARY PINNING OF THE RADIUS

Thomas Earley

Indications

Intramedullary pinning of the radius is indicated in fracture fixation of the radius.

Anesthesia

General anesthesia is required.

Patient Positioning

The animal can be placed in either dorsal or lateral recumbency.

Operative Preparation

Special Draping. An impermeable drape should be applied to the paw but not above the base of the metacarpals.

Specialized Instruments. The instruments required are a hand chuck, a Steinmann pin, a pin cutter, and a Gigli saw.

Incision and Exposure

A longitudinal skin incision over the distal third of the radius is made, and the bone is exposed between the extensor carpi radialis and the common digital extensor tendons. A Gigli saw is passed around the radius, and an osteotomy is performed. A second skin incision may be made over the distal third of the ulna, and a similar osteotomy may be performed.

Figure 9–6A. A third skin incision over the dorsal radial metaphyseal region is made to expose the area for pin insertion.

Details of Procedure

The point of pin insertion is a slightly raised bony area located between the tendon sheaths of the extensor carpi radialis and the common digital extensor muscles (Fig. 9–6A). With the antebrachiocarpal joint in slight flexion, the pin is driven proximally until it is well seated. The pin is then cut off close to the distal radius, and the subcutaneous tissue and skin are sutured over the end of the pin. The other incisions should also be sutured.

Because the intramedullary canal of the radius has an oval shape, a pin that fills the cranial-caudal diameter will not contact the medial or lateral cortices. (Fig. 9–6B). This may result in motion at the fracture site. The fixation should be tested for rotational stability. The reason for inserting the pin into the distal fragment first is to prevent interference with the function of the antebrachiocarpal joint (Fig. 9–6C).

Postoperative Considerations

The activity of the dog should be restricted to leash and house or kennel confinement until the fracture has healed. If rotational instability exists, additional fixation is indicated.

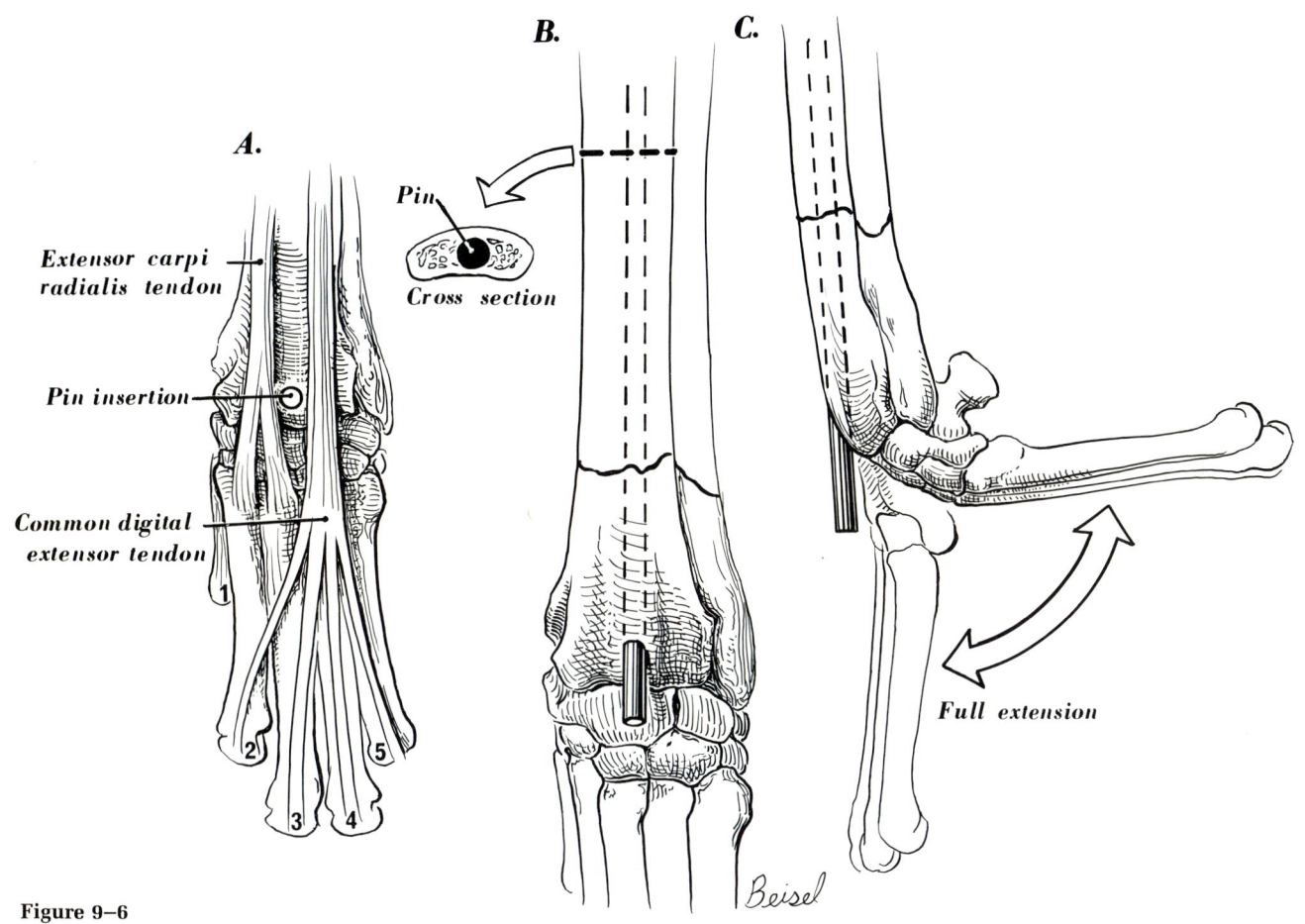

ORTHOPEDIC SURGERY 191

A.
- Extensor carpi radialis tendon
- Pin insertion
- Common digital extensor tendon
- 1, 2, 3, 4, 5

B.
- Pin
- Cross section

C.
- Full extension

Beisel

Figure 9-6

NOTES:

9–7 FEMORAL HEAD OSTECTOMY

Roger A. Rehmel

Indications

Femoral head ostectomy is indicated for those patients in which (1) irreversible damage due to trauma has occurred to the femoral head and/or neck, or (2) a disease process or syndrome has resulted in pain or abnormality of the femoral head and/or neck to such an extent that proper use of the limb is significantly impaired.

Anesthesia

General anesthesia is required.

Patient Positioning

The patient is placed in lateral recumbency.

Operative Preparation

Special Draping. Draping should allow for manipulation of the entire limb.

Specialized Instruments. The instruments required are an osteotome, a bone file, and an orthopedic hammer.

NOTES:

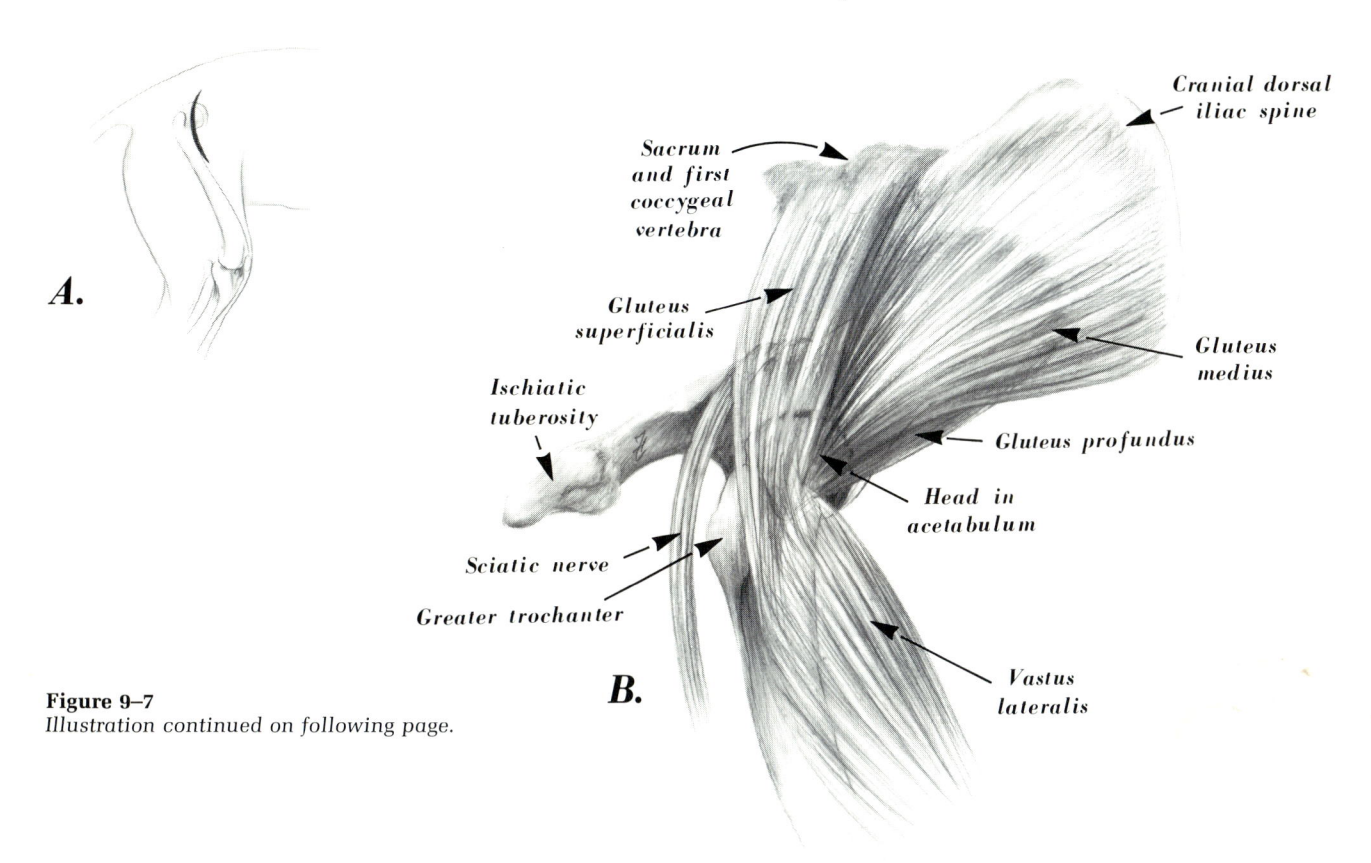

ORTHOPEDIC SURGERY 193

Femoral Head Ostectomy

Figure 9–7
Illustration continued on following page.

Incision and Exposure

Tenotomy of the gluteal muscles is one of several approaches to the canine coxofemoral joint that allows adequate exposure for femoral head ostectomy.

Figure 9–7A. A curved incision is created that arches from a point cranial and dorsal to the greater trochanter, passes over the greater trochanter itself, and terminates along the cranial border of the proximal third of the femur.

Figure 9–7B. From a lateral aspect, only the gluteal muscles inserting upon the greater trochanter obscure direct visualization of the coxofemoral joint. Tenotomy of those muscles combined with proper traction provides good craniodorsal exposure of the canine hip joint.

NOTES: (Continued)

Femoral Head Ostectomy

Labels on upper figure (C): Gluteus superficialis; Greater trochanter; Gluteus medius; Vastus lateralis

Labels on lower figure (D): Gluteus superficialis; Greater trochanter; Gluteus medius; Gluteus profundus; Vastus lateralis

Figure 9–7
Illustration continued on opposite page.

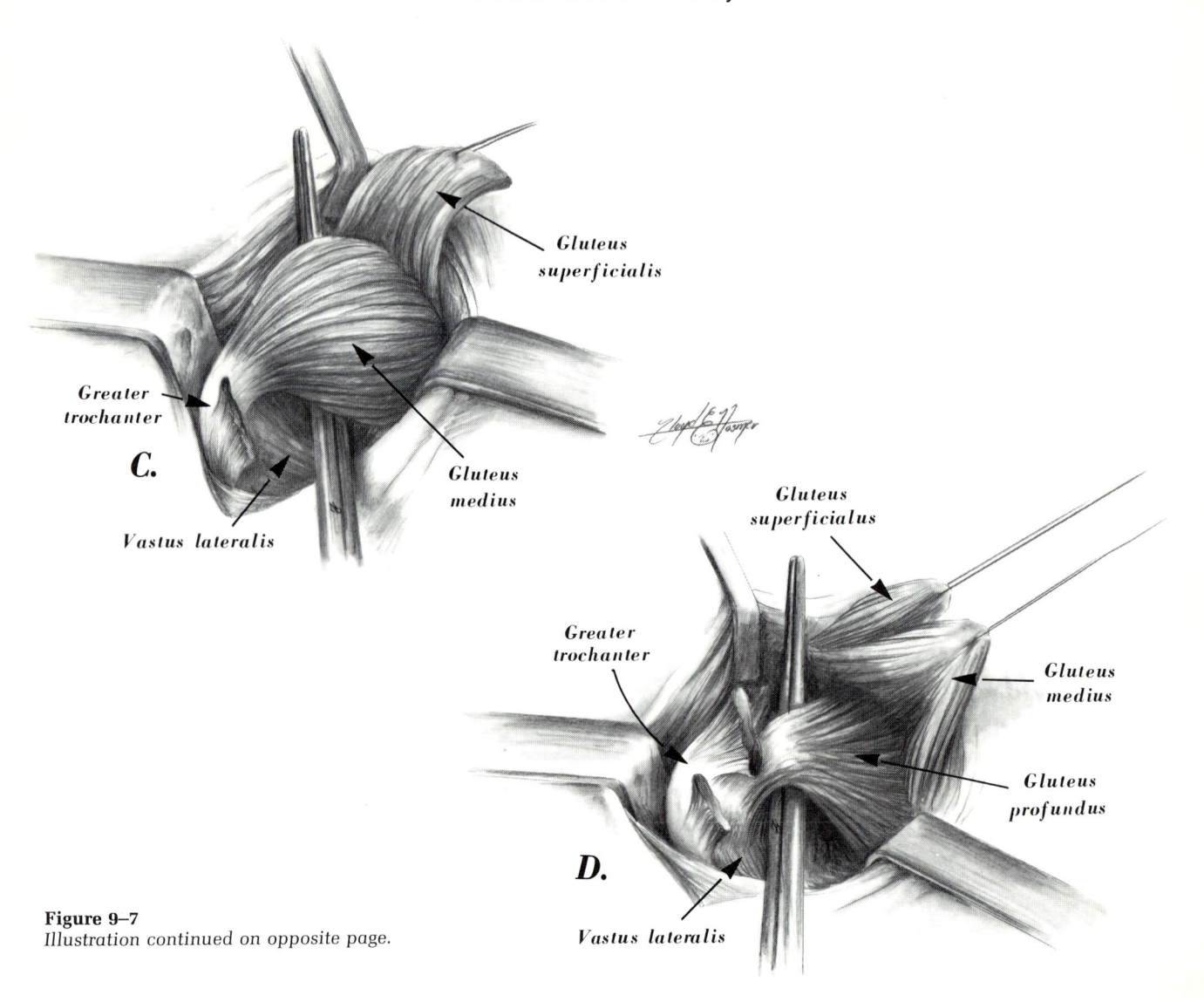

<u>Figures 9–7C, 9–7D, and 9–7E.</u> In turn, the gluteus superficialis, medius, and profundus muscles are each isolated and tenotomized at their insertions on the greater trochanter. The gluteal muscles are temporarily tagged with suture material and retracted dorsally. The underlying joint capsule is identified, and a stab incision is made through it into the coxofemoral joint (Fig. 9–7E). The capsular opening is enlarged with Mayo scissors parallel to the curvature of the acetabulum.

NOTES: (Continued)

ORTHOPEDIC SURGERY

Femoral Head Ostectomy

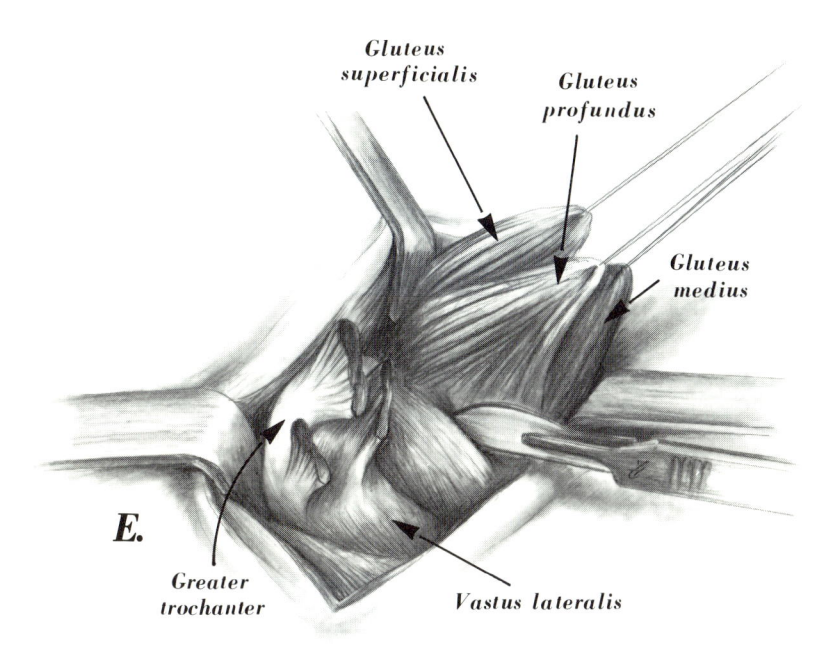

Figure 9–7 Continued
Illustration continued on following page.

NOTES: *(Continued)*

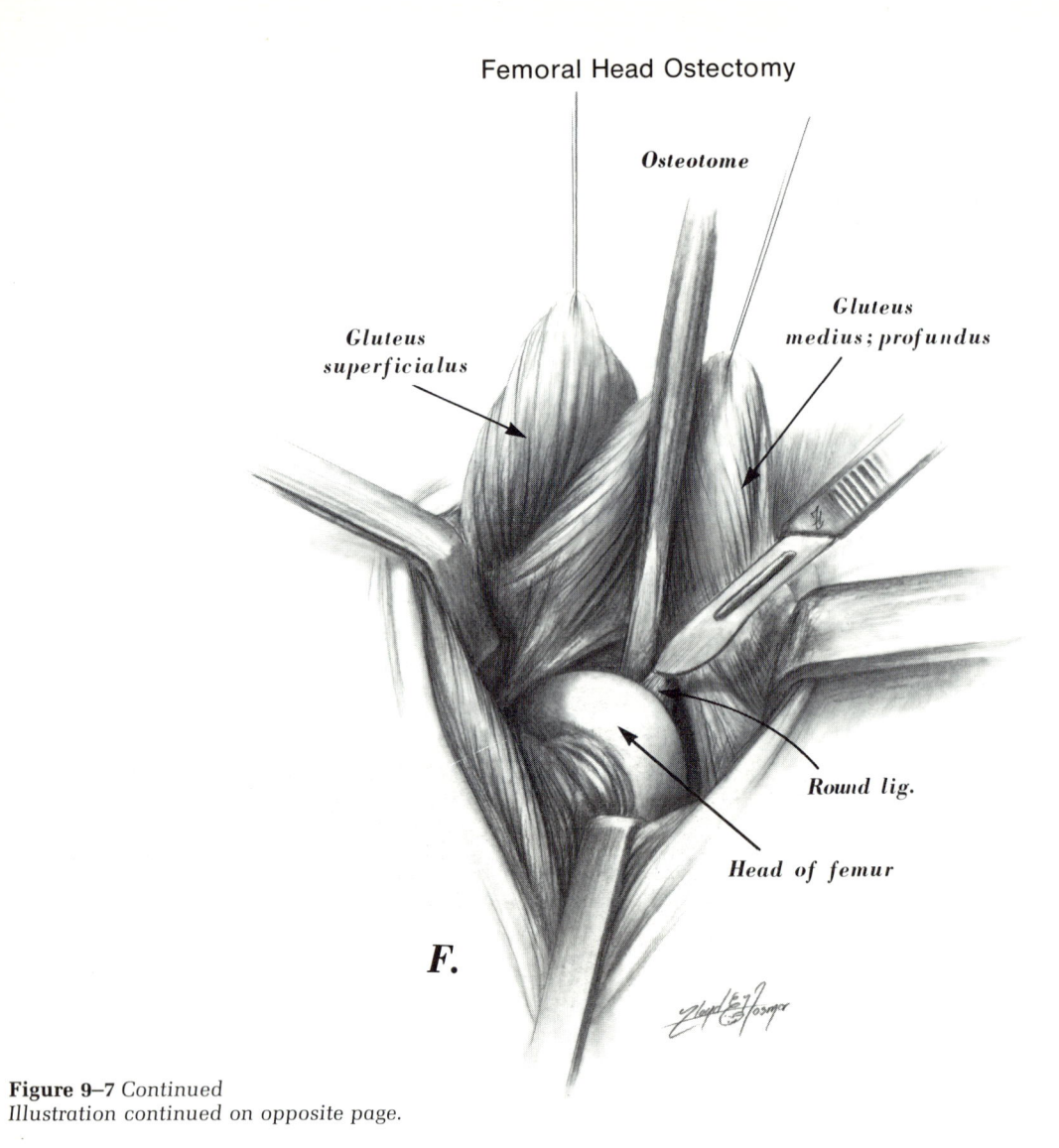

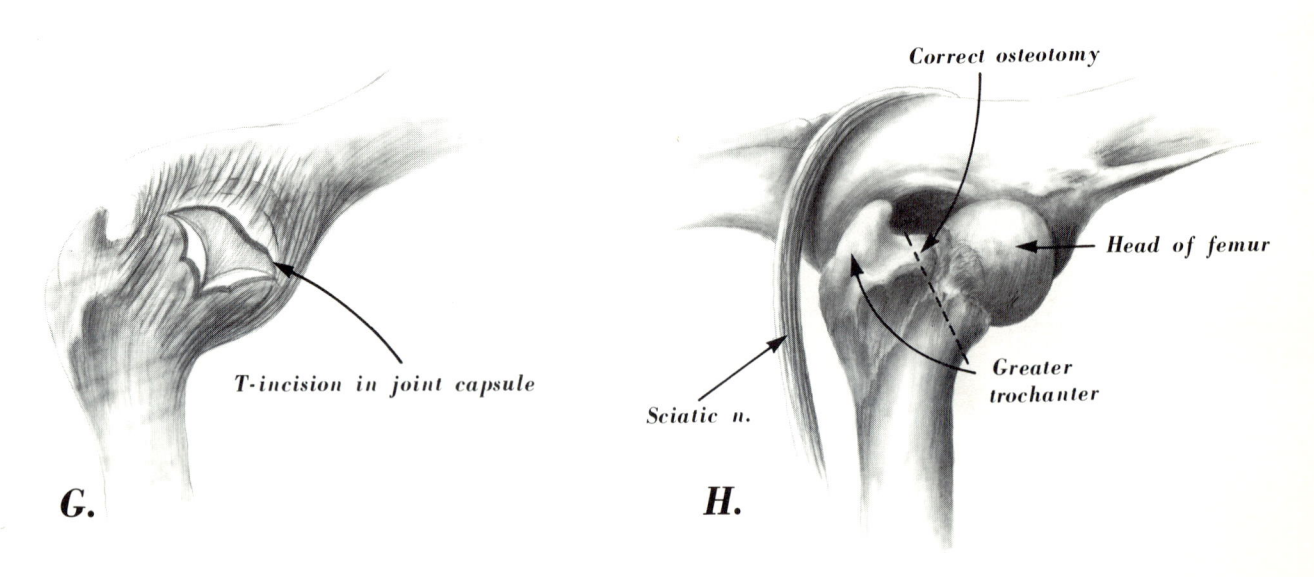

Figure 9–7 Continued
Illustration continued on opposite page.

196

Femoral Head Ostectomy

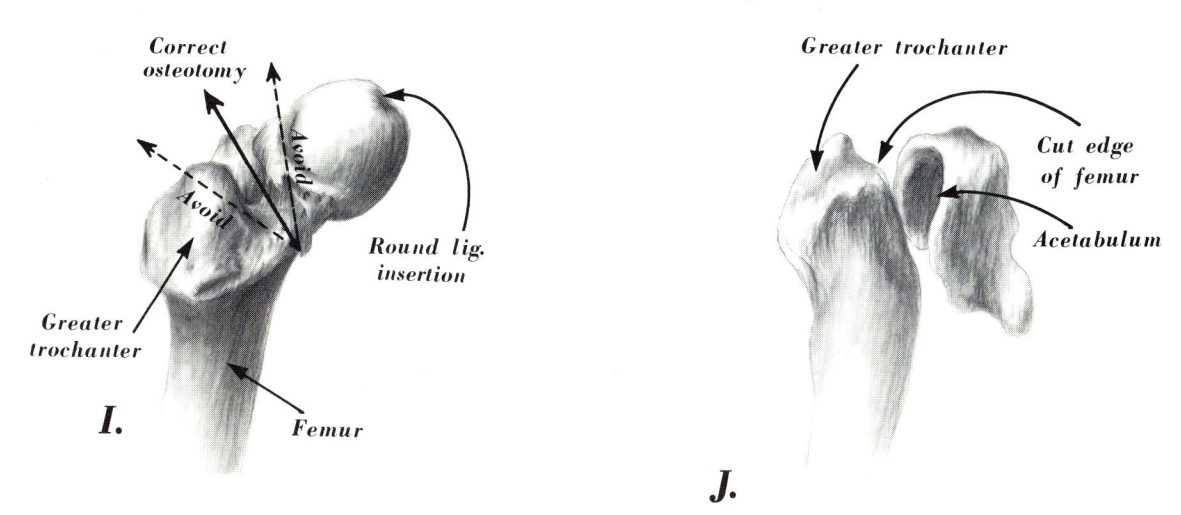

Figure 9-7 Continued

Details of Procedure

Figure 9-7F. An instrument, such as an Adson periosteal elevator, is placed between the acetabulum and femoral head caudal to the round ligament. The instrument is utilized to create a cranial-ventral coxofemoral subluxation that exposes the now taut round ligament. The round ligament is sharply incised.

Figure 9-7G. An incision perpendicular to the first capsular incision is made in the reflection of the joint capsule on the femoral neck. As much of the capsular attachment to the femur as possible is elevated free to expose the entire femoral neck.

Figures 9-7H and 9-7I. Visualization of the femoral head and neck can be increased by subluxating the femur and externally rotating it 90 degrees from its normal position. The correct line of osteotomy can now be determined so that the entire head and neck can be removed with a single cut. The present position and exposure of the femoral head allow the osteotomy to be performed with either a Gigli wire, bone cutter, or osteotome without endangering surrounding soft tissue — especially the sciatic nerve.

Once the ostectomy has been performed and the femoral head and neck have been removed, the remaining bone should be made absolutely smooth with a bone file.

Figure 9-7J. The femur is derotated and allowed to assume its new position in relation to the pelvis.

The gluteal muscles are apposed in turn to their insertions with the appropriate size absorbable suture material, utilizing a horizontal mattress pattern. The remainder of the closure is routine, keeping in mind to eliminate all dead space.

Postoperative Considerations

Sutures are removed in seven to ten days. For the first five weeks, use of the operated leg is to be encouraged but should be restricted to walking. Manipulation of the joint by the client while the patient is in lateral recumbency is good physiotherapy.

9–8 INTRAMEDULLARY PINNING OF THE FEMUR

THOMAS EARLEY AND MELVYN J. POND

Indications

Intramedullary pinning of the femur is indicated in fracture fixation of the femur.

Patient Positioning

The patient is placed in lateral recumbency, with the leg hung upward.

Operative Preparation

Special Draping. An impermeable drape is applied from the paw to include the distal half of the tibia.

Specialized Instruments. The instruments required are a Gigli wire, a hand chuck, and a Steinmann pin (unthreaded).

Incision and Exposure

A lateral skin incision is made over the mid-shaft femur to expose the fascia lata (Fig. 9–8A). The fascia lata is incised to retract the vastus lateralis muscle cranially and the biceps femoris muscle caudally, thus exposing the femur (Fig. 9–8B).

Details of Procedure

A Gigli wire is passed around the diaphysis of the femur, and a short oblique osteotomy is performed (Figs. 9–8C and 9–8D). Using the hand chuck, the Steinmann pin is inserted into the proximal fragment

NOTES:

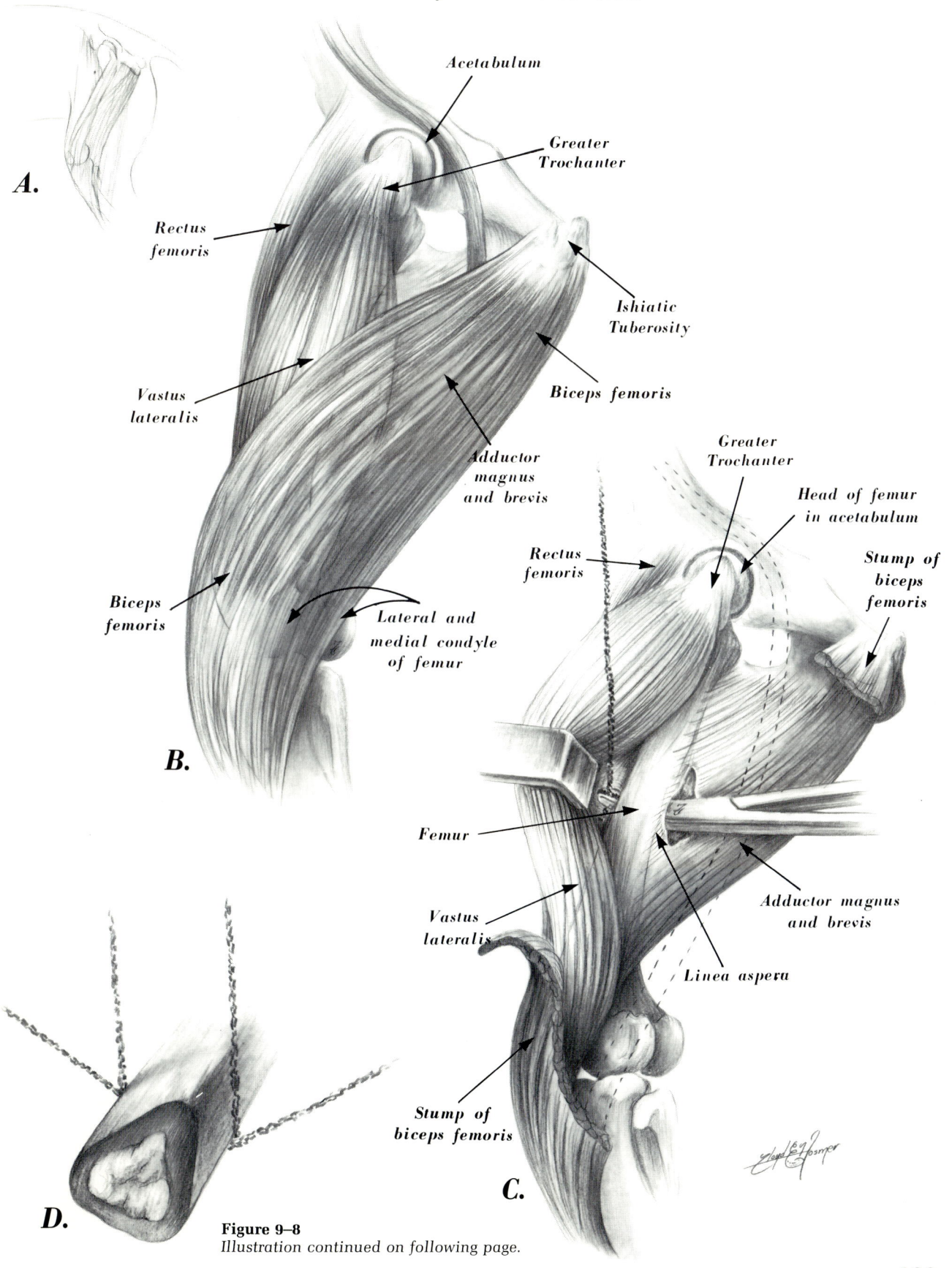

Intramedullary Pin-Fractured Femur

A.

Acetabulum
Greater Trochanter
Rectus femoris
Ishiatic Tuberosity
Vastus lateralis
Biceps femoris
Adductor magnus and brevis
Biceps femoris
Lateral and medial condyle of femur

B.

Greater Trochanter
Head of femur in acetabulum
Rectus femoris
Stump of biceps femoris
Femur
Vastus lateralis
Adductor magnus and brevis
Linea aspera
Stump of biceps femoris

C.

D.

Figure 9–8
Illustration continued on following page.

199

Intramedullary Pin-Fractured Femur

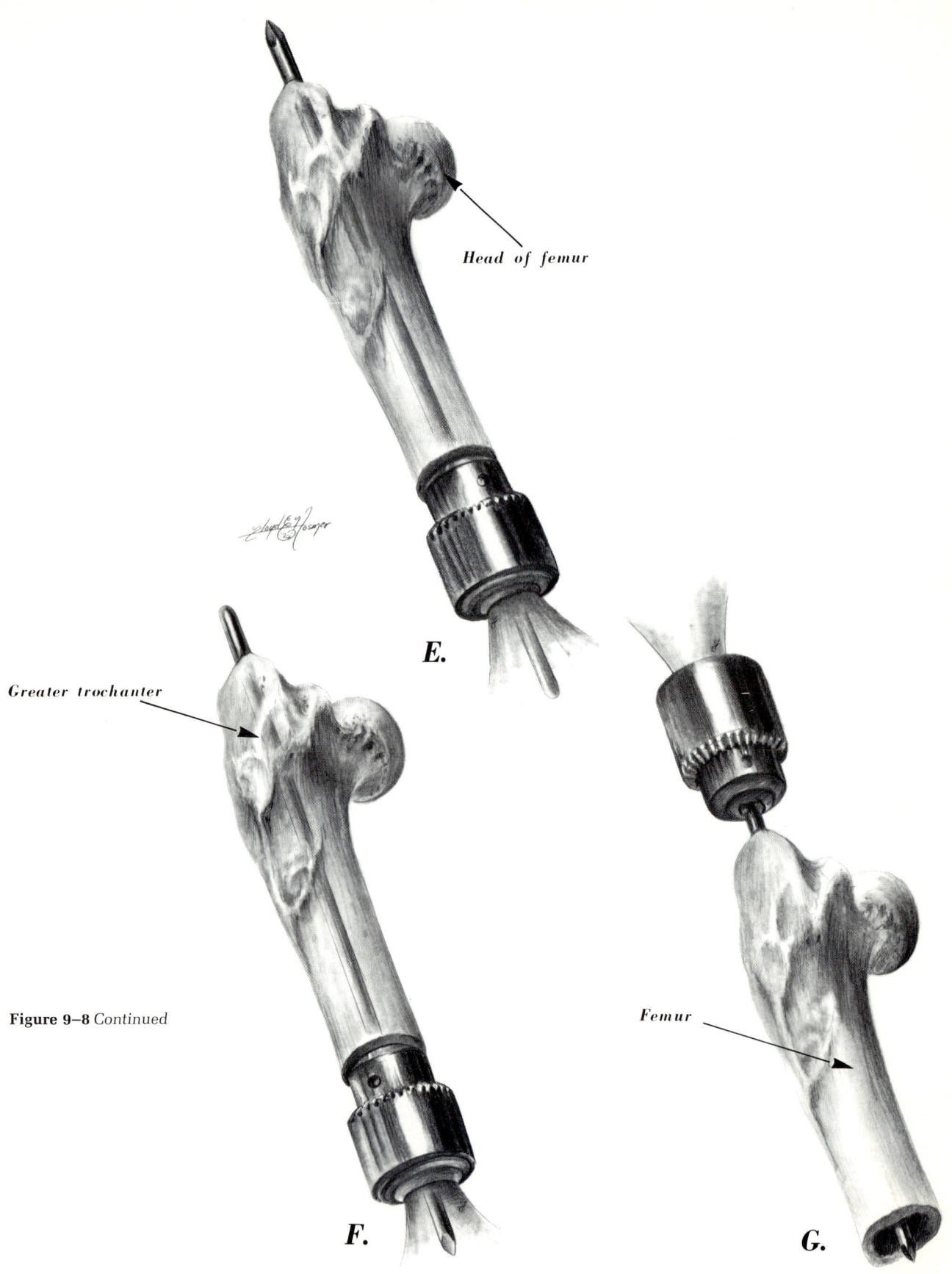

Head of femur

E.

Greater trochanter

Figure 9–8 Continued

F.

Femur

G.

(retrograde pinning) (Fig. 9–8E). With the proximal fragment slightly adducted and the hip joint extended, the pin is driven out of the trochanteric fossa and through the skin (Fig. 9–8F). This maneuver protects the sciatic nerve from injury during pin penetration. The proximal end of the pin is then grasped with the chuck and pulled until the distal point is flush with the osteotomy site. The fracture is then reduced (using bone clamps), and the pin is introduced and seated into the distal fragment (Fig. 9–8G). A pin of identical length should be used to estimate the depth of penetration of the intramedullary pin. The exposed proximal end of the pin is cut off with a pin cutter.

The fascia lata is sutured, and the subcutaneous tissue and skin are closed routinely.

Postoperative Considerations

Leash activity when outside and house or kennel confinement at other times is recommended until the fracture has healed. Passive flexion and extension of the hock and stifle are recommended until 75 per cent weight bearing is resumed to aid in circulation, reduce edema, and prevent joint stiffness. The pin should be removed (extracted from the top through a small skin incision) when the fracture has healed.

NOTES: *(Continued)*

9–9 LUXATING PATELLA: TROCHLEAR ARTHROPLASTY AND TIBIAL CREST TRANSPLANTATION

Roger A. Rehmel

Indications

Trochlear arthroplasty and tibial crest transplantation are two procedures that are employed to correct a medial patellar luxation in the dog.

Anesthesia

General anesthesia is required.

Patient Positioning

The patient is placed in lateral recumbency.

Operative Preparation

Special Draping. Draping should allow for complete manipulation of the involved limb.

Specialized Instruments. The instruments required are an Adson periosteal elevator, a bone cutter, and an appropriate size rat-tail file and bone rongeur.

Incision and Exposure

Using a surgical knife, an incision of sufficient length is made through the skin and subcutaneous tissue of the lateral stifle. A similar incision is made through the fascial planes and joint capsule.

Details of Procedure

Figure 9–9A. Patients with medial patellar luxation usually have a shallow trochlea. Trochlear arthroplasty restores correct shape, depth, and width. The surgeon begins by carefully making parallel cuts in the articular cartilage to accommodate the width of the patella. The cartilage between the cuts is removed with either a surgical knife or a bone rongeur. Subchondral bone is removed to a depth corresponding to the thickness of the patella. A fine rat-tail file is used to smooth the bottom and sides and to form the final shape of the trochlea.

Figure 9–9B. The completed trochlea in cross section should mimic the shape of the patella in cross section ("U" shape). It should also be wide enough to allow the patella to nestle into the trochlea. There is often the tendency to make the trochlea too narrow and unnecessarily deep.

Figure 9–9C. Patients with medial patellar luxation often have an abnormally aligned tibial crest. Tibial crest transplantation is designed to correct this fault.

The tibial crest is identified, and a surgical knife is used to make an incision along its lateral border. This allows the cranial tibial muscle to be partially elevated and retracted laterally. The tuberosity on the tibial crest is delineated without disturbing the insertion of the patellar ligament on the crest. An osteotome or bone cutter is then used to leave the attachment of the patellar ligament to the crest intact.

The osteotomized tibial tuberosity is swung laterally underneath the cranial ti-

ORTHOPEDIC SURGERY 203

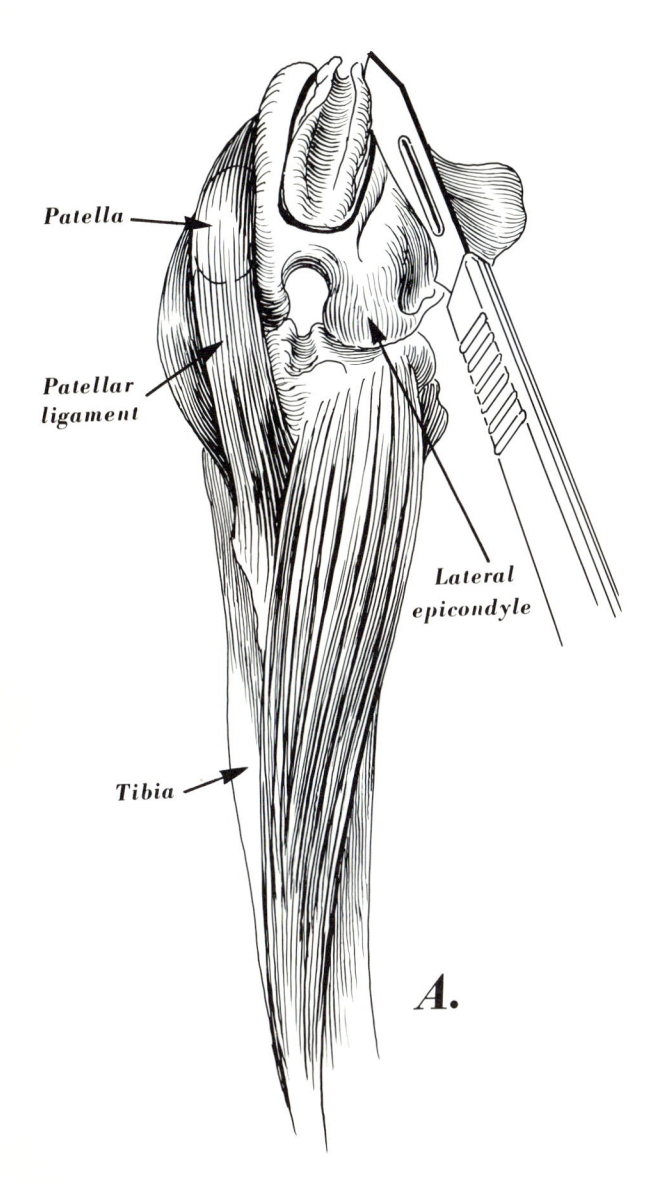

bial muscle to lie in contact with the lateral aspect of the tibial crest. This new position is stabilized by employing the appropriate Kirschner wire or intramedullary pin as shown in the diagram. Excess pin is removed, and the cranial tibial muscle is sutured in place with appropriate size Dexon or chromic catgut. Joint capsule and overlying fascial planes, subcutaneous tissue and skin are closed in a routine manner.

Postoperative Considerations

Skin sutures are removed in 10 to 14 days. Only limited activity (walking) should be allowed over the next 4 weeks.

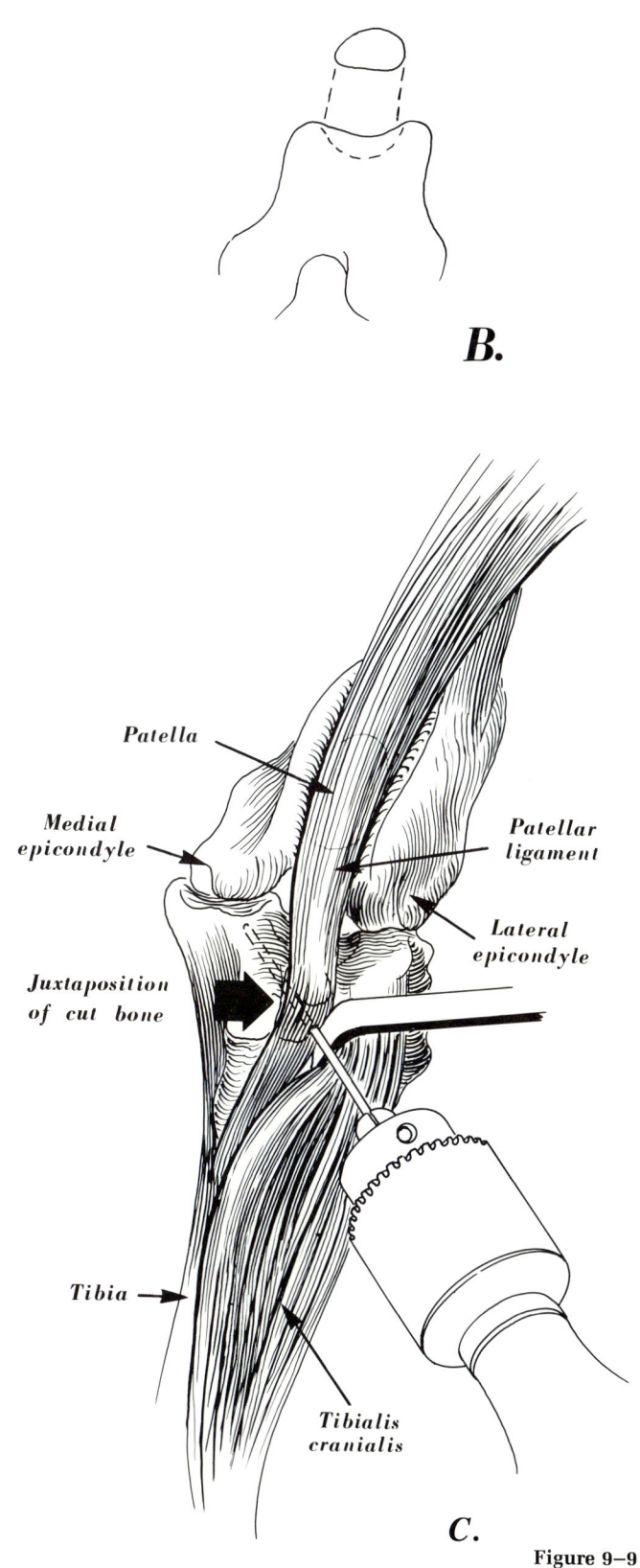

Figure 9–9

9–10
INTRAMEDULLARY PINNING OF THE TIBIA

Thomas Earley

Indications

Intramedullary pinning of a fractured tibia is an acceptable means of internal fixation.

Anesthesia

General anesthesia is required.

Patient Positioning

The animal may be placed in lateral or dorsal recumbency, with the leg hung upward in preparation for a medial approach to the tibia.

Operative Preparation

Special Draping. An impermeable drape is applied to the paw and should extend to the tibial-tarsal joint.

Specialized Instruments. The instruments required are a Gigli saw, an intramedullary pin, and a hand chuck.

Incision and Exposure

A medial approach to the tibia is made. The tibia lies close to the surface, and only the skin and subcutaneous tissues require incision. Near the distal third of the tibia, the median branch of the saphenous artery, vein, and nerve will be encountered, which should not be severed.

A midshaft fracture is created across the tibia and fibula by passage of the Gigli saw around these bones.

Figure 9–10A. Because retrograde pinning of the tibia often interferes with stifle function, insertion of the pin at the proximal end is recommended. The site of insertion on the proximal tibial plateau bisects a line that connects the medial condyle with the tibial tuberosity.

Figure 9–10B. When inserting a large diameter pin in the tibia of some achondroplastic dogs, it may be necessary to prebend the pin to accommodate the caudal bow of the diaphysis.

The incision is closed with simple interrupted sutures in the subcutaneous tissues and routine closure of the skin.

Postoperative Considerations

Exercise is restricted for four to six weeks. When the fracture has healed, the pin is removed.

ORTHOPEDIC SURGERY 205

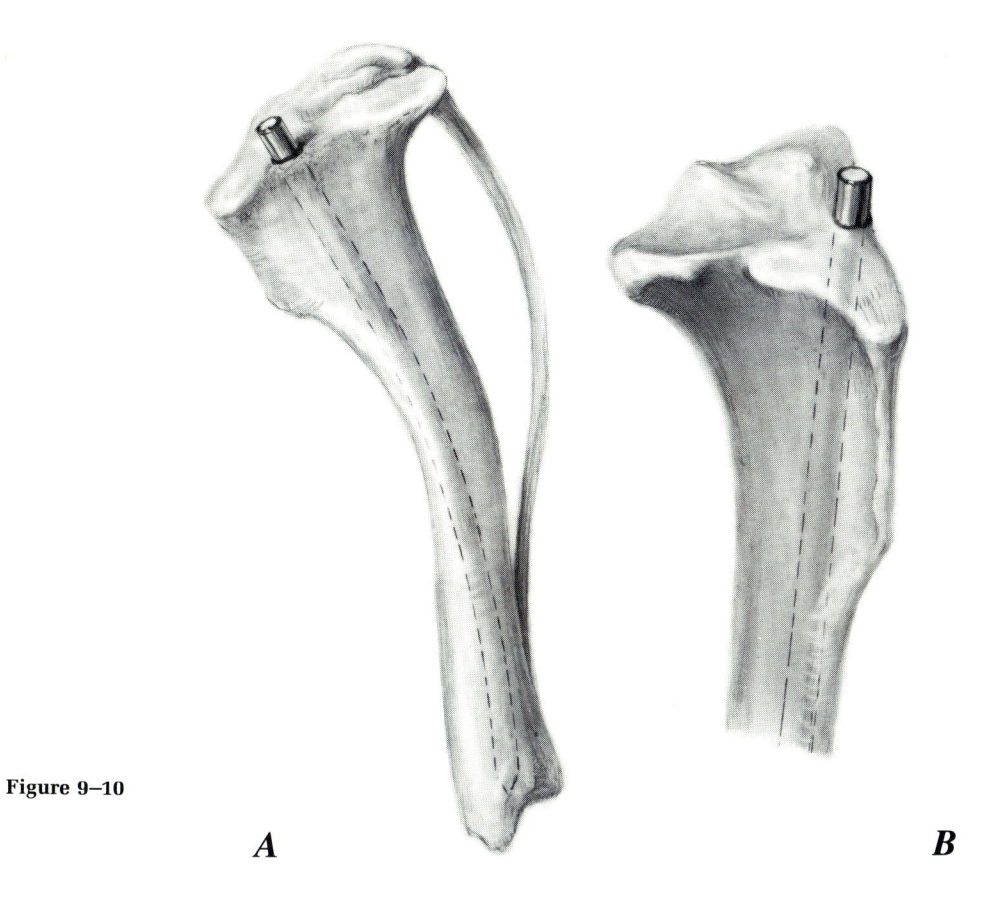

Figure 9–10

A

B

NOTES:

9–11 FRACTURED TIBIA — FULL KIRSCHNER APPLICATION

Thomas Earley

Indications

The Kirschner apparatus is used primarily in fracture fixation and joint immobilization. This procedure demonstrates its use in reduction and stabilization of a simple mid-diaphyseal fracture of the tibia.

Anesthesia

General anesthesia is required.

Patient Positioning

The animal can be placed in either lateral or dorsal recumbency, with the rear leg hung upwards.

Operative Preparation

Special Draping. An impermeable wrap should cover the paw but not extend beyond the proximal metatarsals.

Specialized Instruments. The following instruments are required:

—four fixation pins (⅛ inch in diameter)
—two short connecting rods (³⁄₁₆ inch in diameter)
—long connecting rod (³⁄₁₆ inch in diameter)
—four single clamps
—two double clamps
—open-end or spintite wrench (⁵⁄₁₆-inch)
—hand chuck
—pincutter
—Gigli wire

Incision and Exposure

Mid-diaphyseal tibial and fibular fractures are created with a Gigli wire through a medial skin incision (Fig. 9–11A). The fragments are then displaced, producing some overriding.

Details of Procedure

Figure 9–11 B. With the skin gathered toward the fracture site, two fixation pins should be pushed through the skin and then driven (lateral to medial or medial to lateral) in each fragment at approximately 25 to 30 degrees to each other. This gathered skin facilitates reduction of the overriding fragments.

Figure 9–11 C. A short connecting rod carrying a double clamp is secured to each fragment with single clamps. The single clamps should remain approximately ¼ inch above the skin surface. It is important to offer a counterforce when tightening the nuts on all clamps so that no movement of the Kirschner apparatus or the bone fragment occurs. Excess lengths of the fixation pins should be cut off at this time.

Figure 9–11 D. After the surgeon has reduced the fracture, the assistant slides a long connecting rod into the remaining hole in each double clamp, using the fixation pins as handles. Making sure that the flat side of the head of the bolt is in the proper position, the double clamps are tightened.

Postoperative Considerations

Restrict activity to leash only for about six weeks. Occasionally, drainage will be observed around some pins; however, occasional removal with a sterile gauze sponge is adequate. The apparatus should be removed when the fracture has healed.

ORTHOPEDIC SURGERY 207

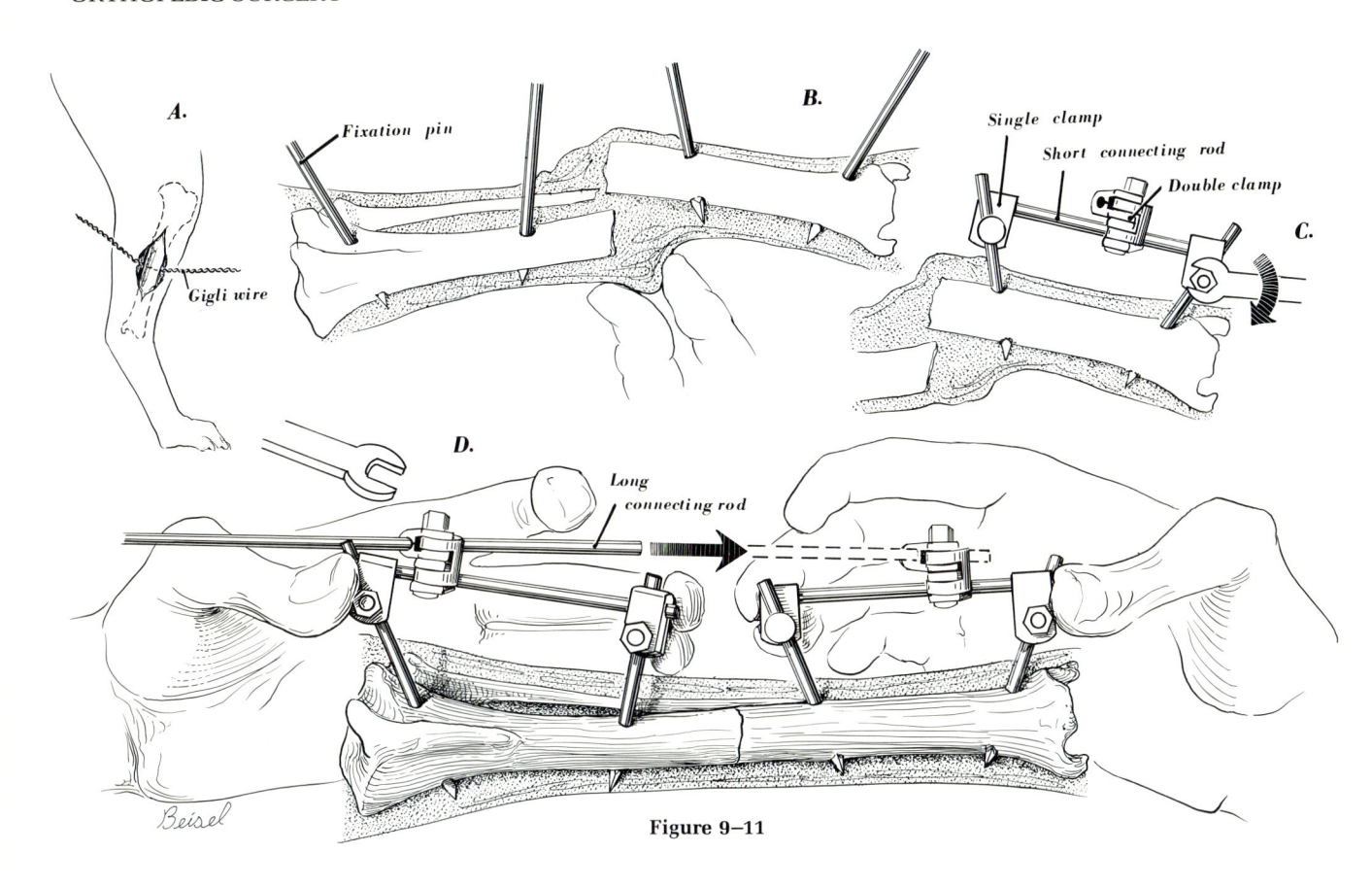

Figure 9-11

NOTES:

9–12 FELINE ONYCHECTOMY

Clarence A. Rawlings

Indications

Onychectomy is indicated as an elective procedure to prevent furniture mutilation by house cats.

Anesthesia

General anesthesia is indicated.

Patient Positioning

The patient is placed in lateral recumbency.

Operative Preparation

Specialized Instruments. A Rescoe nail trimmer is necessary for the described procedure, or a No. 11 Bard-Parker blade can also be used to amputate the third phalanx.

Details of Procedure

Figure 9–12 A. The normal relation of the phalanges and foot pad are demonstrated. The entire third phalanx (P-3) should be removed.

Figure 9–12 B. The feet should be surgically scrubbed but not clipped. A tourniquet is placed above the elbow.

The Rescoe nail trimmer is positioned snugly onto the dorsal surface between P-2 and P-3. During clipper positioning, the nail should be pulled cranially. As little skin as possible should be excised.

Figure 9–12 C. The cutting edge of the Rescoe nail trimmer is positioned at the cranial edge of the foot pad. As the cutting edge is advanced, the pad is moved caudally while rotating the nail dorsally and caudally. The third phalanx is then excised by the Rescoe nail trimmer. Avoid cutting the foot pad or leaving any portion of P-3.

Figure 9–12 D. A single suture is used to close the defect. After applying a snug foot bandage, the tourniquet is removed. The foot bandage may be removed after 24 hours.

Postoperative Considerations

Foot bandages are removed 24 hours after surgery, and the animal is observed for several more hours prior to discharge from the hospital.

NOTES:

ORTHOPEDIC SURGERY 209

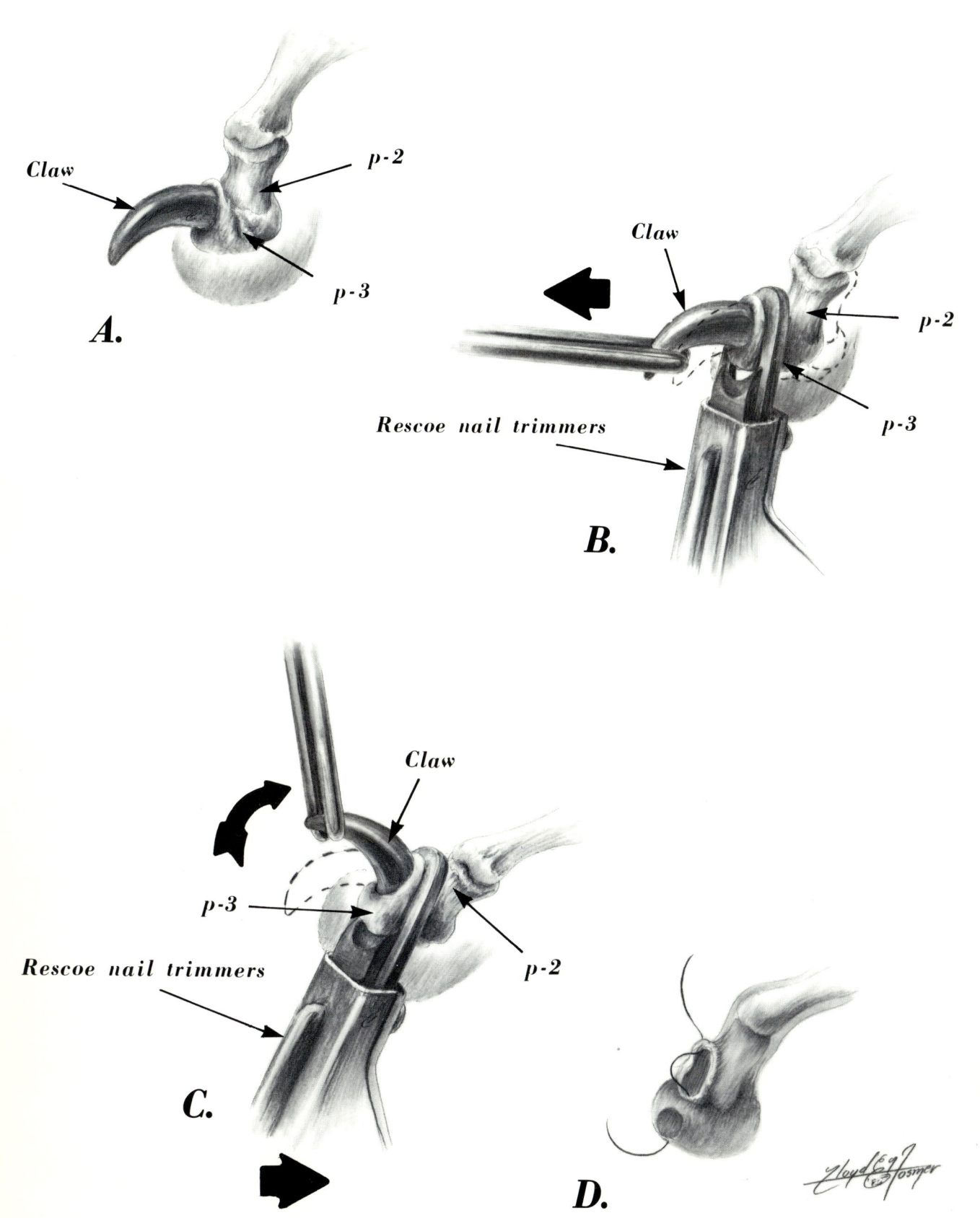

Figure 9–12

9–13 CAUDECTOMY

Roger A. Rehmel

Indications

Caudectomy is performed when irreversible damage to the tail has occurred or for acceptable cosmetic purposes. The procedure subsequently described is not the method of choice for three- to seven-day-old pups of breeds whose tails are traditionally docked.

Anesthesia

General anesthesia is required. If the patient is placed in declining sternal recumbency, intermittent positive pressure ventilation is recommended.

Patient Positioning

Placing the patient in declining sternal recumbency of about 15 degrees aids the operative procedure.

Operative Preparation

Special Draping. It is advisable to place a pursestring suture in the anal area to avoid fecal contamination.

Specialized Instruments. Although not necessary, electrocautery is desirable.

Suture Material. Major vessels are ligated with the appropriate size of polyglycolic acid or chromic catgut.

Details of Procedure

The site of caudectomy is determined by lesion, client preference, or breed standard. If possible, it should occur at a coccygeal joint. Aseptic technique in patient preparation, draping, and surgery is paramount.

Figure 9–13 A. A bilateral, symmetrically curved incision is made on the dorsal surface of the tail at the appropriate distance distal to the desired length. A connecting, straight ventral incision is made while the tail is held at a 45 degree angle from the body. The incision made as described and illustrated will insure enough skin to comfortably cover the end of the last remaining coccygeal vertebra in all positions of tail carriage. Note that the curved dorsal incision extends proximal to the straight ventral incision.

Figure 9–13 B. The superficial lateral coccygeal artery (one on each side) is identified and ligated with absorbable suture material cranial to the caudectomy site. Access to and identification of the arteries is facilitated by the proximal extension of the curved dorsal incision, mobilization of the skin cranially, and careful dissection of overlying tissues.

Figure 9–13 C. To complete the caudectomy, a surgical knife is passed dorsal to ventral through the predetermined joint space. If the preferred caudectomy site dictates division of a coccygeal vertebra, then a bone cutter can be employed.

NOTES:

ORTHOPEDIC SURGERY

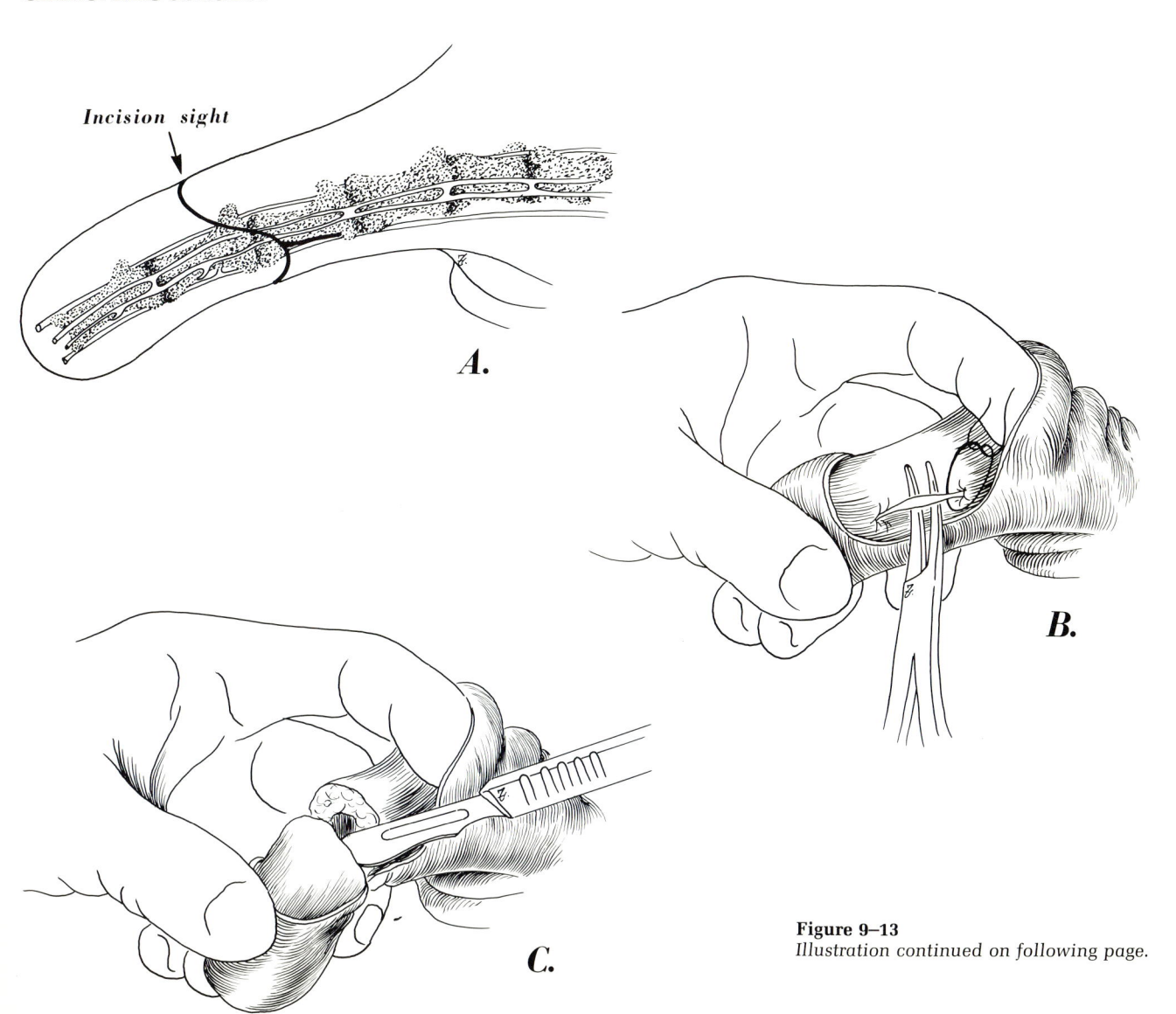

Incision sight

A.

B.

C.

Figure 9–13
Illustration continued on following page.

Figure 9–13 Continued

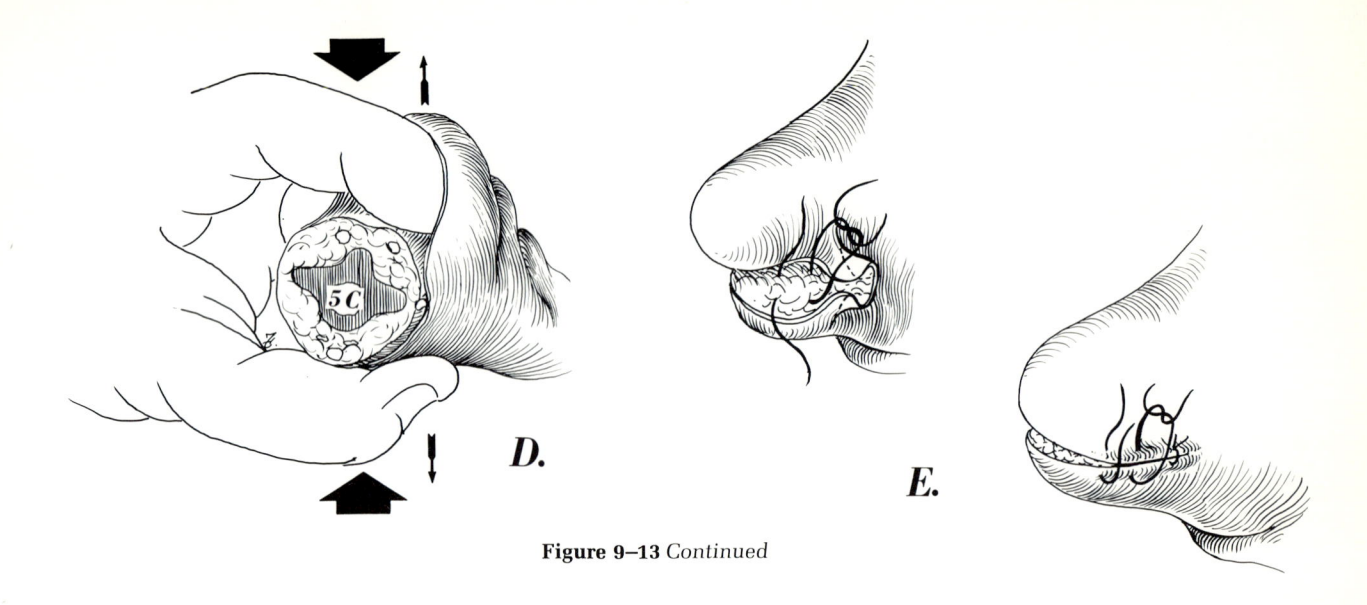

Figure 9–13 D. The distal portion of the tail is discarded, and the remaining proximal portion is held between the thumb and forefinger. Application of digital pressure controls hemorrhage, which can then be eliminated by electrocautery or ligation. A bloodless field is imperative if hematoma or seroma formation is to be avoided.

Figure 9–13 E. An absorbable suture material is utilized to place simple interrupted stitches in the subcutaneous tissue of each skin flap, being careful to achieve accurate alignment and apposition. NOTE: Subcutaneous suture should not include any tissue overlying the vertebrae. Any "dog ears" (puckered excess skin) at the commissures of the joint skin flaps are excised. Nonabsorbable suture material is used to place simple interrupted stitches in the skin.

Postoperative Considerations

Total control of hemorrhage and meticulous closure help to insure an uncomplicated postoperative period and the desired cosmetic result. Some patients may require the remaining tail to be bandaged and/or an Elizabethan collar to be worn. Sutures should remain in place for 10 to 14 days.

NOTES: (Continued)

ANESTHETIC DRUG DOSAGES

Appendix 1

CLARENCE A. RAWLINGS

JOHN I. TAYLOR

DOG

Sedation

GENERIC NAME	TRADE NAME	SOLUTION (mg/ml)	DOSAGE RANGE OR RATE (mg/lb)	PREFERRED ROUTES
Acepromazine maleate	Acepromazine	10	0.05–0.5	S/Q, I.M.
Chlorpromazine	Thorazine	25	0.25–1.0	S/Q, I.M.
Promazine	Sparine	50	1.0–2.0	S/Q, I.M.
Xylazine[1]	Rompun	20	0.5	I.V.
			0.5–1.0	I.M.
Morphine sulfate	Morphine and atropine	16 + 0.4	0.05–3.0	S/Q
Oxymorphone[1,2]	Numorphan	1	0.05–1.0	S/Q, I.V., I.M.
Fentanyl citrate and Droperidol[1]	Innovar-Vet	0.4 / 20	1.0 ml/15–60 lbs	I.M., I.V.

[1] Must be preceded by administration of atropine (dosage = 0.02 mg/lb).
[2] May be preceded with phenothiazine derivative tranquilizer to produce neuroleptanalgesia.

General Anesthesia
PREANESTHETICS

GENERIC NAME	TRADE NAME	SOLUTION (mg/ml)	DOSAGE RANGE OR RATE (mg/lb)	PREFERRED ROUTES
Atropine sulfate	Atropine	0.5	0.02	S/Q, I.M., I.V.
Meperidine HCl	Demerol	50	1.0–1.5	S/Q, I.M.
Oxymorphone	Numorphan	1	0.03–0.05	S/Q, I.M.
Pentazocine	Talwin	30	1.0–2.0	S/Q, I.M., I.V.
Fentanyl citrate and droperidol	Innovar-Vet	0.4 } 20	1.0 ml/25–60 lb	I.M.
Diazepam	Valium	5	0.5–1.0	S/Q, I.M., I.V.
Acepromazine maleate	Acepromazine	10	0.03–0.05	S/Q, I.M., I.V.
Phenobarbital sodium		120 (vial)	1.0–3.0	I.M.

INDUCTION
Intravenous

GENERIC NAME	TRADE NAME	SOLUTION (mg/ml)	DOSAGE RANGE OR RATE (mg/lb)	PREFERRED ROUTES
Thiamylal sodium[1,2]	Surital	25 (2.5%)	8.0	I.V.
Thiopental sodium[1]	Pentothal	25 (2.5%)	10.0	I.V.
Methohexital sodium	Brevital	10 (1%)	1.5–3.0	I.V.
Oxymorphone	Numorphan	1	0.1	I.V. (slow)
Fentanyl citrate and droperidol	Innovar-Vet		1.0 ml/20–40 lbs	I.V. over 3–5 min.

[1]If preceded by a narcotic analgesic or tranquilizer, reduce dosage by one third to one half.
[2]May be combined with 20% lidocaine as 1 mg : 1 mg ratio to reduce Surital dosage by one half and prolong effect. *Note:* Do not exceed 4.0 mg/lb lidocaine.

Inhalation (Mask Induction)

Halothane (Fluothane)
  Method Preoxygenation: 100% O$_2$ for 2–5 min.
  Incremental (0.5%) increase in concentration from 0.5% to effect up to 4% (if animal is healthy and sedated, may start with higher concentration).

Halothane and nitrous oxide
  Method Preoxygenation: 100% O$_2$ for 2–5 min.
  Start N$_2$O at 2:1 ratio with O$_2$. Initiate halothane at 0.5% and incrementally (0.5%) increase to effect up to maximal of 3%.

APPENDIX 1

Maintenance

Halothane (Fluothane)
Following thiobarbiturate induction, try not to exceed 3% concentration and maintain on 0.5–2%.

Methoxyflurane (Metofane, Penthrane)
Following thiobarbiturate induction, set at 1–3% concentration, then maintain at 0.03–1.5%.

Halothane and nitrous oxide
Note: During maintenance, the minimum O_2 concentration should not be below 30%.
A safe range is 50–66% N_2O in O_2 (i.e., 1:1 or 1:2 ratio $O_2 : N_2O$).

Balanced anesthetic regimens
Example: Supplementation of Innovar-Vet induction with oxymorphone (0.025 mg/lb increments), nitrous oxide, and muscle relaxant.

Muscle Relaxation

GENERIC NAME	TRADE NAME	SOLUTION (mg/ml)	DOSAGE RANGE OR RATE (mg/lb)	PREFERRED ROUTES
Succinylcholine chloride	Sucostrin[1]	20	0.1–0.5	I.V.
Gallamine	Flaxedil[1,2]	20	0.5 (0.2–1.0)	I.V.
Pancuronium bromide	Pavulon[1,2]		0.1	I.V.

[1]Repeat dosage in half initial dosage.
[2]To reverse nondepolarizing relaxants, give atropine (dosage = 0.04 mg/lb) and neostigmine methyl sulfate (Stiglyn) (dosage = 0.03 mg/lb).

Local Anesthesia

Caudal or epidural lidocaine (dosage = 1 ml or 20 mg/7–10 lb)
The lidocaine may be supplemented with epinephrine.

Intravenous block: Baer block
Method (1) I.V. catheter; (2) exsanguinate with leg wrap; (3) tourniquet; and (4) reinfuse with 1% lidocaine until veins are distended (maximum dosage of 4 mg/lb).
Note: Release tourniquet slowly.

Intravenous Fluids

Lactated Ringer's solution (dosage = 5 ml/lb/hr up to a maximum of 40 ml/lb given to effect). Replace 1 cc of blood loss with 3 cc of lactated Ringer's solution, unless a low packed-cell volume indicates whole blood transfusion.)

Narcotic Antagonists

GENERIC NAME	TRADE NAME	SOLUTION (mg/ml)	DOSAGE RANGE OR RATE (mg/lb)	PREFERRED ROUTES
Nalorphine[1]	Nalline	5	0.5	S.Q., I.M., I.V., (1 mg/20 mg meperidine)
Naloxone HCl[2]	Narcan	0.4	0.4–1.25	I.M., I.V.

[1]Dosage rate varies, depending upon the potency of the narcotic analgesic used.
[2]Antagonizes all commonly used narcotics as well as pentazocine.

CAT

Sedation

GENERIC NAME	TRADE NAME	SOLUTION (mg/ml)	DOSAGE RANGE OR RATE (mg/lb)	PREFERRED ROUTES
Acepromazine maleate	Acepromazine	10	0.025–0.1	S.Q., I.M.
Xylazine	Rompun	20	0.05–1.0	S.Q., I.M.
Ketamine HCl[1]	Ketaset	100	5.0–12.5	S.Q., I.M.
			1.0–5.0	I.V.

[1]May be used in combination with Acepromazine, xylasine, diazepam, pentazocine, oxymorphone.

General Anesthesia
PREANESTHETICS

GENERIC NAME	TRADE NAME	SOLUTION (mg/ml)	DOSAGE RANGE OR RATE (mg/lb)	PREFERRED ROUTES
Atropine sulfate	Atropine	0.5	0.02	S.Q., I.M., I.V.
Acepromazine maleate	Acepromazine	10	0.025–0.1	S.Q., I.M. only
Ketamine HCl	Ketaset	100	5.0	I.M.
Meperidine HCl	Demerol	50	1.0	S.Q., I.M.

APPENDIX 1

INDUCTION

Intravenous

GENERIC NAME	TRADE NAME	SOLUTION (mg/ml)	DOSAGE RANGE OR RATE (mg/lb)
Thiamylal sodium[1]	Surital	25 (2.5%)	8.0
Thiopental sodium[1]	Pentothal	25 (2.5%)	10.0
Ketamine HCl	Ketaset	100	2.0–4.0

[1] If preceded by a tranquilizer, reduce dosage by one third to one half.

Intramuscular

GENERIC NAME	TRADE NAME	DOSAGE RANGE OR RATE (mg/lb)
Ketamine	Ketaset	12.5
Xylazine	Rompun	0.25

Inhalation

Halothane ±nitrous oxide

Mask induction method: (1) Preanesthetize (optional); (2) apply maximal or minimal restraint; (3) preoxygenate: 100% O_2 for 2 min; (4) introduce $N_2O:O_2$ ratio 1:1; and (5) incremental (0.5%) increase in concentration to effect.

Chamber induction method (1) Preanesthetize (optional); (2) connect T-piece to inlet; (3) flow N_2O 4 liters: O_2 1.5 liters with halothane to highest concentration (approximately 5%); and (4) induce in 2–5 minutes.

MAINTENANCE

Halothane
Halothane and nitrous oxide } Same as for dog, except that a nonrebreathing system should be used.
Methoxyflurane

SUTURE MATERIALS — Appendix 2

Introduction

Choice of Suture Material

Based upon
Type of wound
Chemical and physical characteristics of the suture material
Biologic reactions of the various suture materials
The suture material should be as strong as the normal tissues through which it passes.
If biologic processes reduce the strength of the suture material, the loss of suture strength must be proportional to the gain in wound strength.

Suture size
The strength of the suture material needs to be no greater than the strength of the tissue on which it is used.
Oversized suture material does not add strength to the repaired wound. It may weaken the wound through excessive tissue reactions.
Small suture material
Causes less tissue trauma
Allows smaller knots to be tied
Forces the surgeon to handle the suture material more gently
Is less likely to strangulate tissues

Two Groups of Suture Material

Absorbable suture material
Characteristics
Digested and assimilated by the body during the healing process
Replaced by healthy tissues through the action of macrophages
Absorbed more rapidly in the presence of an abundant blood supply, sepsis, or naturally occurring enzymes (i.e., those of the pancreas and the small intestine)
Types
Animal
Synthetic

Indications
> When nonabsorbable suture material might act as a nidus for stone formation (urinary bladder)
> When contamination cannot be eliminated (G.I. tract)
>> Minimal bacteria-harboring characteristics
> Where it is desirable to have the body remove the suture material (liver, spleen)
> Where subcutaneous sutures are required

Contraindications and reservations
> For infected wounds
> For grossly contaminated wounds
> For skin

Nonabsorbable suture material
> Characteristics
>> Not absorbed or digested by the tissues
>> Becomes encapsulated when buried
>> High tensile strength
>> Low tissue reactivity
> Three types of nonabsorbable suture material
>> Metallic
>> Natural
>> Synthetic
> Indications
>> Desire for high tensile strength and/or low tissue reactivity
>> Presence of infection
>>> Use monofilamentous nonabsorbable material
>>>> More difficult to handle
>>>> Holds knots less securely
>> Multifilamentous nonabsorbable material has following properties
>>> Tends to support bacteria
>>> Produces greater tissue reactivity
>>> Easier to handle
>>> Holds knots better
> Usually less expensive than absorbable suture material

Absorbable Suture Material

Surgical Gut (Catgut)

Description
> Derived from submucosa of sheep intestines
> Classified by its degree of tanning or chromatization with chromic acid
>> Type A — Plain, untreated catgut
>> Type B — Mild treatment
>> *Type C — Medium treatment ("chromic")
>> Type D — Prolonged treatment
> Available sizes — No. 7–0 to No. 3–0

---

*Most frequently used catgut in veterinary surgery.

Tissue reactivity
  Stimulates an inflammatory reaction when buried, which results in its absorption
  Broken down by enzymatic degradation and phagocytosis
Absorption
  Plain catgut — absorbed after 3–5 days — intense tissue reactivity
  Medium chromic catgut — absorbed after 10–15 days
    Loses 60% of its strength within 7 days after placement
    All catgut swells from the absorption of tissue fluids
      Must contain three square throws *and* must be cut with 1/4″ ends to prevent untying
Indications
  Apposition of mucosal surfaces within the G.I. tract
  Ligation of ovarian and uterine stump
  Ligation of spermatic cord
  Deep sutures in parenchymal organs (liver, spleen)
  Repair of mucous membranes where minerals or salts may precipitate (gall bladder, urinary bladder)
  General abdominal closure
  Ligation of small vessels
Contraindications
  For skin
  Where minimal inflammation is desirable (cardiovascular system)
  Where prolonged suture strength is required (tendons)

Polyglycolic Acid (Dexon)

Description
  Synthetic suture material
  Has greater tensile strength and better handling characteristics than surgical gut
    Polyglycolic acid is more expensive than surgical gut, and surgeon's knots or multiple throws are required to prevent slippage of knots
Tissue reactivity
  Almost inert
  Produces considerably less tissue inflammation than surgical gut
Absorption
  Absorbed by enzymatic digestion
  Loses 40% of its strength within 7 days after placement and is completely gone within 60 days
Indications
  Suture material of choice in all urinary tract surgery
  Indications similar to those for surgical gut
Contraindications
  Contraindications similar to those for surgical gut

APPENDIX 2

Nonabsorbable Suture Material

Metals

Types of metal
  Tantalum — nontoxic, noncorrosive, and inert *in vivo* but tends to fragment
  *Stainless steel
    Available as multifilament and monofilament
    Nontoxic, noncorrosive, inert, high tensile strength, easily sterilized, relatively inexpensive
    Difficult to handle, kinks easily, lacks elasticity, produces bulky knots
    Twisting should be avoided to prevent strangulation of tissue
  Metal clips (hemoclips)
    Noncorroding metals
    Used to ligate small vessels and approximate wound edges
    Require special equipment for application
Tissue reactivity — inert, least tissue reaction of any suture material
Indications
  General closure
  Tendons
  Contaminated wounds
  Skin

Natural Nonabsorbable Suture Materials

Silk
  Description
    Derived from the cocoon of silk moth larvae
    Excellent handling characteristics, holds knots securely, retains tensile strength well, inexpensive, and readily sterilized
  Tissue reactivity — low
    Usually becomes encapsulated but may form cysts that may open and form fistulas
  Indications
    Vessel ligation
    Ophthalmic surgery
    Cardiovascular surgery
    Gastrointestinal surgery
    Some urologic surgery (perineal urethrostomy)
  Contraindications
    Should not penetrate the lumen of hollow organs (may cause abscess or serve as nidus for calculi formation)
  Skin — causes pustules
    Contaminated wounds — multifilament, capillary action, ability to harbor organisms

---

*Most frequently used metallic suture material in veterinary surgery.

Cotton
: Less irritating than gut, silk, or linen, low cost, and easily sterilized
: Indications — similar to those for silk
: Contraindications — similar to those for silk
: : Has marked capillary action
: : Tends to stick to wet gloves and is electrostatic, making handling more difficult

Synthetic Nonabsorbable Suture Materials

Types
: Polymerized caprolactam (Vetafil)
: : Twisted synthetic fibers enclosed within a smooth "proteinaceous" outer coat
: : Popular for use in skin closure
: : Chemical sterilization does not render the material sufficiently sterile to be safely buried
: : : Heat-sterilized Vetafil may be buried under *aseptic* conditions.
: : : Heat sterilization renders material more difficult to handle.
: : Available in 0.3 mm (00), 0.4 mm (0), 0.6 mm, and 1.0 mm sizes.
: Braided polyester fibers
: : Types
: : : Braided Dacron — Mersilene (Ethicon)
: : : Teflon-impregnated Dacron — Tevdek (Deknatel)
: : : Dacron coated with Teflon — "silk" Polydek (Deknatel)
: : : Dacron-impregnated with Teflon — "cottony" Dacron (Deknatel)
: : Advantages — strong, somewhat elastic, little tissue reactivity, good handling characteristics, high tensile strength, noncapillary, easily sterilized
: : Disadvantages — poor knot holding, capillary if outer coating is broken, fray easily
: : Indications
: : : Skin
: : : General closure
: : : Cardiovascular surgery
: : : Tendons
: : : G.I. surgery penetrating the lumen
: : Contraindications
: : : Contaminated wounds
: Nylon
: : Monofilament or braided multifilament
: : High tensile strength, little tissue reactivity
: : Low coefficient of friction, so knots tend to slip easily and are difficult to tie
: : Used primarily for skin closure

Polypropylene (Prolene)

- Characteristics that make it a very desirable suture material
  - Strength
  - Knot security
  - Low tissue drag
  - Low tissue reactivity
  - Nonabsorbable
  - Resistance to suture infection (monofilament)
- Indications
  - All types of tissue
  - Contaminated wounds

Index

Page numbers in *italics* indicate illustrations.
Page numbers followed by (t) indicate tables.

Abdomen, approach to and opening of, 50-52, *50, 52*
  closure of, 51, *53-54*
Absorbable suture material. See *Suture material, absorbable.*
Acepromazine maleate (Acepromazine), effect of, 9
Acidemia, 9
Acidosis, metabolic, correction of, 7
    indication of, 7
    treatment of, 12
Alkalosis, respiratory, 9
Allis tissue forceps, 26, *26*
  application of, and trauma, 1
Ammonium compounds, quaternary, 16
Anal sac, extraction of, 104-105, *104, 105*
Anastomosis, esophageal, 55-61, *56-58, 60*
  intestinal, 100-103, *100, 102*
Anesthesia, 5-13. See also under specific operative
    procedures.
  administration of, equipment preparation for, 8
  and cardiac disease, 8-9
  and hepatic disease, 9-10
  and pulmonary disease, 9
  and renal disease, 10-11
  choice and techniques of, importance of, 5
  complications associated with, 13
  drug therapy prior to, 6
  effect of, on cardiac output and contractility, 8
  effect of antibiotics on, 6
  effect of antihistamines on, 6
  effect of vitamins on, 6
  evaluation of patient prior to, 5
  fluid administration during, 12
  general, for cats, dosages of, 216-217(t)
    induction, inhalation, 217(t)
      intramuscular, 217(t)
      intravenous, 217(t)
    maintenance, 217(t)
    preanesthetics in, 216(t)
  for dogs, dosages of, 214-215(t)
    for muscle relaxation, 215(t)
    induction, inhalation, 214(t)
      intravenous, 214(t)
    maintenance, 215(t)
    preanesthetics in, 214(t)
  history session before, 5
  hypertension and, 11
  hypotension and, 11
  induction of, in cardiac disease patients, 9

Anesthesia (*continued*)
  in hepatic disease patients, 10
  in pulmonary disease patients, 9
  in renal disease patients, 10-11
  local, for dogs, 215
  management of patient under, 12
  monitoring of patient under, 11-12
  phenothiazine tranquilizers and, 6
  physical examination of patient prior to, 5
  response of patients under drug therapy to, 6
  withdrawal of organophosphate insecticides prior to, 6
Anesthesia machine, checking of, 8
Anesthetics, for cats, dosages of, 216-217(t)
  for dogs, dosages of, 213-216(t)
Anesthetized patient, oxygen supply to, 12
Antagonists, narcotic, for dogs, 216(t)
Antibiotics, effect of, on anesthesia, 6
Antibiotic therapy, prior to surgery, 7-8
Anticonvulsant drugs, administration of, prior to surgery, 6
Antihistamines, effect of, on anesthesia, 6
Arthroplasty, trochlear, in correction of patellar luxation,
    202-203, *203*
Asepsis, 1
Atelectasis, after thoracotomy, reduction of, 45
Atlantoaxial subluxation, stabilization of, 156-159, *157-159*
Attire, in operating room, 15-16

Backhaus towel clamps, 23, *23*
Bard-Parker scalpel handle, 23, *23*
Bicarbonate, administration of, 7
Blood, transfusion of, 7
Brown-Adson tissue forceps, 23, *23*
Bulla, osseous, osteotomy of, 160-163, *161, 162*

Calculi, cystic, removal of, 112-115, *113, 114*
  urethral, removal of, 116-117, *116*
Canine castration, 145-147, *145, 146*
Cardiac contractility, effect of anesthesia on, 8
Cardiac disease, anesthesia and, 8-9
  characteristics of, 8
  induction of anesthesia in patients with, 9
Cardiac output, effect of anesthesia on, 8
  effect of halothane (Fluothane) on, 8

225

Cardiac output (continued)
  effect of thiobarbiturates on, 8
  thermodilution, 12
Carmalt forceps, 24, 25
Castration, canine, 145–147, 145, 146
  feline, 148–150, 148, 150
Catgut, 2, 219–220
Caudectomy, 210–212, 211, 212
Cerclage wiring, of fractured humerus, 184–185, 185
Cervical disks, fenestration of, 164–168, 165–168
Cervical ventral decompression, 169–171, 170
Cesarean section, 138–141, 138, 140
  anesthetic regimens in, 139
Chest, drainage of, 71–73, 71, 72
Chest drain, use of, after repair of diaphragmatic rupture, 83
Chest tube, use of, after pulmonary lobectomy, 79
Cholinergic drugs, withdrawal of, prior to anesthesia, 6
Clamps, Backhaus towel, 23, 23
Closure, abdominal, 51, 53–54
  interrupted sutures and, 3
  number of stitches in, 3
Condyle, lateral, of fractured humerus, lag screw application to, 188–189, 189
Congestion, hypostatic, reduction of, after surgery, 13
Conjunctival flora, reduction of, 38
Connell stitch, in gastrotomy closure, 88, 89
Cornea, laceration of, repair of, 39–41, 40
Corticosteroids, administration of, prior to surgery, 6
Cystotomy, 112–115, 113, 114

Decompression, cervical ventral, 169–171, 170
Diaphragm, rupture, of, repair of, 80–83, 81, 82
Diarrhea, results of, 6
Digitalis, administration of, prior to surgery, 6
Disks, cervical, fenestration of, 164–168, 165–168
  intervertebral, fenestration of, thoracolumbar hemilaminectomy and, 172–175, 173, 174, 175
Distichiasis, lid-splitting procedures for, 43–44, 43
Diuretics, administration of, prior to surgery, 6
Drain(s), chest, 71–73, 71, 72
  Penrose, in salivary gland excision, 65
Draping, 18–20, 18, 19
  fenestrated, 18, 18
  four corner, 18–20, 19
Draping materials, 18
Drug therapy, continuation of, prior to surgery, 6
  response of patients under to anesthesia and surgery, 6
Ductus arteriosus, patent, ligation of, 74–76, 75, 76

Ear, lateral, resection of, 151–155, 152, 154
Edema, pulmonary, caused by left heart failure, treatment of, 9
Elective procedures, evaluation of young animals for, 5
Electrocardiogram, 12
Electrolyte losses, evaluation of, 6–7
  therapy for, 7
Enterotomy, 97–99, 98
Enzyme levels, and anesthesia, for hepatic disease patients, 10
Epithelialization, of keratectomy site, 39
Esophageal anastomosis, 55–61, 56–58, 60
Esophagotomy, 55–61, 56–58, 60
Eye, globe of, immobilization and exposure of, 36–37, 37
  lesions of, removal of, 38–39, 38
  rotation of, under anesthesia, 36
Eyelashes, ectopic, removal of, 43–44, 43
Eyelid, third, flap using, 41–42, 42

Fasting, of patient, prior to surgery, 5, 14
Feedings, tube, preparation of, 67
Feline castration, 148–150, 148, 150
Feline onychectomy, 208–209, 209
Feline perineal urethrostomy, 120–124, 121–124
Femur, fractured, intramedullary pinning of, 198–201, 199–200
  head of, ostectomy of, 192–197, 193–197
Fenestration, of cervical disks, 164–168, 165–168
  of intervertebral disks, thoracolumbar hemilaminectomy and, 172–175, 173, 174, 175
Flap, third eyelid, 41–42, 42
Flora, conjunctival, reduction of, 38
Fluid(s), administration of, during anesthesia, 12
  intake of, in old animals, prior to surgery, 5–6
  intravenous, for dogs, 215
  loss of, evaluation of, 6–7
    replacement of, 7
    routes for, 6
    therapy for, 7
Fluid volume, evaluation of, 11
Fluothane. See Halothane.
Food, withholding of, prior to surgery, 14
Forceps, Allis tissue, 26, 26
  application of, 1
  Brown-Adson tissue, 23, 23
  Carmalt, 24, 25
Foreign matter, addition of, and healing, 1
Fracture, of femur, intramedullary pinning of, 198–201, 199–200
  of humerus, cerclage wiring of, 184–185, 185
    intramedullary pinning of, 182–183, 183
    lateral condyle of, lag screw application to, 188–189, 189
  of radius, intramedullary pinning of, 190–191, 191
  of tibia, application of full Kirschner apparatus to, 206–207, 207
    intramedullary pinning of, 204–205, 205

Gastropexy, permanent, 91–93, 92, 93
Gastrotomy, 84–90, 85–90
Germicidal rinse, 20–21
Germicidal solutions, for cleansing of operative site, 16
Gland, salivary, excision of, 61–65, 62, 63, 64
Globe. See Eye, globe of.
Gloving, closed method, 21–22, 21
Gowning, of surgeon and operative team, 21

Hair, removal from operative site, 1, 16, 16
Halothane (Fluothane), and hepatic disease patients, 10
  contraindications to, 8–9
  effect on cardiac output, 8
Halsted mosquito hemostat, 24, 25
Halsted suture pattern, in gastrotomy closure, 89–90, 89, 90
Healing, addition of foreign matter and, 1
  delayed, reasons for, 1
  morphologic changes in, 1
Heart. See under Cardiac.
Hemilaminectomy, thoracolumbar, and intervertebral disk fenestration, 172–175, 173, 174, 175
Hemostasis, in application of sutures, 3
Hemostat, Halsted mosquito, 24, 25
  Kelly, 24, 25
Hepatic disease patients, anesthesia and, 9–10
  halothane and, 10
Hernia, diaphragmatic, repair of, 80–83, 81, 82
Hexachlorophene, 16, 20

INDEX

Humerus, fractured, cerclage wiring of, 184–185, *185*
    intramedullary pinning of, 182–183, *183*
    lateral condyle of, lag screw application to, 188–189, *189*
Hyperkalemia, treatment of, 7
Hypertension, and anesthesia, 11
Hypostatic congestion, reduction of, after surgery, 13
Hypotension, and anesthesia, 11
Hypothermia, and tissue perfusion, 11
Hypoxemia, 9

Insecticides, organophosphate, withdrawal of, prior to anesthesia, 6
Instruments, 23–26, *23–26*
    care in use of, 1
Intervertebral disks, fenestration of, thoracolumbar hemilaminectomy and, 172–175, *173, 174, 175*
Interrupted sutures. See *Sutures, interrupted.*
Intestinal anastomosis, 100–103, *100, 102*
Intramedullary pinning, of fractured femur, 198–201, *199, 200*
    of fractured humerus, 182–183, *183*
    of fractured radius, 190–191, *191*
    of fractured tibia, 204–205, *205*
Intravenous fluids, for dogs, 215
Intravenous route, establishment of, 8

Kelly hemostat, 24, *25*
Keratectomy, site of, epithelization time of, 39
    superficial, 38–39, *38*
Kirschner apparatus, application of, to fractured tibia, 206–207, *207*
Knot, granny, 30, *31*
    half-hitch, 30, *31*
    Miller's, 30, *31*
    square, 30, *31*
    surgeon's, 30, *31*

Laceration, corneal, repair of, 39–41, *40*
Lag screw, application of, to fractured humerus, lateral condyle of, 188–189, *189*
Lateral condyle, of fractured humerus, lag screw application to, 188–189, *189*
Ligation, knots used for, 30–31, *31*
    pinpoint, of bleeding vessels, 1
    simple, 30, *31*
Liver, decreased function of, tests for, 10
Lobectomy, pulmonary, 77–79, *78*
Luxation, of patella, correction of, 202–203, *203*

Mask, surgical, proper application of, 15–16
Mastectomy, 142–144, *142, 144*
Mathieu retractor, 23, *23*
Mayo scissors, 24, *25*
Mayo-Heger needle holder, 26, *26*
Medication, postoperative, 13
    preinduction, 6
Methoxyflurane (Metofane), effect of, on cardiac output, 8
Metofane, effect of, on cardiac output, 8
Metzenbaum scissors, 24, *24*
Monitoring, of anesthetized patient, 11–12
Muscle relaxation, of dogs, anesthesia for, 215(t)

Narcotic antagonists, for dogs, 216(t)
Nasolacrimal apparatus, irrigation of, 33–34, *34*
Needle holder, Mayo-Heger, 26, *26*
Needles, holding of, 26
    withdrawal of, 26
Nephrectomy, 109–111, *110*
Nephrotomy, 109–111, *110*
Neurological surgery, 156–175. See also under specific procedures.
Nonabsorbable suture material. See *Suture material, nonabsorbable.*

Olecranon, ostectomy of, and tension band wiring, 186–187, *187*
Onychectomy, feline, 208–209, *209*
Operating room, and its equipment, cleaning and disinfection of, 14–15
    attire in, 15–16
Operative site, preparations of, 16–20, *17*
    removal of hair from, 16, *16*
Operative time, prolonged, risks in, 2
    reduction of, 2
Ophthalmic surgery, 33–44. See also under specific procedures.
Organophosphate insecticides, withdrawal of, prior to anesthesia, 6
Orthopedic surgery, 177–212. See also under specific procedures.
Ostectomy, of femoral head, 192–197, *193–197*
    of olecranon, and tension band wiring, 186–187, *187*
Osteotomy, of osseous bulla, 160–163, *161, 162*
Ovariohysterectomy, 133–137, *134, 136*
Oxygen, supply of, to anesthetized patient, 12

Patella, luxating, correction of, 202–203, *203*
Patent ductus arteriosus, ligation of, 74–76, *75, 76*
Patient, evaluation of, prior to anesthesia and surgery, 5
    management of, during administration of anesthesia, 12
        postoperative, 12–13
        preoperative and operative, 14–22
    preanesthetized, common abnormalities of, 6
    preparation of, for surgery, 5–8, 14
PDA. See *Patent ductus arteriosus.*
Penrose drain, in salivary gland excision, 65
Pharyngostomy, 65–67, *66*
Phenothiazine tranquilizers, and anesthesia, 6
Pinning, intramedullary, of fractured femur, 198–201, *199, 200*
    of fractured humerus, 182–183, *183*
    of fractured radius, 190–191, *191*
    of fractured tibia, 204–205, *205*
Pinpoint ligation, of bleeding vessels, 1
Polyglycolic acid, 2, 218
Polyuria, results of, 6
Potassium, administration of, 7
    low level of, correction of, 7
Povidone-iodine scrub, 16, 20
Preanesthesia, for pulmonary disease patients, 9
Preanesthetics, for cats, dosages of, 216(t)
    for dogs, dosages of, 214(t)
Preanesthetized patients, common abnormalities of, 6
Preinduction medications, 6
Preparation solutions, application of, 17, *17*
    for cleansing of operative site, 16
Prolapse, urethral, correction of, 130–131, *131*
Pulmonary disease, anesthesia and, 9
    characteristics of, 9

Pulmonary edema, caused by left heart failure, treatment
of, 9
Pulmonary lobectomy, 77–79, 78
Pyloromyotomy, 94–97, 94, 96

Quaternary ammonium compounds (Zephiran), 16

Radius, fractured, intramedullary pinning of, 190–191, 191
Recovery facility, 13
Renal disease, anesthesia and, 10–11
Resection, lateral ear, 151–155, 152, 154
    tarsoconjunctival, 43–44, 43
Respiratory alkalosis, 9
Retractor, Mathieu, 23, 23
Rupture, diaphragmatic, repair of, 80–83, 81, 82

Salivary gland, excision of, 61–65, 62, 63, 64
Scalpel, Bard-Parker, 23, 23
Scissors, Mayo, 24, 25
    Metzenbaum, 24, 24
    Sharp-Sharp, 24, 24
    wire suture, 24, 24
Scrub solutions, 20
    for cleansing of operative site, 16
Scrotal urethrostomy, 118–119, 118
Sedation, of cats, agents for, 216(t)
    of dogs, agents for, 213(t)
Sedative agents, use of, prior to surgery, 6
Sharp-Sharp scissors, 24, 24
Shock, antibiotic therapy prior to surgery for
    prevention of, 7–8
Shoulder, approach to, 176–181, 176, 179–180
Silk sutures. See Suture material(s), silk.
Soft tissue surgery, 45–155. See also under specific
    procedures.
Splenectomy, 106–109, 107, 108
Sterilization. See Castration and Ovariohysterectomy.
Subconjunctival injection, 35–36, 36
    drugs and dosages used in, 35(t)
Subluxation, atlantoaxial, stabilization of, 156–159, 157–159
Surgery, "clean," 38
    continuation of drug therapy prior to, 6
    evaluation of patient prior to, 5
    fasting of patient prior to, 5, 14
    neurological, 156–175. See also under specific procedures.
    ophthalmic, 33–44. See also under specific procedures.
    orthopedic, 176–212. See also under specific procedures.
    patient preparation for, 5–8, 14
    principles of, 1–3
    response of patients under drug therapy to, 6
    soft tissue, 45–155. See also under specific procedures.
    water intake of patient prior to, 14
Surgical environment, preparation of, 14–16
Surgical scrub, equipment for, 20
    technique for, 20
Surgical team, preparations of, 20–22, 21
Surital. See Thiamylal sodium.
Sutures, application of, hemostasis in, 3
    interrupted, and closure, 3
    size(s) of, 2, 30, 31, 218
        guidelines for selection of, 2(t), 218
    transfixion, 3
Suture material(s), 2–3, 218–223
    absorbable, 2–3
        characteristics of and indications for, 2–3, 218–219
        polyglycolic acid (Dexon), 220
        surgical gut, 219–220
    application of, 2

Suture material(s) (continued)
    Halsted principles for, 3
    as foreign matter, 1–2
    choice of, 2, 218
    effects of tying of, 2
    ideal, characteristics of, 2
    nonabsorbable, characteristics and indications for, 3, 219
        metals, 221
        natural, 221–222
        synthetic, 222–223
    response of body to, 1–2
    silk, 3, 221
    size of, 2, 2(t), 30, 31, 218
    types of, 2–3, 218, 219
Suture pattern(s), 27–31, 27, 28, 29, 30, 31
    Connell, in gastrotomy closure, 88, 89
    Halsted, in gastrotomy closure, 89–90, 89, 90
    Lembert, 28, 29
    mattress, 30, 30
    simple continuous, 27, 27
        continuation of, 28, 28
        finishing knot for, 28, 28
        preferred placement method for, 27, 27
    simple interrupted, 28, 29

Tarsoconjunctival resection, 43–44, 43
Tension band wiring, of olecranon, 186–187, 187
Thermodilution cardiac output, 12
Thiamylal sodium (Surital), contraindications to, 8–9
Thiobarbiturates, effect of, on cardiac output, 8
Third eyelid, flap using, 41–42, 42
Thoracolumbar hemilaminectomy, and intervertebral disk
    fenestration, 172–175, 173, 174, 175
Thoracotomy, 45–49, 46, 47, 48
Tibia, crest of, transplantation of, in correction of patellar
    luxation, 202–203, 203
    fractured, application of full Kirschner apparatus to,
        206–207, 207
    intramedullary pinning of, 204–205, 205
Tissue perfusion, hypothermia and, 11
Toweling, of hands and forearms of operative team, 21
Tracheotomy, 68–70, 68, 70
Tracheotomy assembly, 70, 70
Tranquilizers, phenothiazine, and anesthesia, 6
Transfixion sutures, 3
Transolecranon approach, 186–187, 187
Transplantation, of tibial crest, in correction of patellar
    luxation, 202–203, 203
Trauma, tissue, 1
Trochlear arthroplasty, in correction of patellar luxation,
    202–203, 203
Tube feedings, preparation of, 67

Urethra, prolapse of, correction of, 130–131, 131
    ruptured, repair of, 125–129, 126, 128
Urethrostomy, feline perineal, 120–124, 121–124
    scrotal, 118–119, 118
Urethrotomy, 116–117, 116
Urinary bladder, state of, prior to surgery, 6

Vessels, bleeding, pinpoint ligation of, 1
Vitamins, effect of, on anesthesia, 6
Vomiting, results of, 6

Water, patient intake of, prior to surgery, 14
Wire suture scissors, 24, 24
Wiring, cerclage, of fractured humerus, 184–185, 185
    tension band, of olecranon, 186–187, 187

Zephiran, 16